Essential Public Health
Theory and Practice

LIVERPOOL JMU LIBRARY

3 1111 01411 4068

Essential
Public Health

Theory and Practice

**Stephen Gillam, Jan Yates and
Padmanabhan Badrinath**

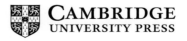

CAMBRIDGE UNIVERSITY PRESS
Cambridge, New York, Melbourne, Madrid, Cape Town,
Singapore, São Paulo, Delhi, Tokyo, Mexico City

Cambridge University Press
The Edinburgh Building, Cambridge CB2 8RU, UK

Published in the United States of America by Cambridge University Press, New York

www.cambridge.org
Information on this title: www.cambridge.org/9781107601765

© Cambridge University Press 2007, 2012

This publication is in copyright. Subject to statutory exception
and to the provisions of relevant collective licensing agreements,
no reproduction of any part may take place without the written
permission of Cambridge University Press.

First published 2007
Second Edition 2012

Printed in the United Kingdom at the University Press, Cambridge

A catalogue record for this publication is available from the British Library

ISBN 978-1-107-60176-5 Paperback

Additional resources for this publication at www.cambridge.org/9781107601765

Cambridge University Press has no responsibility for the persistence or
accuracy of URLs for external or third-party internet websites referred to
in this publication, and does not guarantee that any content on such
websites is, or will remain, accurate or appropriate.

Every effort has been made in preparing this book to provide accurate and up-to-date
information which is in accord with accepted standards and practice at the time of publication.
Although case histories are drawn from actual cases, every effort has been made to disguise
the identities of the individuals involved. Nevertheless, the authors, editors and publishers can
make no warranties that the information contained herein is totally free from error, not least
because clinical standards are constantly changing through research and regulation. The
authors, editors and publishers therefore disclaim all liability for direct or consequential damages
resulting from the use of material contained in this book. Readers are strongly advised to pay
careful attention to information provided by the manufacturer of any drugs or equipment that
they plan to use.

Contents

Contributors

JENNY AMERY
Chief Professional Officer Health and Education, UK Department for International Development, London

PADMANABHAN BADRINATH
Associate Clinical Lecturer, Department of Public Health and Primary Care, University of Cambridge, and Consultant in Public Health Medicine, NHS Suffolk

CAROL BRAYNE
Director, Institute of Public Health, Addenbrooke's Hospital, Cambridge

RACHEL CROWTHER
Public Health Consultant, Oxford

STEPHEN GILLAM
Director of Public Health Teaching, School of Clinical Medicine, University of Cambridge, and Visiting Professor, University of Bedfordshire, and General Practitioner, Luton

RICHARD LEWIS
Director, Health Advisory Practice, Ernst & Young UK

KIRSTEEN L. MACLEOD
Public Health Registrar, Bedfordshire

DAVID PENCHEON
Director, NHS Sustainable Development Unit (England)

CHRISSIE PICKIN
Deputy Director of Public Health, Tasmanian Department of Health and Human Services, Tasmania, Australia

JENNIE POPAY
Professor of Sociology and Public Health, Faculty of Health and Medicine, Division of Health Research, Lancaster University

VEENA RODRIGUES
Clinical Senior Lecturer in Public Health, Norwich Medical School, University of East Anglia, Norwich

LINCOLN SARGEANT
Public Health Consultant, NHS Cambridgeshire

NICHOLAS STEEL
Clinical Senior Lecturer in Primary Care, Norwich Medical School, University of East Anglia, Norwich and Public Health Consultant, NHS Norfolk Primary Care Trust

SARAH STEWART-BROWN
Chair of Public Health, School of Medicine, Warwick University, Coventry

JAN YATES
Public Health Consultant, NHS Midlands and East

Foreword to the second edition

All health professionals need an understanding of the determinants of good health at population level. This has been recognised both nationally in guidance to medical and nursing schools and internationally by the World Health Organization. To help their patients through and beyond the episodes of illness that bring them into surgeries and hospitals, doctors need to understand the factors that propel patients there in the first place. Moreover, as the costs of health care increase across the globe, tomorrow's health professionals need a sound understanding of population-based approaches to promoting health and preventing ill health.

The first edition of this book was highly commended and the second edition begins with a section covering core public health knowledge and skills. I am pleased to see that the first chapter considers public health leadership. This is crucially important for being, in the jargon of the times, 'distributed'. All of us working in the UK National Health Service, at one level or another, share responsibility for leadership, whether clinical or managerial, and for ensuring that priority is given to preventive care or to improving the curative services we offer.

I note that the second half of the book adopts the same life-course approach to improving population health as was used in the recent White Paper on public health: 'Healthy Lives, Healthy People'. That too stresses the importance of multi-sectoral working to tackle the main causes of mortality and morbidity from infancy onwards.

A textbook of this nature, which brings together both principles and practice in a user-friendly format, is particularly timely. Public health in England is undergoing a dramatic transformation with much of the workforce moving to local government. The issues we face as public health practitioners, such as obesity, climate change and an ageing population, become even more challenging during such transitions. This book should be valuable to students of medicine and other health professions but also to public health practitioners in other countries. The second edition, like the first, will help prepare you to tackle some of the tough health challenges we face today.

Dame Sally C. Davies
Chief Medical Officer and Chief Scientific Advisor
Department of Health
London

Foreword to the first edition

Myriad challenges face international health today, from the prospect of hundreds of millions of tobacco-related deaths in the twenty-first century, to the devastation of sub-Saharan Africa by AIDS, to the rise of cardiovascular and metabolic diseases in many countries still laid low by ancient communicable diseases. The tide of the tobacco epidemic is turning in Britain and in some other industrialised countries, but in these places further progress depends on greater use of proven life-saving interventions (such as those in the prevention of vascular diseases) as well as on appropriate responses to challenges posed by ageing populations, unhealthy lifestyles and major – but comparatively neglected – sources of disability such as mental and musculo-skeletal diseases.

The editors of this book have produced a lucid and thoughtful account of critical perspectives and tools that will enable students and practitioners to understand and tackle such prevailing problems in public health. This book's appeal to health-care professionals from many different backgrounds should help to advance the interdisciplinary approach to health promotion and disease prevention that the editors themselves wisely advocate.

John Danesh
Professor of Epidemiology and Medicine
University of Cambridge

Foreword to the first edition

Public health knowledge and practice is derived from a number of different academic fields. This makes the specialty very stimulating but immediately confronts the student with a dilemma: breadth versus depth. This book strikes the right balance between the need for coverage of several relevant disciplines with the detail required to understand specific public health challenges. We all need to use the frameworks described here to locate our learning and practice.

The three-domains model of public health practice described in the introduction has utility for all health workers – and we need to reflect on the location of information we use at the intersection of the three domains. Modern information technology provides assistance to health practitioners, e.g. through search engines and internet resources, but the growth in information and specialised knowledge characteristic of modern health systems can be overwhelming. For practitioners dedicated to improving public health there is always a 'population of interest'. For example, for the health visitor deprived families in her locality, for the general practitioner a practice population, for the director of public health a whole population and for the paediatrician or children's lead manager a subset of that population.

The community diagnostic model and the life-course structure is welcome. This book is written to assist learning for students from many disciplines studying public health. They will benefit from the clarity of the authors' approach, the wisdom distilled here and the recognition of our global and local public health challenges.

Tony Jewell
Chief Medical Officer, Wales

Acknowledgements

The authors would like to thank family, friends and colleagues for their encouragement and ideas – and, of course, our students. In particular, we thank Jayshree Ramsurun for her unstinting support.

Introduction

Stephen Gillam

Historical background

Until recently it was a commonly held view that improvements in health were the result of scientific medicine. This view was based on experience of the modern management of sickness by dedicated health workers able to draw on an ever-growing range of diagnostics, medicines and surgical interventions. The demise of epidemics and infectious disease (until the manifestation of AIDS), the dramatic decline in maternal and infant mortality rates and the progressive increase in the proportion of the population living into old age coincided in Britain with the development of the National Health Service (established in 1948). Henceforth, good-quality medical care was available to most people when they needed it at no immediate cost. Clearly there have been advances in scientific medicine with enormous benefit to humankind, but have they alone or even mainly been responsible for the dramatic improvements in mortality rates evident in developed countries in the last 150 years? What lessons can we learn from how these improvements have been brought about?

Public health has been defined as '*the science and art of preventing disease, prolonging life and promoting health through the organised efforts of society*' [1]. In Europe and North America, four distinct phases of activity in relation to public health over the last two hundred years can be identified. The first phase began in the industrialised cities of northern Europe in response to the appalling toll of death and disease among working-class people who were living in abject poverty. Large numbers of people had been displaced from the land by landlords seeking to take advantage of the agricultural revolution. They had been attracted to growing cities as a result of the industrial revolution and produced massive changes in population patterns and the physical environment in which people lived [2].

The first Medical Officer of Health in the UK, William Duncan (1805–63), was appointed in Liverpool. Duncan surveyed housing conditions in the 1830s and discovered that one third of the population was living in the cellars of back-to-back

Essential Public Health, Second Edition, ed. Stephen Gillam, Jan Yates and Padmanabhan Badrinath.
Published by Cambridge University Press. © Cambridge University Press 2012.

houses with earth floors, no ventilation or sanitation and as many as 16 people to a room. It was no surprise to him that fevers were rampant. The response to similar situations in large industrial towns was the development of a public health movement based on the activities of medical officers of health, sanitary inspectors and supported by legislation.

The public health movement, with its emphasis on environmental change, was eclipsed in the 1870s by an approach at the level of the individual, ushered in by the development of the 'germ theory' of disease and the possibilities offered by immunisation and vaccination. Action to improve the health of the population moved on first to preventive services targeted at individuals, such as immunisation and family planning, and later to a range of other initiatives including the development of community and school nursing services. The introduction of school meals was part of a package of measures to address the poor nutrition among working-class people, which had been brought to public notice by the poor physical condition of recruits to the army during the Boer War at the turn of the twentieth century.

This second phase also marked the increasing involvement of the state in medical and social welfare through the provision of hospital and clinic services [2]. It was in turn superseded by a 'therapeutic era' dating from the 1930s with the advent of insulin and sulphonamides. Until that time there was little that was effective in doctors' therapeutic arsenal. The beginning of this era coincided with the apparent demise of infectious diseases on the one hand and the development of ideas about the welfare state in many developed countries on the other. Historically, it marked a weakening of departments of public health and a shift of power and resources to hospital-based services.

By the early 1970s, the therapeutic era was itself being challenged by those, such as Ivan Illich (1926–2002), who viewed the activities of the medical profession as part of the problem rather than the solution. Illich was a catholic priest who had come to view the medical establishment as a major threat to health. His radical critique of industrialised medicine is simply summarised [3]. Death, pain and sickness are part of human experience and all cultures have developed means to help people cope with them. Modern medicine has destroyed these cultural and individual capacities, through its misguided attempts to deplete death, pain and sickness. Such 'social and cultural iatrogenesis' has shaped the way that people decipher reality. People are conditioned to 'get' things rather than do them. 'Well-being' has become a passive state rather than an activity.

The most influential body of work belonged to Thomas McKeown (1911–88). He demonstrated that dramatic increases in the British population could only be accounted for by a reduction in death rates, especially in childhood. He estimated that 80 to 90% of the total reduction in death rates from the beginning of the eighteenth century to the present day had been caused by a reduction in those deaths due to infection – especially tuberculosis, chest infections and water- and food-borne diarrhoeal disease [4].

Most strikingly, with the exception of vaccination against smallpox (which was associated with nearly 2% of the decline in the death rate from 1848 to 1971), immunisation and therapy had an insignificant effect on mortality from infectious diseases until well into the twentieth century. Most of the reduction in mortality from TB, bronchitis, pneumonia, influenza, whooping cough and food- and water-borne diseases had already occurred before effective immunisation and treatment became available. McKeown placed particular emphasis on raised nutritional standards as a consequence of rising living standards. This thesis was challenged in turn by those who stress the importance of public health measures [5].

The birth of a 'new public health' movement dated from the 1970s [6]. This approach brought together environmental change and personal preventive measures with appropriate therapeutic interventions, especially for older and disabled people. Educational approaches to health promotion have proved disappointingly ineffective. Contemporary health problems are therefore seen as being societal rather than solely individual in their origins, thereby avoiding the trap of 'blaming the victim'.

The intriguing truth is that the role of knowledge as a determinant of health is as yet ill defined. Scientific advances in our understanding of how to improve health are embodied in the evolving panoply of medical interventions – new drugs, vaccines, diagnostics, etc. These new insights are, in turn, assimilated more informally by health professionals and the general public. How to harness new knowledge more effectively, for example, through the exploitation of new information technologies and marketing techniques is a topic of growing interest to students of public health [7].

Restoring knowledge to a central role in recent health trends is consistent with explanations of trends in other times and in other populations. In the early twentieth century the decline of childhood mortality was powerfully determined by the propagation to parents of new bacteriological knowledge [8]. Over the last three decades, increased access to knowledge and technology has accounted for as much as two-thirds of the annual decline in under-5 mortality rates in low- and middle-income countries [9].

In any event, what is needed to address society's health problems are rational health-promoting public policies with a sound basis in epidemiology: the study of the distribution and determinants of disease in human populations.

Health care's contribution in context

Health professionals have long lived with the ambiguities of their portrayal in literature and the media: on the one hand as compassionate modern miracle-workers, on the other as self-interested charlatans. The implications of McKeown and Illich's work were largely ignored by clinicians. However, powerful counter-arguments have been mounted in their defence.

Attempts have been made to estimate the actual contribution of medical care to life extension or quality of life [10]. Estimating the increased life expectancy attributable to the treatment of a particular condition involves a three-step procedure:

- calculating increases in life expectancy resulting from a decline in disease-specific death rates,
- estimating increases in life expectancy when therapy is provided under optimal conditions (using the results of clinical trials, using life tables), and
- estimating how much of the decline in death rates can be attributed to medical care provided in routine practice.

Bunker credits 5 of the 30 years increase in life expectancy since 1900, and half the 7 years of increase since 1950, to clinical services (preventive as well as therapeutic). In other words, compared with the large improvements in life expectancy gained from advancing public health, the contribution of medical care *was* relatively small but is *now* a more significant determinant of life expectancy. The continuing inequalities in health by social class point to further potential for improvement. The net effect of social class on life expectancy of the whole population is 3 years of which about a third can be charged against the use of tobacco and possibly a third against poorer access to medical care. Bunker estimates that the population would gain up to 2½ years of life expectancy if everyone assumed the lifestyle of the fittest [11].

There are thus three main approaches to improving the health of the population as a whole and national policy must take into account their strengths and limitations. Increasing investment in medical care may make the most predictable contribution to reducing death and suffering but its impact is limited. The benefits of health promotion and changing lifestyles are less predictable. Redistribution of wealth and resources addresses determinants of glaring health inequalities but is of still more uncertain benefit.

Domains of public health

Public health in the NHS has undergone dramatic changes in recent years. All health professionals require some generalist understanding in this field. Rather fewer will need more advanced skills in support of aspects of their jobs (health visitors, general practitioners, commissioning managers, for example). This group also includes non-medical professions such as environmental health and allied agencies such as charities and voluntary groups. A small number of individuals will specialise in public health but this group is expanding. Directors of public health increasingly hail from non-medical backgrounds.

Nowadays, public health is seen as having three domains: health improvement, health protection and improving services (Figure 1). All these domains are covered within this book. Each has its own chapter and examples from all three are used to demonstrate how the skills underpinning public health are put into practice.

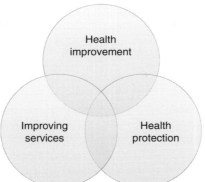

Figure 1 Three domains of
Public Health (UK Faculty of
Public Health).

Health improvement	Health protection	Improving services
• Improving and promoting health • Reducing inequalities • Tackling broader determinants such as employment and housing • Family/community health • Education • Lifestyle/health education • Surveillance of specific diseases	• Clean air, water and food • Infectious disease surveillance and control • Protection from radiation, chemicals and poisons • Preparedness and disaster response • Environmental health hazards • Prevent war and social disorder	• Health systems policy and planning • Quality and standards • Evidence-based health-care • Clinical governance • Efficiency • Research, audit and evaluation

The disciplines that underpin public health include medicine and other clinical areas, epidemiology, demography, statistics, economics, sociology, psychology, ethics, leadership, policy and management. Public health specialists typically work with many other disciplines whose activities impact on the population's health. These might, for example, include health service managers, environmental health officers or local political representatives.

The science of public health is concerned with using these disciplines to make a diagnosis of a population's, rather than an individual's, health problems, establishing the causes and effects of those problems, and determining effective interventions. The art of public health is to create and use opportunities to implement effective solutions to population health and health-care problems. This book intends to capture both the art and the science.

Throughout their careers health-care and allied professionals are presented with opportunities to help prevent disease and promote health. Doctors and nurses need to look beyond their individual patients to improve the health of the population. Later in

Table 1 Individual and population health

Individual	Population
Examination of a patient	Community health surveys
Drawing up diagnostic possibilities	Assessing health-care needs: setting priorities
Treatment of a patient	Preventive programmes, service organisation
Continuing observation	Continuing monitoring and surveillance
Evaluation of treatment	Evaluation of programmes/services

their careers, many will be involved in health service management. Health professionals with a clear understanding of their role within the wider context of health and social care can influence the planning and organisation of services. They can help to ensure that the development of health services really benefits patients.

This book seeks to develop for its readers a 'public health perspective' asking such questions as:

- What are the basic causes of this disease and can it be prevented?
- What are the most cost-effective approaches to its clinical management?
- Can health and other services be better organised to deliver the best models of practice such as health-care delivery?
- What strategies could be adopted at a population level to ameliorate the burden of this disease?

As we have seen, population approaches to health improvement can be portrayed as in opposition to clinical care. This dichotomy is overstated and, in many respects, clinical and epidemiological skills serve complementary functions. There are parallels between the activities of health professionals caring for individuals and public health workers tending populations (Table 1).

Public health and today's NHS

For the last 40 years in the UK, public health specialists have operated primarily from within the health sector. However, recent reforms have returned directors of public health to the local authorities from whence they originally evolved. (The first medical officers of health began discharging their responsibilities from municipalities in the middle of the nineteenth century). This places them closer to those responsible for upstream influences on health, e.g. in housing, transport, leisure and the environment. They are supported by Public Health England, a dedicated, new service set up as part of the Department of Health to strengthen emergency preparedness and protect people from infectious diseases and other hazards (see Chapter 10).

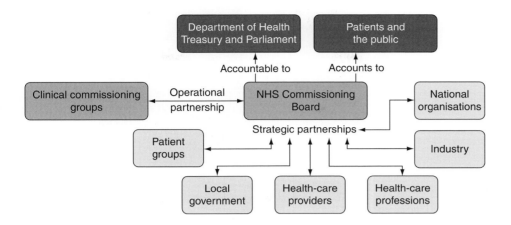

Figure 2 The UK National Health Service.

As well as specialised public health practitioners within these settings, many other professionals include an element of public health within their role, e.g.:

- Environmental health officers – tackling food safety, communicable disease control, healthy environments.
- Health visitors – child health-care includes important public health work such as encouraging breast feeding and promoting smoking cessation.
- District nurses – care of the elderly includes areas such as ensuring adequate heating and safety in the home.
- Voluntary organisations – for example, mental health charities carry out mental health promotion.
- Information analysts, epidemiologists, researchers and librarians – these people are key to the ability of public health specialists to use information and evidence to measure and improve health.
- Occupational health officers – essential to manipulating the risks to health from our working environments and making individual and structural changes to minimise these.

Health services are in constant flux. The structure of today's NHS in England is shown in Figure 2. The policy process and rationale for recent reforms are described in Chapter 16. The impact of NHS reorganisations have often disappointed, tending to reaffirm the limited impact of health services on population health.

The structure of this book

Following this introductory chapter, the book falls into two main sections. The first section takes readers round a cycle (see Figure 3). Diagnosing the public health challenges facing a community could be considered to start the cycle but the toolkit of public health skills a practitioner needs to acquire are added to at each stage and are

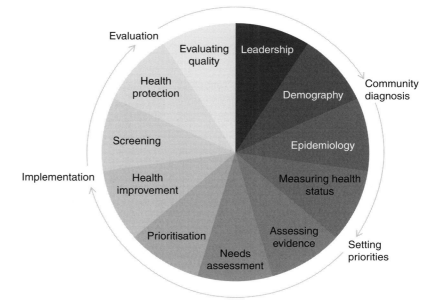

Figure 3   The public health toolkit.

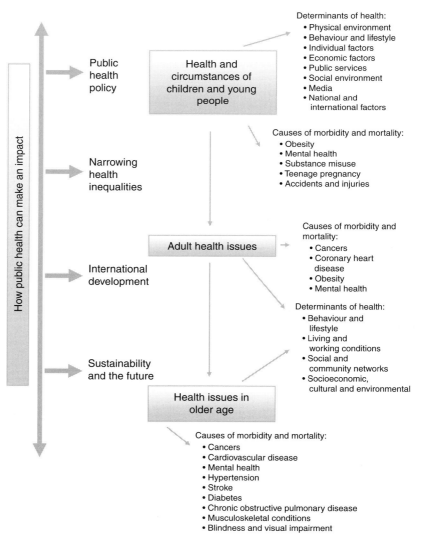

Figure 4   The challenges of public health and the context in which it is practised seen through the lens of a life-course approach.

rarely useful in isolation. Following an assessment of needs, interventions are defined, prioritised, implemented and evaluated for their impact on those same needs. The foremost of these disciplines is epidemiology, the subject of a companion book in this series and a major chapter within this book.

The second half of the book will consider the main challenges that public health practitioners are facing and the contexts within which they work. We use a life-course approach to do this, considering first the challenges of child public health before moving on to the health of adults and older people. Next, we consider the impact of working in public health on the narrowing of health inequalities, policy development, improving the quality of health-care and on international development. Figure 4 demonstrates how these public health challenges are connected. The final chapter examines future challenges.

Alongside this book there is an Internet Companion (www.cambridge.org/ 9781107601765) where the reader will find suggestions for further reading, additional material, interactive exercises and self-assessment questions. We recommend you go online to explore this now.

The practice of public health is about change. Thus, the first chapter considers the role of public health practitioners as leaders and managers.

REFERENCES

1. Department of Health, *Public Health in England. Report of the Committee of Inquiry into the Future Development of the Public Health Function.* Department of Health, London, 1988.

2. C. Hamlin, The history and development of public health in high-income countries. In R. Detels, R. Beaglehole, M. A. Lansang and M. Gulliford, *Oxford Textbook of Public Health*, 5th edn., Oxford, Oxford University Press, 2009, ch. 1.2.

3. I. Illich, *The Limits to Medicine. Medical Nemesis: The Expropriation of Health*, London, Penguin, 1976.

4. T. McKeown, *The Modern Rise of Population*. London, Edward Arnold, 1976.

5. S. Szereter, The importance of social intervention in Britain's mortality decline 1850–1914: a re-interpretation of the role of public health. In B. Davey, A. Gray and C. Seale (eds.), *World Health and Disease: A Reader*, 3rd edn., Milton Keynes, Open University Press, 2002.

6. J. Ashton, Public health and primary care: towards a common agenda. *Public Health* **104**, 1990, 387–98.

7. National Social Marketing Centre for Excellence, *Social Marketing. Pocket Guide*, London, Department of Health, 2005.

8. D. C. Ewbank and S. H. Preston, Personal health behaviour and the decline in infant and child mortality: the United States, 1900–1930. In J. C. Caldwell, S. Findley, P. Caldwell *et al.* (eds.), *What We Know About Health Transition; The Cultural, Social and Behavioural Determinants of Health: Proceedings of an International Workshop, Canberra, May 1989*, Canberra, Australian National University, 1989, pp. 116–49.

9. D. T. Jamison, Investing in health. In D. T. Jamison, J. G. Breman, A. R. Measham *et al.* (eds.), *Disease Control Priorities in Developing Countries*, 2nd edn., Washington, DC and New York, NY, The World Bank and Oxford University Press, 2006, pp. 3–36.

10. J. Powles, Public health policy in developed countries. In R. Detels, R. Beaglehole, M. A. Lansang and M. Gulliford, *Oxford Textbook of Public Health*, 5th edn., Oxford, Oxford University Press, 2009, ch. 3.2.

11. J. Bunker, The role of medical care in contributing to health improvement within society. *International Journal of Epidemiolology* **30**, 2001, 1260–3.

Part 1

The public health toolkit

Management, leadership and change

Stephen Gillam and Jan Yates

Key points

- Management and leadership are separate theoretical domains but are often conflated
- The delivery of improved population health outcomes requires practitioners to develop and use management and leadership skills
- Different styles of leadership and management are appropriate to different circumstances
- Effective health professionals understand that their services are constantly evolving and need to be able to manage change

The nature of management

Management in health-care – like medicine – is about getting things done to improve the care of patients. Most front-line practitioners work closely alongside managers, but often do not fully understand what managers actually do, and do not see them as partners in improving patient care. This lack of understanding is one source of the tensions that can arise between doctors and managers.

Classical management theories evolved out of military theory and were developed as advanced societies industrialised. While they recognised the need to harmonise human aspects of the organisation, problems were essentially seen as technical. Early theories made individuals fit the requirements of the organisation. Later theories, borrowing on behavioural psychology and sociology, suggest ways in which the organisation needs to fit the requirements of individuals. New management theories tend to layer new (and sometimes contradictory) concepts and ideas on top of older counterparts rather than replace them. A summary of the main schools of management theory is included in the Internet Companion.

Essential Public Health, Second Edition, ed. Stephen Gillam, Jan Yates and Padmanabhan Badrinath.
Published by Cambridge University Press. © Cambridge University Press 2012.

What do you think managers do?

We can think about management in terms of the tasks or actions a manager needs to perform (see Box 1.1 [1]) but it is also useful to think of management as having several different dimensions:

- **Principles**: management is about people, securing commitment to shared values, developing staff and achieving results. These help determine the culture of organisations.
- **Theories**: management is underpinned by a plethora of different theories and frameworks. These, in turn, shape the language – and jargon – of management.
- **Structures**: the way organisations are set up, e.g. as bureaucracies, open systems, matrices, networks, etc.
- **Behaviours**: personal and organisational.
- **Techniques**: including communication skills, management by objectives, finance, accounting, planning, marketing, project management and quality assurance.

Box 1.1 Management tasks

- **Defining the task**. Break down general aims into specific manageable tasks.
- **Planning**. Be creative: think laterally and use the ideas of others. Evaluate the options and formulate a working plan. Turn a negative situation into a positive one by creative planning.
- **Briefing**. Communicate the plan. Run meetings, make presentations, write clear instructions. The five skills of briefing are: preparing, clarifying, simplifying, vivifying (making the subject alive), being yourself.
- **Controlling**. Work out what key facts need to be monitored to see if the plan is working, and set standards to measure them against. To control others, you need also to be able to control yourself, e.g. managing your time to best effect.
- **Evaluating**. Assess the consequences of your efforts. Some form of progress report and/or debriefing meeting will enable people to see what they are achieving. The people as well as the task need evaluating, and the techniques of appraisal are important tasks for the leader of the team.
- **Motivating**. Simple ways often work best. Recognition, for instance, of someone's efforts, be it by promotion, extra money or, more frequently, by personal commendation, seldom fails. Success motivates people and communicates a new sense of energy and urgency to the group.
- **Organising**. See that the infrastructure for the work is in place and operating effectively.
- **Setting an example**. Research on successful organisations suggests that key factors are the behaviour, the values, and the standards of their leaders. People take more notice of what you are and what you do than what you say.

- **Communicating**. Be clear and focused. Who needs to know what to get your aims realised?
- **Housekeeping**. Manage yourself – your time and other resources. Have coping strategies for recognising and dealing with pressure for yourself and others.

Theories of leadership

There are a variety of theories on leadership. Early writers tended to suggest that leaders were born, not made, but no-one has been able to agree on a particular set of characteristics required. The following are commonly listed as leadership qualities:

- above-average intelligence;
- initiative or the capacity to perceive the need for action and do something about it;
- self-assurance, courage and integrity;
- being able to rise above a particular situation and see it in its broader context (the 'helicopter trait');
- high energy levels;
- high achievement career-wise;
- being goal-directed and being able to think longer term;
- good communication skills and the ability to work with a wide variety of people.

Modern theories have proposed two types of leadership: transactional and transformational. Transactional leadership attempts to preserve the status quo while transformational leadership seeks to inspire and engage the emotions of individuals in organisations. They are distinguished by different values, goals and the nature of follower–manager relations. Transactional leadership concentrates on exchanges between leaders and staff, offering rewards for meeting particular standards in performance. Transformational leadership highlights the importance of leaders demonstrating inspirational motivation and concentrates on relationships [2].

Another popular concept to emerge in more recent literature on leadership is that of 'emotional intelligence' [3]. This is the capacity for recognising our own feelings and those of others, motivating ourselves and managing emotions well in ourselves. In their description of health leadership, Pointer and Sanchez highlight that [4]:

- leadership is a process, an action word which manifests itself in doing;
- the locus of leadership is vested in an individual;
- the focus of leadership is those who follow;
- leaders influence followers – their thoughts, feelings and actions;
- leadership is done for a purpose: to achieve goals;
- leadership is intentional not accidental.

What qualities characterise the leaders you have encountered?

In health-care, increasing consideration is being given to the organisational context within which people work and what is required of a leader in that work situation. Note that leadership and management are not synonymous. A manager is an individual who holds an office to which roles are attached whereas leadership is one of the roles attached to the office of manager. Just because you are in a senior position will not make you a leader, and certainly not an influential one. Both leaders and managers wield power and must have the ability to influence others to achieve organisational aims.

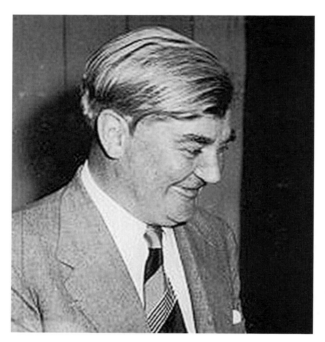

Aneurin Bevan (1897–1960). Founder of the NHS.

Classical views of leadership emphasised charisma as personified in an unbroken line of political figures going back before Alexander the Great – Julius Caesar, Napoleon, Hitler, John Kennedy and Nelson Mandela. Military models underline a heroic view of leaders able to inspire devotion and self-sacrifice. We can see, however, from Box 1.2 that a post-heroic view of leadership recognises a more appropriate (and less masculine) set of virtues and skills for the modern health service. Leading with an appropriate style is more effective than simply command-ing or directing.

Therefore, how you carry out your managerial functions and the way you exercise power and authority – your management or leadership style – is central. To be success-ful, it must be appropriate to the situation. Different styles are needed at different times

Box 1.2 Sources of power

Power based on the position of the individual	Power based on the individual
Positional power Vested in individuals by virtue of the position they hold eg 'Team leader'	**Expert power** Specialist expertise such as that of an NHS consultant
Resource power Control over staff, funds or other resources	**Personal power** What an individual brings personally such as style, charisma, skills

and in different organisational contexts. All of us have preferred styles conditioned by personality and experience. The ability to adapt your approach to different circumstances is a major determinant of effectiveness, just as communication skills with individual patients require versatility according to circumstances.

You are likely to have a preferred way of exercising influence which reflects your own predispositions – your value systems and sense of what is important. Some people are naturally authoritarian; others more laissez-faire. Some are dominating; others prefer a more participative approach. Your preferred style is that to which you will naturally default unless you consider that some other style would be more appropriate.

So how do we determine what style is appropriate in what circumstance? The very attributes that might define a leader in one context may be inappropriate in other circumstances. Winston Churchill was famously rejected as Prime Minister by peacetime Britons. According to contingency theories of leadership, four variables have to be taken into account when analysing contingent circumstances. Unsurprisingly, the one over which you have most control is 'you'!

- the manager (or leader) – his or her personality and preferred style;
- the managed (or led) – the needs, attitudes and skills of his or her subordinates or colleagues;
- the task – requirements and goals of the job to be done;
- the context – the organisation and its values and prejudices.

What might the consequences be of managers or leaders with power lacking the management and leadership skills to wield it 'well'?

Before we move to leading and managing change, it is important to remember that not everyone will want to be or be able to be a leader. Leaders cannot lead unless there are people to follow. Followership theory is less well developed than that for leadership, with the concept introduced in 1988 [5], but it is clear that styles of followership are an important consideration for leaders and managers in achieving their goals (see Box 1.3 [6]).

Box 1.3 Four types of follower

- **Implementers**. Take and carry out orders in support of the leader but with little questioning.
- **Partners**. Respect the leader's position and will provide intelligent challenge when they feel it necessary.
- **Individualists**. Prefer to think for themselves and may not be easy to lead.
- **Resources**. Blind followers who do what is requested but no more.

Theories of change

Surveying most health systems, two features are immediately apparent. The first is the extraordinary complexity, as ever more sophisticated technology is developed to meet an ever expanding range of health problems. A second feature of modern health-care is how fast new technologies and services are evolving. Leaders and managers in this environment are therefore concerned with understanding the needs for and managing change.

There are many management tools which can be used to analyse change and the forces which might support or hinder it. For example, a PESTLE analysis [7] can be used to consider the context within which a specific change is occurring. The PESTLE acronym covers the influences on an organisation (Box 1.4).

Introducing a new service or changing an existing service in response to the kind of drivers identified by using a tool such as PESTLE is difficult. Many people will initially resist change even if the results are likely to benefit them. The process of change involves helping people within an organisation or a system to change the way they work and interact with others in the system. Leaders need to understand how people respond to change in order to plan it.

Think about your organisation or a health-care system. You could use the whole of the NHS. Use the PESTLE model to analyse what is driving change in that system.

Box 1.4 PESTLE analysis

Political

What is happening politically which could affect your organisation?

E.g. government policy

Environmental

What environmental issues affect your organisation?

E.g. carbon reduction requirements

Social

How do social factors affect your organisation?

E.g. population growth, ageing

Technological

How does changing technology impact on your organistion?

E.g. new drugs, medical devices

Economic

What are the implications of finances and economics for your organisation?

E.g. taxes, payment models

Legal

What legal factors influence your organisation?

E.g. medico-legal requirements, registration

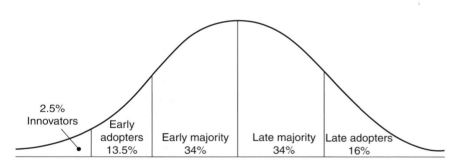

Figure 1.1   Diffusion of innovation.

2.5% Innovators

Early adopters 13.5%

Early majority 34%

Late majority 34%

Late adopters 16%

The psychology of change

Everett Rogers' classic model (Figure 1.1) of how people take up innovation is one model which can help us to understand different people's responses to change [8]. This was based on observations on how farmers took up hybrid seed corn in Iowa. The model describes the differential rate of uptake of an innovation, in order to target promotion of the product, and labels people according to their place on the uptake curve. Rogers' original model described the 'late adopters' as 'laggards' but this seems a pejorative term when there may be good reasons not to take up the innovation. How soon after their introduction, for example, should nurses and doctors be prescribing new, usually more expensive, inhalers for asthma?

Individuals' 'change type' may depend on the particular change they are adopting. This depends on the perceived benefits, the perceived obstacles, and the motivation to make the change. People are more likely to adopt an innovation:

- that provides a **relative advantage** compared to old ideas;
- that is **compatible** with the existing value system of the adopter;
- that is readily understood by the adopters (**less complexity**);
- that may be experienced on a limited basis (**more trialability**); and
- where the results of the innovation are more easily noticed by other potential adopters (**observability**).

Pharmaceutical companies use this model in their approaches to general practitioners. The local sales representatives know from the information they have about GPs in their area whether a GP is an early adopter. Early adopters are often opinion leaders in a community. Early on in the process of promotion they will target those GPs with personal visits, whereas they may send the late adopters an information leaflet only, as those GPs will not consider change until more than 80% of their colleagues have taken up the new product.

Anyone hoping to change people's behaviour is looking for the 'tipping point' [9]. This is the point or threshold at which an idea or behaviour takes off, moving from uncommon to common. You see it in many areas of life, new technologies like the uptake of mobile phones, fashion garments or footwear, books or television programmes. The pharmaceutical industry looks for that point for GPs to prescribe their pharmaceutical product, or for customers to choose their product when buying over the counter. The change in behaviour is contagious like infectious disease epidemics, a social epidemic. Using the model of diffusion, the tipping point comes at the point between the early adopters and the early majority. It applies equally to changing behaviour of professionals and the public.

This same technique can be used with staff going through a process of change. It is important to identify change types and opinion leaders. Knowing likely opponents is important because if they can be persuaded to support the change they are likely to become important advocates. Understanding people's psychological reaction to change is a key to helping overcome their resistance.

Organisational behaviour and motivation

It is important to understand how people operate within the organisation in which they work. Organisational behaviour can be studied at three levels: in relation to individuals, to teams and to organisational processes [10]. Managers everywhere are interested in how such concepts as job satisfaction, commitment, motivation and team dynamics may increase productivity, innovation and competitiveness.

Box 1.5 Handy's types of organisational culture

Power culture

Power is held by a few and rediates out from the centre like a web
Few rules and bureaucracy mean that decisions can be swift

Role culture

Hierarchical bureaucracy where power derives from a person's position

Task culture

Power derives from expertise and structures are often matrices with teams forming as necessary

Person culture

All individuals are equal and operate collaboratively to pursue the organisational goals

In what type of organisation do you think you work? How does this influence your ability to do your job?

What factors affect the behaviour of staff and teams in your workplace?

Types of organisation

How organisations function is a combination of their culture and structures. Organisational culture has been described as a set of norms, beliefs, principles and ways of behaving that together give each organisation a distinctive character [11]. Culture and structure can be analysed. In a simple and early model, Charles Handy built on his own and earlier work to define types of organisations [12] (see Box 1.5).

Types of team

We can see from this simple model of organisational culture that the type of teams which operate within an organisation may be determined by the type of organisation. However, all organisations may at some point form various types of team to carry out specific functions. Teams are often described as:

• **Vertical or functional**. Teams which carry out one function within an organisation such as an infection control team within a hospital.

- **Horizontal or cross-functional**. Teams which are made up of members from across an organisation. These may be formed for specific projects such as managing the introduction of a new service which might need operational, clinical and financial input or can be long-standing teams such as an executive team running an organisation.
- **Self-directed**. Teams which do not have dedicated leadership or management. These may generate themselves within an organisation to achieve aims or they can be specifically designed to give employees a feeling of ownership.

Tuckman's model [13] (see Figure 1.2) explains how teams develop over time and can be used to consider how individuals, including the leader, behave over time within those teams.

Organisational psychologists identify three components of our attitudes to work: cognitive (what we believe, e.g. my boss treats me unfairly), affective (how we feel, e.g. I dislike my boss) and behavioural (what we are predisposed to do, e.g. I am going to look for another job). Attitudes are important as they influence behaviour.

An early and still widely quoted theory of job satisfaction was elaborated by Herzberg [14] – see Figure 1.3. In this theory, 'hygiene' factors are those which individuals need to be satisfied in a job but do not themselves lead to motivation (e.g. a good relationship with peers, working environment, status and security). 'Motivating' factors are related to the job itself and include recognition, advancement, responsibility and personal growth. The message for managers was that taking care of hygiene factors was a basic prerequisite, a focus on motivating factors would maximise job satisfaction.

In marked contrast, dispositional models of job satisfaction assume it to be a relatively stable characteristic of individuals that changes little in different situations – due to genetic or personality factors. Some long-term studies have indeed found that individuals are consistent in their attitudes to work in different settings. In any event, selecting employees with the 'right attitude' does seem crucial to maintaining a satisfied workforce. Certainly, studies from industry suggest that higher levels of job satisfaction are associated with higher levels of job performance, with lower levels of employee turnover and absenteeism – and more satisfied customers [15].

One other factor which may influence your job satisfaction is your expectations. This may be relevant in health-care. For example, negative attitudes among newly qualified doctors may relate to the mismatch between the expectations generated by medical students and the harsh realities of life as a junior doctor [16].

The importance of positive reinforcement, setting goals and clarifying expectations is stressed in leadership-based theories. Job enrichment to give more control over content, planning and execution can help motivate employees. David McClelland considered the importance of matching people and job-related rewards, recognising three different sorts of personal need (Table 1.1 [17]).

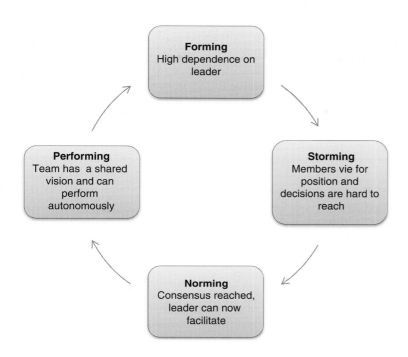

Figure 1.2 Bruce Tuckman's team-development model.

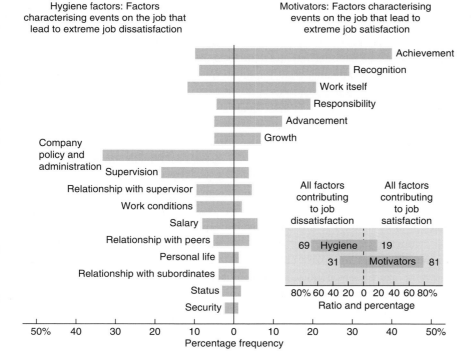

Figure 1.3 Herzberg's two-factor theory of job satisfaction.

Table 1.1 McClelland's motivational needs theory

Need	Description
Need for achievement	The need to accomplish goals, excel and strive continually to do things better
Need for power	The need to influence and lead others, and be in control of one's environment
Need for affiliation	The desire for close and friendly interpersonal relationships

How much do you think you will need achievement, power and affiliation in your future work?

Professional and clinical leadership

Leadership and management are not, of course, the same thing though they are often conflated. Clinicians' roles as leaders and managers are not theirs by right – though they are often assumed. Leadership skills help doctors become more actively involved in planning and delivery of health services but also support roles in research, education and health politics. Clinicians differ significantly from other managers in (usually) continuing to deliver hands-on clinical services. This provides an understanding of how management decisions impact on clinical practice and the care of patients, and can help translate national initiatives into local practice as effectively as possible.

Management competencies are important to health professionals for three overriding reasons. They help to:

• improve efficiency – make best use of always limited resources;
• ensure systems are in place to monitor and maintain quality of care, the stuff of 'clinical governance', which is concerned with patient safety and quality;
• cope constructively with change as health services continually evolve and develop. The current reforms to the NHS, which are supposed to transfer significant power to clinical commissioning groups, have highlighted the role of clinicians, especially doctors, as both leaders and managers. The UK Leadership Council's NHS Leadership Framework [18] is built on a concept of shared leadership and sets out the competencies doctors and other NHS professionals need to run health-care organisations and improve quality of care. The domains of this framework are shown in Figure 1.4 (see Internet Companion).

The concept of professionalism is relevant here as the framework describes leadership in four stages from one's own professional practice and the self-leadership required for that through leading services and teams to leading whole organisations

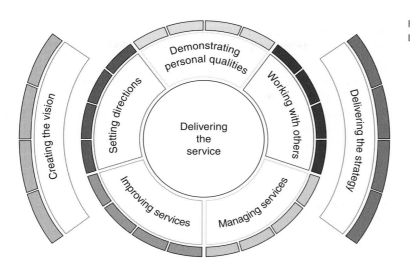

Figure 1.4   The UK NHS
Leadership Framework.

and systems. Hallmarks of professions are monopoly and autonomy [19]. In other words, there is a defined set of activities over which professionals have a licensed monopoly of practice and within which they have considerable autonomy to operate. Health professionals see themselves as accountable in at least four ways: to their peers, to managers where they work, to patients and to their professional body. Health professionals will consider themselves answerable to their professional body (e.g. UK General Medical Council, Medical Board of Australia, UK Nursing and Midwifery Council, US States Boards of Nursing) as much as to their employing organisation. Indeed, if their registration with their professional body lapses or is withdrawn they cannot be employed anywhere as a member of that profession. They constitute a distinct type of employee because they have their own source of authority in addition to the usual managerial line of command. This is not usually an issue, since the organisation employs them to deliver services that can only be provided by a member of that profession and, therefore, their professional and managerial accountabilities align. However, management and professional account-abilities can sometimes conflict and this issue needs to be taken into account when professionals exercise their various forms of power. This can be a particular issue for public health practitioners where professional independence and the pro-vision of expert advice may conflict with organisational duties such as financial balance.

Management, leadership and change in public health practice

We have described a number of theories relating to management, leadership and change. But how can these be used in the field of public health? Public health

Table 1.2 The leadership and management of strategy development

Strategic question	How do we achieve this?
How do we make the case for change?	• Assess local needs taking account of national strategies (see Chapter 6 on assessing need) • Define and account for the drivers for and against change (e.g. PESTLE analysis)
What are we aiming to do?	• Clarify aims, objectives and desired outcomes – a leader/manager needs to bring the vision to life • Define local standards and set targets
How can we make change happen?	• Understand the principles of change management and plan to address the factors that might resist change • Include a description of the actions that are required, and an assessment of the resource implications of putting the new service into place with clear financial plans • Consider the organisational context and how you need teams and individuals to operate in the new system
How do we engage with partners including patients and public?	• Involve all those who are affected by the strategy including clinicians and managers • Identify who will support and who will oppose it; develop an approach to overcoming this opposition. Consider who has the power in these relationships and how that affects the strategy development
How do we know we have done what we wanted to do?	• Evaluate impact by demonstrating achievement against the standards and targets through monitoring routine data and special studies (see Chapter 11 for evaluating the impact of services)
How do we make successful change become normal practice?	• The change in practice needs to be sustained to ensure that it becomes routine, as people tend to revert to their old ways of working • This requires individuals to change the way they do things. Continuing education, appropriate management strategies, alterations to the work environment with a process of on-going monitoring/audit/feedback may all be required • Consider what motivates people and how to use leadership and management skills to build a culture of continuous improvement

practitioners often occupy leadership positions, often exercising power without direct managerial accountability for outcomes. They drive the changes they believe, on the basis of evidence and experience, will result in improved population health. Strategy is at the heart of the change process and we can use the development of a strategy as a good example of how leadership and management skills can be applied in practice. Table 1.2 outlines the questions posed in strategy development and how the skills we have outlined in this chapter need to be applied at each stage, in conjunction with the core public health skills described in the next few chapters.

Conclusion

The skills needed for leadership and management vary across an individual's career and must be assessed and developed over time. Leadership and management behaviours can be learned but continuous improvement requires an open-minded approach to assessing our own skills level, an ability to seek and accept constructive feedback on our performance and a willingness to change. How can we lead and manage change if we are unwilling to lead, manage and change ourselves?

How you would go about managing a new service or change that would require leadership and management to deliver?
You can use the questions in Table 1.2 and the theory outlined in this chapter to consider how you would go about managing that change.

REFERENCES

1. S. Gillam, *Leadership and Management for Doctors in Training*, London, Radcliffe Publishing, 2011.
2. W. Bennis and B. Nanus, *Leaders*, New York, NY, Harper Collins, 1996.
3. D. Goleman, *Emotional Intelligence.* London, Bloomsbury Publishing, 1996
4. D. Pointer and J. P. Sanchez, Leadership in public health practice. In F. D. Scutchfield and C. W. (eds.), *Principles of Public Health Practice*, New York, NY, Thomson Delmar Learning, 2003.
5. R. Kelley, In praise of followers. *Harvard Business Review*, November, 1988
6. I. Chaleff, *The Courageous Follower*, San Francisco, CA, Berrett-Koehler, 1995
7. Chartered Institute of Personnel and Development (CIPD), *PESTLE analysis factsheet*, November 2010.
8. E. Rogers, *The Diffusion of Innovation*, 4th edn., New York, NY, Free Press, 1995.
9. M. Gladwell, *The Tipping Point. How Little Things Can Make a Big Difference*, London, Abacus, 2000.
10. J. Greenberg and R. Baron, *Behaviour in Organisations: Understanding and Managing the Human Side of Work*, 2nd edn., Boston, Allyn & Bacon, 1990.
11. A. Brown, *Organisational Culture*, London, Pitman Publishing, 1995.
12. C. B. Handy, *Understanding Organizations*, 3rd edn., Harmondsworth, Penguin Books, 1985.
13. B. Tuckman, Developmental sequence in small groups. *Psychological Bulletin* **63**(6), 1965, 384–99.
14. F. Herzberg, *Work and the Nature of Man*, Wenatchee, WA, World Publishing Company, 1966.
15. S. Robbins and T. Judge, *Organizational Behaviour*, 12th edn., Upper Saddle River, NJ, Prentice Hall, 2007.
16. M. Goldacre, T. Lambert, J. Evans and G. Turner, Preregistration house officers' views on whether their experience at medical school prepared them well for their jobs: national questionnaire survey. *British Medical Journal* **326**, 2003, 1011–12.

17. D. McClelland, *Human Motivation*. Englewood Cliffs, NJ, General Learning Press, 1973.

18. Academy of Medical Royal Colleges & Institute for Innovation and Improvement, *Medical Leadership Competency Framework. Enhancing Engagement in Medical Leadership*, 3rd edn., Warwick, NHS Institute for Innovation and Improvement, University of Warwick, 2010.

19. E. Friedson, *Profession of Medicine: A Study of the Sociology of Applied Knowledge*, Chicago, IL, University of Chicago Press, 1970.

2

Demography

Padmanabhan Badrinath and Stephen Gillam

Key points

- Demography is the scientific study of human populations.
- It is important to understand the structure of a population in order to plan health and public health interventions; population structures can be represented as age pyramids.
- Population growth or decline depends upon fertility, mortality and migration.
- The concepts of demographic, epidemiological and health transitions help explain dramatic shifts in population structure and patterns of disease that have taken place in most countries.
- The measurement of demographic statistics is difficult and modelling is used to provide comparable data across the world.

Introduction

Demography is the scientific study of human populations. It involves analysis of three observable phenomena: changes in population size, the composition of the population and the distribution of populations in space. Demographers study five processes: fertility, mortality, marriage, migration and social mobility. These processes determine populations' size, composition and distribution. Basic understanding of demography is essential for public health practitioners because the health of communities and individuals depends on the dynamic relationship between the numbers of people, the space which they occupy and the skills they have acquired. The main sources of demographic information vary between countries and they are well developed in the western hemisphere.

Essential Public Health, Second Edition, ed. Stephen Gillam, Jan Yates and Padmanabhan Badrinath.
Published by Cambridge University Press. © Cambridge University Press 2012.

Population structure

Understanding the structure of a population in terms of the numbers and proportions of men and women in different age groups informs the planning of preventive and health-care interventions. One way of depicting the structure of a population is a population pyramid or age pyramid. This is a graphical way of presenting population data by sex and age group. Pyramids provide a simple way to compare population structures across countries and can provide an indication of the state of development of each country. As an illustration, Figures 2.1 and 2.2 show the data for India and the UK. India is typical of a developing country with a broad base tapering at the top. In developed countries such as the UK, the pyramid generally shows a bulge in the middle and has a narrower base.

Use the two pyramids in Figures 2.1 and 2.2 to describe in words the population structure of India and the UK.

In India, there are larger numbers of young people and, as age increases, the population within each age band decreases. This tapering shape is typical of a developing country where fertility is high but mortality in childhood is high and fewer people live to older ages. In the UK, there is a bulge in the numbers of people around 35–54 years. Fertility has recently been lower but more people survive into middle age. The pyramid is also reflective of the life expectancy at various ages. In developed countries such as the UK life expectancy at 65 is much higher than in developing countries. In the UK the life expectancy at 65 is 18 and 20 years for men and women respectively. In India it is 14 and 15 years.

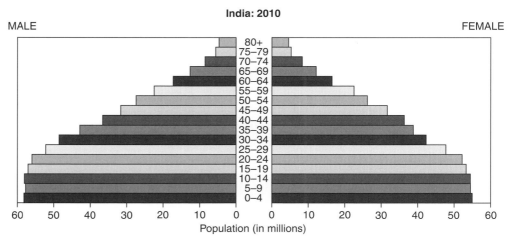

Figure 2.1   Population pyramid for India, 2010. Source: US Census Bureau, International Data Base.

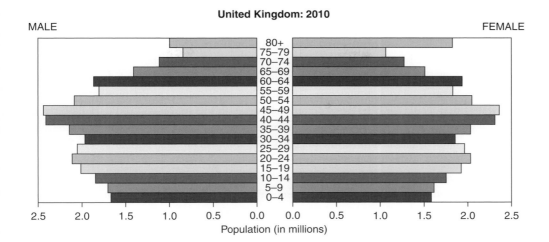

Population trends

World population trends available from the United Nations (UN) show that while the population at the global level continues to increase, that of more-developed regions as a whole is hardly changing. Virtually all population growth is occurring in the less-developed regions with rapid population growth being a characteristic of the 50 least-developed countries. Collectively, these regions will grow 58 per cent over the next 50 years, as opposed to 2 per cent in more-developed regions. Less-developed regions will account for 99 per cent of the expected growth in world population over this period. For example, the population is projected to triple between 2005 and 2050 in many countries including Afghanistan, Liberia, Mali, Niger and Uganda. The population of 51 countries including Germany, Italy, Japan, the Baltic states and most of the former Soviet Union is expected to be lower in 2050 than in 2005 and population growth in less-developed regions is eventually expected to slow down [1].

Figure 2.2   Population pyramid for United Kingdom, 2010. Source: US Census Bureau, International Data Base.

Reasons for population trends

These overall population trends are underpinned in the main by distinct changes in *fertility* and *mortality* across the globe. *Migration* also plays a part when large numbers of people move from one country to another.

Fertility

Fertility refers to the actual bearing of children, the child-bearing performance of a woman, couple or population. As a simple measure of fertility the crude birth rate of a population can be used (with either live or all births as the numerator and person-time at risk as the denominator). A more sophisticated measure of fertility is the general fertility ratio (the number of births per 1000 women of child-bearing age, generally 15–44 or 49 years) but this requires more detailed population data and may not always be available. At a further level of complexity fertility rates may be standardised to account for differences in the age structures of populations and this is termed the total fertility rate. Total fertility rate is defined as the number of children that would be born per woman if she were to live to the end of her child-bearing years and bear children at each age in accordance with prevailing age-specific fertility rates. The total fertility rate in 2008 varied from 1.0 for Singapore to 7.34 in Mali and for the world is estimated to be 2.5 children per woman [2]. In more-developed regions people bear insufficient children to replace those people who die and this trend, termed below-replacement fertility, is expected to continue to 2050. Conversely, fertility is still high in most of the least-developed countries; it is expected to show some decline but still remain higher than the rest of the world. Fertility is influenced by various factors. In the developing countries these include universality of marriage, lower age at marriage, low level of literacy, poor standard of living, limited use of contraceptives and traditional ways of life.

Mortality

Mortality describes the death rates due to a range of causes. The ways in which mortality is measured are detailed in Chapter 4. Trends in mortality have been shifting over time and still vary across the globe. Most people nowadays live longer on average than the wealthiest people did a century ago. Despite these gains there remains a huge preventable burden of premature death and disease worldwide. The dramatic reduction in death rates over the last two centuries can be explained by changes in the social and economic determinants of health and to a lesser extent by public health interventions. 'High-tech' medical interventions, if narrowly defined, explain only a small amount. Medical interventions can be defined more broadly to include technologies such as oral rehydration solutions that are widely used both by professionals and lay people. These have certainly had more impact in recent decades, especially on child mortality in low-income countries.

In 2009, there were approximately 56 million deaths worldwide, and over three quarters occurred in less-developed regions of the world (World Health Organization data). A quarter of all deaths occur in children under five; almost all of these deaths occur in low-income countries. There are striking differences in the pattern of death between high- and low-income regions (see Chapter 17). Communicable diseases are responsible for over 40% of deaths in low-income regions but non-communicable diseases account for a rising proportion of deaths also.

Since 1990, the global under-5 mortality rate has fallen by a third – from 89 deaths per 1000 live births in 1990 to 60 in 2009 [3]. All regions except sub-Saharan Africa, southern Asia and Oceania have seen reductions of at least 50%. The highest rates of child mortality continue to be in sub-Saharan Africa, where 1 child in 8 dies before the age of 5 – nearly 20 times the average of 1 in 167 for developed regions. About half of global under-5 deaths in 2009 occurred in only five countries: India, Nigeria, Democratic Republic of the Congo, Pakistan and China. Of under-5 deaths, 40% occur within the first month of life, and some 70% occur within the first year of life. The two biggest killers of children under age 5 are pneumonia (18% of deaths) and diarrhoeal diseases (15%). Progress on the millennium development goals is described in Chapter 17. In wealthy countries, child mortality is dominated by sudden infant death syndrome, congenital disorders and injury. These too are increasingly preventable. Child public health is considered in detail in Chapter 12.

The maternal mortality rate (actually the ratio of pregnancy-related deaths to live births) has reduced dramatically over the last two centuries, especially in the developed world, as a result of reforms of obstetric practice and the reduction in puerperal sepsis. By contrast, over 700 mothers die for every 100,000 births in sub-Saharan Africa where the lifetime risk of maternal death is about 1 in 20. In western Europe, less than 10 mothers die for every 100,000 births. In 2008, the lifetime risk of a maternal death was 1 in 11 in Afghanistan as opposed to 1 in 14,300 in Austria.

Can you think of ways of reducing maternal mortality? The provision of extended family-planning services, the availability of safe abortion and improved services for antenatal and obstetric care illustrate the importance in this area of technical interventions.

Adults make up about one half of the world's population and 70% of all deaths occur in adults. About half of these deaths are premature. The chance of an adult dying prematurely varies about ten-fold among countries. In the US context, premature death is defined as the number of years of potential life lost prior to age 75 per 100,000 population. This is an indication of the number of useful years of life that are not available to a population due to early death. Differences in the risk of adult death between regions are largely explained by variation in non-communicable disease death rates and death rates from injury. The death rates from heart disease, diabetes and smoking-related illness are increasing globally. The assessment of the relative importance of cause of death depends upon the indicator used. When potential years of life lost (YLL – see Chapter 4) before the age of 75 years are used, conditions that affect younger adults such as injuries, tuberculosis and maternal mortality assume greater importance. As mortality rates from cardiovascular disease have declined, the proportion of deaths due to cancer has increased and now exceeds the former in many wealthy countries. Reasons for changing patterns of mortality are discussed further below.

Migration

Due to advances in transport, communication and trade the world is experiencing ever-increasing movements of people. As many as 200 million people are living outside their countries of origin, more than double the number from 35 years ago. This movement occurs not only from developing countries to developed countries but also from one developed country to another, as well as between developing countries. There are benefits and risks to increasing migration, which can:

- increase educational levels, or decrease them as young people take up unskilled positions abroad or those educated abroad fail to return home.
- have a positive effect on income (for example, through remittances as migrants send funds home to families). Migration may also increase socio-economic inequity as some individuals, communities or countries benefit more than others; or it may have a negative effect on an economy by potentially reducing external competitiveness.
- increase poverty and inequity within countries where rural-to-urban migration is high (for example China). In rural areas the poorest cannot afford to move and those who move into cities tend to be the more educated.
- increase personal vulnerability due to the potential for illegal migration and 'human trafficking'. For example, women recruited as domestic labour may be vulnerable to sexual exploitation.
- lead to racism and isolation.
- lead to a reduction in the human capital needed to deliver key services at home. For example, only 9 of the 47 sub-Saharan African countries have the World Health Organization (WHO) recommended level of physicians (20 doctors per 10,000 people). lead to population structural imbalances, for example as those unable to move, such as the elderly, concentrate in one place.

Information on migration may be derived from censuses, surveys and other administrative-record systems. However, these vary in accuracy across the world.

With declining fertility rates and aging populations many developed countries use managed migration as a way of meeting their demographic, economic-development and labour-market needs. Migration that increases population sizes or alters patterns of infectious diseases may result in changing needs for health-care. Public health professionals need to ensure that local health services are culturally sensitive and accessible to migrants (e.g. through appropriate translation services). Many countries have migrant health screening in place to protect the indigenous population from communicable diseases.

Life expectancy

The decline in death rates has led to major improvements in life expectancy and life expectancy is a key determinant of future population patterns. Life expectancy at birth is the average number of additional years a person could expect to live if current mortality trends were to continue for the rest of that person's life. An important tool, the demographic life table, is used to estimate life expectancy. This uses data on age-specific mortality rates for a specific year to estimate the lifetime experience of a hypothetical cohort (group) of individuals born that year. It assumes that the current mortality rates continue throughout the lifetime of the cohort and, while this is not completely accurate, it does allow the average life expectancy to be calculated. Life tables are an extremely powerful means of summarising the mortality experience in a way that can be compared across populations, and they are also the basis for population projections which predict population growth over time. More complex life tables can be used to estimate the proportion of deaths attributable to different causes, and measures of morbidity can also be introduced to provide estimates of healthy life expectancy.

Global life expectancy at birth is estimated to have risen from 47 years in 1950 to 68 years in 2008. This is expected to keep on increasing to reach 75 years by 2045–2050. While life expectancy at birth has increased in most countries since 1950, there are huge disparities evident between high- and low-income countries. Sub-Saharan Africa, with the advent of HIV/AIDS (acquired immunodeficiency syndrome) has shown a major reversal in life expectancy, and in some countries of central and eastern Europe life expectancy at birth has also been declining over the past decade. This is attributed in part to economic and industrial disruption following dissolution of the Soviet Union, and increasing death rates from heart disease, injuries and alcohol-related illness.

The primary outcome of fertility decline combined with increases in life expectancy is population ageing: the increasing share of older people in a population relative to younger people. Globally, the number of people aged 60 years or over is expected almost to triple, increasing from 672 million in 2005 to nearly 1.9 billion by 2050. As longevity increases, the health experience of older people assumes greater importance both socially and economically. The proportion of people 60 years and over is higher in wealthy countries but more older people live in low-income countries. Projections suggest a four-fold expansion in the global population of older people during the first quarter of this century. The health and social policy challenges this raises are described in Chapter 14.

Preston and colleagues [4] have investigated the relationship between life expectancy and income during the twentieth century (Figure 2.3). The positions of the dots show the relationship between a single country's income and its life expectancy. The different shades refer to the specified years. With the passage of time, the level of life expectancy attainable at a given income has increased. Why? The most fundamental cause is likely to be the advance of knowledge working in two main ways [5]. This knowledge may be formally embodied as medical techniques and interventions. Simultaneously, knowledge informs the actions of both health professionals and the general public. These actions need then to be reinforced by appropriate social policies (Chapter 16). The history of tobacco control provides perhaps the best contemporary illustration [6].

Figure 2.3   The changing relationship between life expectancy and income during the twentieth century [4].

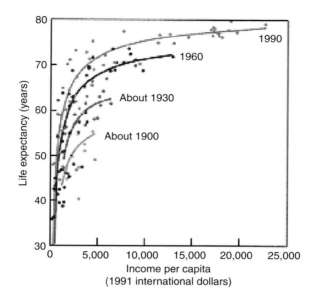

Health transitions

The health transition is a framework for explaining the spectacular shifts in population structure and patterns of disease that have taken place in most countries [7]. It describes the ways in which the world's health needs have changed and will continue to change. The demographic transition describes the change in birth and death rates from high fertility and high mortality rates in more traditional societies to low fertility and low mortality rates in so-called modern societies. Five stages can be identified during a country's demographic transition (Box 2.1).

The epidemiological transition refers to the long-term changes in the patterns of sickness and disability that have occurred as societies have changed their

Box 2.1 Stages of demographic transition

High stationary. High birth rate and high death rate so population remains stationary.

Early expanding. Death rate begins to decline while birth rate remains unchanged.

Late expanding. Death rate declines still further and birth rate tends to fall.

Low stationary. Low birth rate and low death rate so population stationary.

Declining. Birth rate lower than death rate and the population begins to decline.

> **Box 2.2 [10] Impact of non-communicable diseases in developing countries**
>
> The burden of mental illnesses, such as depression, alcohol dependence and schizophrenia, has been seriously underestimated by traditional approaches that take account of deaths and not disability.
>
> Adults under 70 years of age in sub-Saharan Africa today face a higher probability of death from a non-communicable disease than adults of the same age in established market economies.
>
> By 2020, tobacco is expected to kill more people than any single disease, even HIV/AIDS.

demographic, economic and social structures. As originally described, the epidemiological transition consists of three stages [8]:

- The era of pestilence and famine when life expectancy was low. The major causes of death were malnutrition, infectious disease, complications of pregnancy and childbirth.
- The era of receding pandemics, which in western Europe began in the eighteenth century and lasted until the early years of the twentieth century with the great influenza pandemic of 1918–20.
- The era of non-communicable diseases characterised by low fertility rates, population growth and in particular cardiovascular disease and cancer among other so-called degenerative or chronic disease.

A fourth stage has also been proposed [9]:

- The age of delayed degenerative diseases where, as preventive and interventional advances are made, degenerative diseases are postponed. Here, the patterns of mortality remain similar to those in the third stage but are shifted progressively toward older ages; rapid improvements in survival are concentrated among the population in older ages.

Of course, the way this transition has evolved in different countries is highly variable; low-income countries today are not merely replicating the experience of wealthier countries. For example, population growth, poverty, environmental degradation and the demographic trap (constant rapid population growth due to high fertility and low mortality) may prevent the transition from high mortality/fertility to low mortality/fertility in some sub-Saharan African countries. The poorest in developing countries may be experiencing a triple burden of communicable disease, non-communicable disease and socio-behavioural illness (Box 2.2).

The major factors responsible for the health transition are health determinants, demographic changes and therapeutic interventions. Historically, social and economic development, improving nutritional status, sanitary systems and increased literacy among women have been of major importance. Thomas McKeown proposed that improved nutrition beginning in the eighteenth century, together with improvements in water supply and sanitation services and the reduction in birth rates, propelled the health transition (see Introduction). Effective medical measures came too late to make a significant contribution. For example, it has been estimated that only 3.5% of the total decline in mortality in the USA between 1900 and 1973 could be ascribed to medical measures introduced for the major infections (see Chapter 10). On the other hand, targeted public health interventions including vaccination and improved child health-care have had major benefits. These general developments have interacted with more specific public health measures directed towards the control of both infectious and non-communicable disease.

The universal ageing of the population as a result of declining fertility and, to a lesser extent, declining death rates has resulted in the emergence of non-communicable diseases in adulthood with a long latent period. The absolute number of people with these diseases has increased inexorably, even as age- and cause-specific death rates have declined (see Chapter 13).

Factors that tend to reduce the risk of dying once disease has become established include effective health services and higher education levels. The most effective health services are not necessarily those most technologically advanced but rather those which are readily accessible. Historically speaking, the contribution of health services has been small because until recently most medical interventions were ineffective. In low-income countries, however, the therapeutic component has been of greater importance, contributing to the major decline in child mortality seen over the past few decades. While its impact on adult mortality has been smaller, health services are nevertheless important in the relief of suffering. Future gains in health status are most likely to derive from more effective public health measures.

By focusing on the important social and economic causes of changing death rates, the concept of health transition offers potential for understanding health trends and thus improving health in all countries. However, it does not explain all differences in death rates between countries or necessarily predict changes associated with modernisation (as the recent deterioration in life expectancy in some eastern European countries illustrates). Furthermore, the theory does not easily account for marked declines in mortality rates from major non-communicable disease such as heart disease and stroke. In other words, although health transition theory provides a useful descriptive tool, it requires more elaboration to be of much predictive value.

Disease and disability

While mortality is important for the study of demography it does not provide a complete picture to inform public health action. Premature and potentially preventable death represents the most important challenge for public health but death rates alone as an indicator of health status fail to account for the full burden of disease.

A more comprehensive indicator promoted by the World Bank combines losses from premature death with loss of healthy life resulting from disability to calculate the disability-adjusted life year (DALY). These DALYs can be defined as the sum of years of potential life lost due to premature mortality and the years of productive life lost due to disability. The calculation of DALYs involves multiple assumptions and has many limitations. In some regions and for many diseases, the necessary data on disease incidence and duration are unavailable. Nevertheless, DALYs provide a broader measure of the global impact of disease. They help highlight inexpensive and effective ways to reduce dramatically the burden of communicable disease which accounts for 35% of the world total. Tackling the remaining 65% requires more complex policy approaches.

Healthy-life expectancy rises with increasing life expectancy. However, the percentage of life expected to be lived in healthy states declines. Overall, disability rises with age and disability onset becomes more compressed around the average age. Prevalence levels of disability are greater in low socio-economic groups than in higher socio-economic groups. Major inequalities in health are apparent when the population is categorised by social class, income, occupation, education and ethnicity (Chapter 15). Several possible explanations for these have been advanced: misclassification of social class, particularly in women and the retired; downward 'drift' because of ill health; inequalities in the distribution of major risk factors for disease; inequalities in the distribution of income. An important reason for inequalities in health appears to be the distribution of wealth within a country. In countries where income distribution is relatively equal, health inequalities are less than in countries where there are gross disparities in wealth [11]. In short, health inequalities may reflect social policies that neglect the needs of poor people.

Methodological issues in demography

The accuracy with which demographic statistics are collected across the world varies greatly. In order to compare the measures discussed in this chapter data are needed on the numbers of people (population 'stock'), births, deaths, disease and migration. It is a necessary element of demography to collect these data in the best possible way, assess their accuracy and, where necessary, deal with gaps or inaccuracy through estimation.

The data on population stock often come from censuses. A census is defined by the United Nations as 'the total process of collecting, compiling and publishing demographic, economic and social data pertaining at a specified time or times, to all persons in a country or delimited territory.' While the United Nations has worked to improve comparability across the world there will still be variations. As well as numbers of people, censuses may be used to collect data on age, sex, ethnicity, residence, fertility, health and other factors. Censuses are costly to administer and, although crucial in providing the denominator for many demographic and health measures, carry some inherent problems:

- Not all countries carry them out.
- They may not be carried out at the same intervals (decennially is recommended).
- Data become less accurate as time since census elapses.
- Under-enumeration may occur due to, for example, non-response (e.g. of older people), mobility of population (e.g. seasonal migrants).
- Data accuracy may be poor, e.g. for people reporting a digit preference for stating their age (30, 35, 40), inaccurate reporting of marital status or overstatement of age by the elderly.
- Inaccurate assignment of people to geographical areas (e.g. deaths in hospital all reported as from one town but residence being from a much wider area).

Attempts to reduce these inherent errors include validation surveys where intensive efforts are made to contact a sample of respondents to check data.

Vital registration systems collect data on births and deaths. In many countries this is compulsory, which helps ensure data completeness. In much of the developing world, however, birth and death need not be registered so these data can be seriously incomplete. Even with well-established systems inaccuracies are inevitable as they rely heavily on the quality of information and coding being high. In particular, there may be problems with the accuracy of the recording of cause of death. For example, with the increasing age at death of much of the population it is increasingly likely that people die with multiple pathologies; which to state as primary cause of death may be an arbitrary decision. Variations have occurred over time as fashions change, knowledge increases and deaths in countries with well-established systems are better defined (for example, death from bronchopneumonia rather than old age).

Where demographic data are systematically absent an alternative is the application of population surveys, which sample a proportion of the population. For example, the Demographic and Health Surveys (DHS) Project is a worldwide research project to provide data and analysis on the population, health and nutrition of women and children in developing countries [12].

We have seen the importance of fertility in determining population trends but fertility is very difficult to estimate accurately. Estimates of fertility depend, to varying degrees, on the availability of data on births, maternal age and deaths. As we have seen these are of variable accuracy and completeness and this leads to a range of measures being used and potential problems with comparability.

Measuring mortality is similarly problematic. As with fertility, crude measures are possible (number of births or deaths per unit population) but these are highly dependent upon the age structure of the population, so are not comparable. With mortality, age-specific death rates are preferable but not always possible due to data deficiencies. Standardisation is a technique used to apply standard population age-specific mortality rates (for example, the national or regional rates) to the population under study to give an expected number of deaths. This is then used in a ratio with the observed deaths to give a standardised mortality ratio (SMR), which is a useful summary (i.e. an SMR over 100 suggests the mortality experience of this population is worse than that of the standard population) (see Chapter 4). A way of measuring the effectiveness of health-care interventions is 'avoidable mortality' defined as 'all those deaths that, given current medical knowledge and technology, could be avoided by the health-care system through either prevention and/or treatment' [13].

Life tables also rely on accurate demographic data but when there are insufficient data available to construct them they can be modelled with limited mortality rates estimated from global averages. These modelled life tables can then be used to estimate age-specific mortality rates, which are extremely useful in areas where vital registration systems are poor.

Measuring migration can also present particular difficulties. Differences in the size of administrative regions may mean that a short move would count as a migration in one country and a huge move not count in another. Comparability is therefore problematic, especially if boundaries change. It may also be difficult to distinguish temporary migration (e.g. a move to university) from a permanent one. Increasing circular migration where migrants move in and out of a destination also creates problems in measuring migration. If censuses are taken then an estimate of migration can be made by determining the difference in population between two censuses not accounted for by natural increases or depletion. This is termed the 'balancing equation' and estimates net migration (or errors in the data).

Conclusion

The field of demography requires a detailed understanding of various data sources and robust methods to analyse their accuracy and deal with consequent levels of uncertainty. However, demography provides the public health practitioner with some of the most fundamental measures with which to assess the health of a population.

REFERENCES

1. Department of Economic and Social Affairs Population Division, *The World Population Prospects* 2004 Revision, New York, NY, United Nations, 2005. See: http://www.un.org/esa/population/publications/WPP2004/2004Highlights_finalrevised.pdf.
2. The World Bank, Fertility rate, total (births per women) data. See: http://data.worldbank.org/indicator/SP.DYN.TFRT.IN.
3. UNICEF, ChildInfo. Monitoring the situation of children and women. See: http://www.childinfo.org/mortality.html.
4. S. H. Preston, The changing relation between mortality and level of economic development. *Population Studies* **29**, 1975, 231–48.
5. S. Glanz and E. Balbach, *Tobacco War: Inside the California Battles*. Berkeley University, CA, California Press, 2000.

6. J. Powles, Public health policy in developed countries. In R. Detels, R. Beaglehole, M. A. Lansang and M. Gulliford (eds.), *Oxford Textbook of Public Health*, 5th edn., Oxford, Oxford University Press, 2009.

7. R. Beaglehole and R. Bonita, *Public Health at the Crossroads. Achievements and Prospects*, Cambridge, Cambridge University Press, 1997.

8. A. R. Omran, The epidemiologic transition. *Milbank Quarterly* **49** (1), 1971, 509–38.

9. S. J. Olshansky and A. B. Ault, The fourth stage of the epidemiologic transition: the age of delayed degenerative diseases. *Milbank Quarterly* **64** (3), 1986, 355–91.

10. World Health Organization, Health transition. See: http://www.who.int/trade/glossary/story050/en/index.html.

11. R. G. Wilkinson and K. Pickett, *The Spirit Level: Why More Equal Societies Almost Always Do Better*. London, Allen Lane, 2009.

12. MEASURE DHS, Demographic and Health Surveys. See: http://www.measuredhs.com/start.cfm.

13. Centre for Health Economics (CHE), Avoidable mortality: what it means and how it is measured. Research paper 63, 2011, University of York. See: http://www.york.ac.uk/media/che/documents/papers/researchpapers/CHERP63_avoidable_mortality_what_it_means_and_how_it_is_measured.pdf.

3

Epidemiology
Padmanabhan Badrinath and Stephen Gillam

Key points

- Epidemiology concerns the study of the distribution and determinants of disease and health-related states.
- The uses of epidemiology include:
  - determining the major health problems occuring in a community;
  - monitoring health and disease trends across populations;
  - making useful projections into the future to identify emerging health problems;
  - describing the natural history of new conditions, e.g. who gets the disease, who dies from it, and the outcome of the disease;
  - estimating clinical risks for individuals;
  - evaluating new health technologies, e.g. drugs or preventive programmes;
  - investigating epidemics of unknown aetiology.

Introduction

At the core of epidemiology is the use of quantitative methods to study diseases in human populations and how they may be prevented. Thus, epidemiology can be defined as the 'study of distribution and determinants of health-related states and events in the population and the application of this science to control health problems' [1]. It is important to note that epidemiology concerns not only the study of diseases but of all health-related events. For example, we can study the epidemiology of breast feeding or road traffic accidents. Rational health-promoting public policies require a sound basis in epidemiology.

Essential Public Health, Second Edition, ed. Stephen Gillam, Jan Yates and Padmanabhan Badrinath. Published by Cambridge University Press. © Cambridge University Press 2012.

The epidemiological analysis of a disease from a population perspective is vital in order to be able to organise and monitor effective preventive, curative and rehabilitative services. All health professionals and health-service managers need an awareness of the principles of epidemiology. They need to go beyond questions relating to individuals such as 'What should be done for this patient now?' to challenging fundamentals such as 'Why did *this* person get *this* disease at *this* time?', 'Is the occurrence of the disease increasing and, if so, why?' and 'What are the causes or risk factors for this disease?'

In the following pages we look briefly at the origins of epidemiology and then examine some of its key concepts including:

- disease variation;
- the concept of a population;
- measures of disease frequency – rates;
- quantifying differences in risk;
- types of epidemiological study design;
- how to interpret the results of epidemiological studies.

The history of epidemiology

The origins of modern epidemiology can be traced back to the work of English reformers and French scientists in the first half of the nineteenth century. However, writers of the Hippocratic School in the fourth century BC, who stressed the effects of physical factors, such as air, geographical location and water on health and disease [2], are often claimed as prototypic epidemiologists. The Hippocratic corpus underpinned one of two explanatory theories of disease that competed until modern times. Poisonous particles generated by the decomposition of organic matter (miasma) were held responsible for many diseases. Though eventually discredited, the notion of miasma led to important public health interventions – better-ventilated housing and the provision of sanitation. By contrast, contagion theory, which ultimately underpinned germ theory, had its origins in the ancient practice of isolating diseased people.

John Graunt laid the basis of health statistics and epidemiology with his analyses of the weekly bills of mortality in the seventeenth century. Using these data, Graunt described the patterns of mortality and fertility and seasonal variations charting the progress of epidemics, most famously in the plague years. In 1747, James Lind, a British naval surgeon, undertook a study testing his hypothesis of the cause of scurvy and the clinical trial was born (see Box 3.1).

Building on the ideas of Graunt, William Farr institutionalised epidemiology in Victorian England. He developed a system of vital statistics that was to form the basis of disease classification now in its tenth revision. The International Classification of Diseases and Related Health Problems (commonly known by the abbreviation ICD) is designed to promote international comparability in the collection, processing,

Box 3.1 James Lind

In 1747, Lind took 12 seamen with scurvy and, in addition to their normal diet, gave each of six pairs a different dietary supplement for 6 days. The two seamen given oranges and lemons made an almost complete recovery from which Lind inferred that citric acid fruits could prevent scurvy. It was not until 1795 that the British naval authorities accepted his results and included limes in the diet of sailors. Such delays in disseminating evidence were much later to provide the rationale for the evidence-based medicine (EBM) movement (Chapter 5). Only in 1920 were alternative theories eliminated and consensus reached that scurvy resulted from a dietary deficiency.

classification and presentation of morbidity and mortality statistics. Over a long career Farr developed methods for studying the distribution and determinants of human diseases.

Over the last decades, epidemiologists have added to the body of knowledge on disease patterns and their causes in the population by meticulously studying large sections of the population with respect to particular conditions or risk factors. Examples of landmark studies are given later in the chapter.

Time, place, person – disease variation

Epidemiologists seek answers to the following questions:
- How does the pattern of this disease vary over *time* in this population? A decline in disease is as worthy of investigation as a rise.
- How does the *place* in which the population lives affect the disease? International differences in disease patterns mainly, although not wholly, reflect the fact that populations are at different stages in their demographic and epidemiological transitions. International variations are reducing as these transitions take place, just as migrant populations' disease patterns tend to converge towards those of the populations they join.
- How do the *personal characteristics* of people in the population affect the disease's pattern? We can ask 'What is the relative importance of genetic and environmental influences in bringing about population differences in disease?' In large populations, genetic makeup is relatively stable. Changes in disease frequency in large populations over short periods of time are almost wholly due to environmental factors. In individuals, as opposed to populations, genetic makeup is profoundly important in shaping risk of disease, for genetic variation between individuals is great. Disease is, of course, caused by the interaction of the genome and the environment [3].

This is often summarised by describing health states and determinants in terms of 'time, place and person'.

The concept of a population

Epidemiology and public health policy depend on the notion of *population*. Traditionally, health systems have been designed around a population of people with health problems, those who contact the service. Public health specialists, however, have responsibility for the whole population, those who are at risk of health problems and have early stages of disease. This can be seen as the submerged part of the disease 'iceberg' (Figure 3.1). People with symptomatic disease can be further subdivided into those with symptoms not seeking medical help, symptomatic but self-treating, and those who are symptomatic but accessing informal care. Even among the symptomatic only some people seek formal health-care. Below the surface there are a large number who may have latent, pre-symptomatic, undiagnosed disease. However, not all people without symptoms can be described as in perfect health. Many people may have risk factors that make them more prone to various diseases: for example smoking, sedentary lifestyle and obesity, which put them at increased risk of coronary heart disease.

Firstly, we need to define clearly the population we are interested in. This might vary in size from an entire country to a small community. It may also be restricted by the disease in question, e.g. to those suffering from coronary heart disease. When the population is defined we can then consider how the pattern of disease varies. This will allow us to plan services based on the pattern of disease in the population as a whole and not just among users of the service. Secondly, we can then deliver modified services to sub-groups of the population who differ in terms of their needs and are

Figure 3.1   The iceberg of disease.

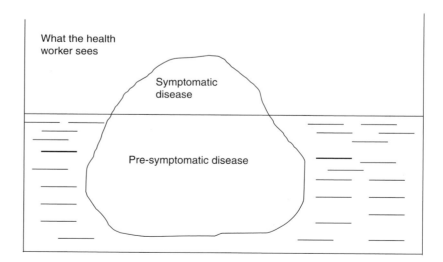

not making effective use of existing services (e.g. homeless, non-native-language-speaking). Thirdly, by using knowledge of population trends and health status we anticipate the need for future services.

Populations may be *stable* or *dynamic*. A stable population is known as a cohort (a group of people with common characteristics). The population is defined at the start of the follow-up period and gradually diminishes in size as its members cease to be at risk of becoming a case (e.g. they die). In contrast, a dynamic population is one in which there is turnover of membership while it is being observed. People enter and leave the population at different times.

Epidemiological variables

Disease patterns are influenced by the interaction of factors (variables) at social, environmental and individual levels. Consideration of these factors aids in the depiction, analysis and interpretation of differences in disease patterns within and between populations. Age, sex, economic status, social class, occupation, country of residence or birth and racial or ethnic classifications may be used to show variations in health status. Most variables used in epidemiology are markers for complex, underlying phenomena that cannot be measured easily. For example, we might measure obesity levels in a population as a marker of the risk of heart disease.

A good epidemiological variable should:
- have an impact on health in individuals and populations;
- be measurable;
- differentiate populations in their experience of disease and health;
- differentiate populations in some underlying characteristics relevant to health, e.g. income or behaviour;
- generate testable aetiological hypotheses;
- help to develop health policy, plan and deliver health-care, prevent and control disease.

Exercise 3.1 Epidemiological variables 1

For each of these qualities, can age be considered a useful epidemiological variable.

Table 3.1 provides some suggestions.

Once we have identified that a disease varies according to such factors as age or social class we can begin to consider how the factor exerts an effect. For example, it is well known that the occurrence of heart disease is more common in men than women. Some of the possible explanations for this include differences in lifestyle factors, occupations and levels of co-existing diseases. Refer to the exercise in the Internet Companion for a detailed discussion of this topic.

Geographical differences in epidemiological variables can also provide important clues to the causes of disease. Figure 3.2 shows the distribution of blood pressure in two populations in two different continents.

Table 3.1 Age as a useful epidemiological variable

Criteria for a good epidemiological variable	Criteria in relation to the factor age
Impact on health in individuals and population	Age is a powerful influence on health as chronological age is related to the general health of the individual
Be measurable accurately	In most populations age is measurable to the day, but in some it has to be guessed, as people are not aware of their exact birth day
Differentiate populations in their experience of disease or health	Large differences by age are seen for most diseases or their determinants
Generate testable aetiological hypotheses, and/or	It is hard to test hypotheses because there are so many underlying differences between populations of different ages
Help in developing health policy, and/or Help to plan and deliver health-care and/or Help to prevent and control disease	Age differences in disease patterns could affect health policy and planning of services. Knowing the age structure of a population is critical to good planning. By understanding the age at which diseases start, preventive and control programmes can be targeted at appropriate age groups

Figure 3.2   The distribution of blood-pressure values in Kenyan nomads and London civil servants [4].

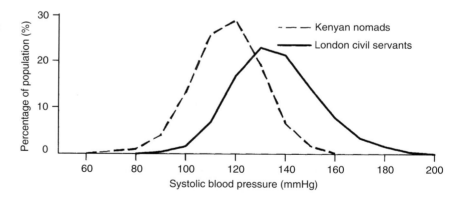

Exercise 3.2   Epidemiological variable 2

Referring to Figure 3.2, answer the following questions:

a. In what ways do the shapes of the distributions differ in the two populations?

b. Roughly, what percentage of the Kenyans and London civil servants have hypertension (assuming a systolic blood pressure over 150 mm Hg is hypertension)?

c. Is there any suggestion from the above figure that the cause of high blood pressure in an individual Kenyan nomad and a London civil servant is likely to differ?

d. What are the possible causes of the different distribution of blood pressure in the two populations?

a. The shape of the distributions of blood pressure is similar – a so-called 'normal' distribution. The Londoners' distribution has shifted rightwards slightly and is therefore called 'skewed'.

b. Five per cent nomads and about 20% of civil servants.

c. No, the cause of high blood pressure in individuals is not presented in the data.

d. The causes of the rightward skew probably include dietary factors, obesity, insufficient exercise, stress and genetic factors.

Measures of disease frequency

One measure of disease frequency is a count of the number of cases of a disease occurring in a population. However, the number of cases alone is not particularly informative. Account must also be taken of the size of the population and usually the length of time over which its members were observed. This gives rise to a comparison between the number of cases in the population and the size of the population over a given time, often expressed as a rate.

The numerator of a rate is the number of 'cases' but defining people as cases can be difficult. For some diseases (e.g. rabies) case definition is clear; for others (such as hypertension) the disease shows a spectrum of severity and arbitrary criteria must be imposed to distinguish diseased from non-diseased.

The denominator of a rate is the 'population at risk' in a defined time period and this too must be carefully defined. The ideal denominator for the pregnancy rate is dependent upon the culture of the population being measured.

In calculating the pregnancy rate what would be the appropriate denominator?

In some cases it is married women in the 15–44 or 15–49 year age groups as these are the only women at risk of becoming pregnant. However, in some cultures this would not be the case and the denominator would not be restricted to married women. This leaves us with a problem if pregnancy rates are compared across populations, as the denominators do not match. When comparing rates across populations it is important to ensure that the same variables are used as numerators and denominators.

Prevalence

A measure of the burden of disease in a population is the *prevalence*. This is the number of cases of disease in a population at a given time and it is frequently used in planning the allocation of health-service resources. Generally, we use the term prevalence to mean a *point prevalence*, which is defined as follows:

$$\text{Point prevalence} = \frac{\text{Number of diseased persons in a defined population at one point in time}}{\text{Number of persons in the defined population at the same moment in time}} \qquad (3.1)$$

Point prevalence is a proportion and does not involve time. *Period prevalence* is the number of cases of disease during a specified time (e.g. a week, month or year). When the period is long the denominator is usually the number of persons at the mid point of the time period (e.g. the mid-year population)

$$\text{Period prevalence} = \frac{\text{Number of diseased persons in a defined population during a specified period of time}}{\text{Number of persons in the defined population over the same period of time}} \qquad (3.2)$$

Incidence

When researching the aetiology of diseases, measures of disease *incidence* are of primary interest. Cases of incident disease in a defined period of time are those which first occur during that time. There are two ways of expressing disease incidence: risk (or cumulative incidence) and incidence rate but in situations where the disease events are rare these give very similar results.

Risk is defined as the number of cases of a disease that occur in a defined period of time as a proportion of the number of people in the population at the beginning of the period. Deaths in the population may be measured rather than the number of cases:

$$\text{Risk in defined period of time} = \frac{\text{Number of persons who become diseased (or die) during the period}}{\text{Number of persons in the population at the beginning of the period}} \qquad (3.3)$$

Risk may also be known as cumulative incidence. It describes the way that populations as a whole experience disease. However, it may also be thought of as the risk an individual has of developing the disease in the specified period of time. Risk is the possibility of harm. In epidemiology, the association between risk of disease and both individual and social characteristics (risk factors) provides the starting point for analysing the causes of disease.

Incidence rate is defined as the number of new cases (or deaths) occurring in a defined period of time in a defined population. The sum of the periods of time for each

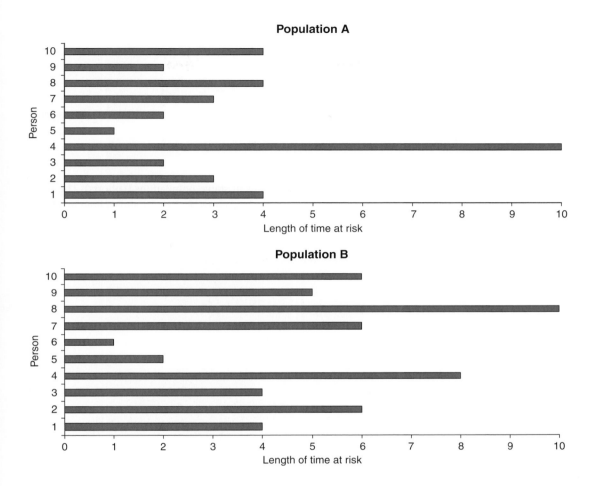

Population A

Population B

individual when he or she is disease-free but may develop the disease is the denom-

Figure 3.3   Populations at risk of death.

inator and is known as the person–time at risk.

$$\text{Incidence rate} = \frac{\text{Number of persons who have become diseased}}{\text{Person–time at risk}} \qquad (3.4)$$

Figure 3.3 shows two populations, A and B, which are observed for 10 years. Over time, members of the populations die. The length of time each person spends alive (and therefore at risk of death) is shown by the bars on the charts. For population A, the person–time at risk, the incidence rate and the risk at 10 years can be calculated:

- Person–time at risk – 10 people with 4 + 3 + 2 + 10 + 1 + 2 + 3 + 4 + 2 + 4 years at risk. Person–time at risk = 35 person years.
- Incidence rate at 10 years = 9 people who died/35 person years at risk = 0.257 people per year (number of cases is 9 as one person remains alive at the end of the period).

- Risk at 10 years = 9 people who died /10 people at the start of the period = 0.9 people per year.

Exercise 3.3 – Risk and incidence

Calculate these for population B

- Person–time at risk – 10 people with 4 + 6 + 4 + 8 + 2 + 1 + 6 + 10 + 5 + 6 years at risk. Person–time at risk = 52 person years
- Incidence rate = 9/52 = 0.173 people per year
- Risk at 10 years = 9/10 = 0.9 people per year

So far we have calculated incidence rates in stable populations (cohorts). The same calculations can be done for dynamic populations. Figure 3.4 shows how incidence might look in a dynamic population.

Exercise 3.4   Incidence in dynamic populations

From Figure 3.4 calculate

a. the person–time at risk at the end of year 7;

b. incidence rate after 7 years; and

c. the risk of the condition at the end of year 3.

a. Person–time at risk = 3 + 4 + 5 + 3 + 5 + 2 + 4 + 3 + 3 + 6 = 38 person years.

b. Incidence rate = 8/38 = 21.1% (two people remain at risk at the end of the period and are not counted in the numerator for incidence rate).

c. The total person years at the end of year 3 is (1 + 1 + 2 + 2 + 1 + 0 + 1 + 3 + 1 + 2 = 14) and person 8 died. Hence the risk of the condition at the end of year 3 is 1/14 i.e. 7.14%.

Sometimes direct measurement of person–time at risk is not possible. This is true for mortality rates where we do not know when each individual became at risk or stopped

Figure 3.4   Incidence in dynamic populations.

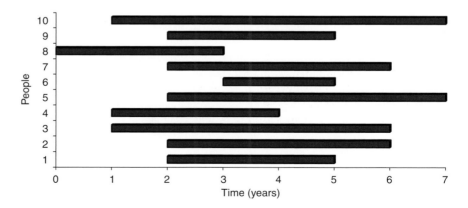

being at risk. Instead, as with estimates of period prevalence, an estimate of the person–time at risk is taken to be the population at the mid-point of the calendar period of interest × the length of the period (usually a year).

For example, the all-cause mortality rate for females in England and Wales for 2005 is defined as:

$$\text{Mortality rate per year} = \frac{\text{Number of female deaths from all causes in England and Wales in 2005}}{\text{Estimate of 2005 mid-year female population of England and Wales}} \qquad (3.5)$$

Relationship between prevalence, incidence and duration of disease

Figure 3.5 (overleaf) shows the prevalent population as the circle on the right and people entering this as incident cases from the non-diseased population on the left. So, in a fixed population, prevalence is approximately equal to the incidence rate (the number of people entering the prevalent population in a defined period of time) multiplied by the duration of the disease (how long they stay there):

$$\text{Prevalence} = \text{Incidence rate} \times \text{Period of follow-up} \qquad (3.6)$$

This means that for conditions with a long duration (e.g. diabetes or heart disease) prevalence is a good estimate of the burden of disease but for conditions with a short duration (e.g. influenza) incidence is a better measure.

Exercise 3.5   Incidence and prevalence

10,000 miners were recruited to a study. At baseline, 50 were found to have lung cancer and were excluded from follow-up. The remainder underwent 6-monthly reviews for 5 years. At the end of 5 years, 9 miners had developed lung cancer.
a. What was the prevalence of lung cancer at baseline?
b. What was the risk of developing lung cancer over five years?
c. What is the approximate incidence rate of lung cancer among miners?
d. Why is it only an approximation?

a. Prevalence at baseline = 50/10,000 = 0.5%.
b. Risk or cumulative incidence over 5 years = 9/9950 = 0.905 per 1000.
c. Incidence rate = 9/(9950 × 5) = 0.181 per 1000 person years.
d. It is assumed that each person contributed a full 5 years of follow-up to the denominator, hence the rate is likely to be underestimated.

Case fatality and survival rates

The terms case fatality and survival rate are often used to compare the killing power of diseases. The case fatality rate is actually a form of risk, which measures the

Figure 3.5   The relationship between prevalence and incidence.

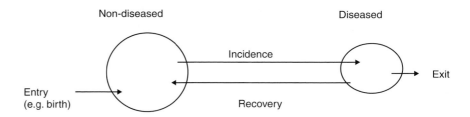

proportion of people with a disease (e.g. cancer) who die within a defined period of diagnosis. If we assume that all cases either die or survive the case fatality rate is related to the survival rate from a disease:

$$\text{Probability (survival)} + \text{Probability (death)} = 1 \tag{3.7}$$

The case fatality and survival rates are not true rates, as they do not measure the rate per unit of time at risk at which death occurs; they are probabilities. The case fatality rate is simply the ratio of deaths to cases.

Quantifying differences in risk

When epidemiologists seek to explain health experiences, they often compare the rates of diseases across populations. These may be populations with different risk factors for disease, or populations who are being treated differently for a disease they already have. In order to do this it is helpful to use measures which compare the risk between the two populations.

Relative Risks

Relative Risk tells us how much more at risk one population is compared to another. For example, we might want to compare how many children with meningitis die if they are treated using antibiotics alone with how many die if they are given steroids as well. To begin, we must define the risk in both populations. There are two main ways of summarising these risks, as either a proportion (a risk as defined earlier in this chapter) or as an odd. For example, if 320 children developed meningitis during one year and 32 died, this can be expressed as a proportion: 32/320 (10%) – i.e. 32 children die for every 320 who get meningitis; or it can be expressed as the odds of dying: 32/288 – i.e. 32 children die for every 288 with meningitis who survive. Then, to compare the risk in two groups we can calculate the ratio between the risk measured in one group and the risk measured in the other group (i.e. divide the risk in one group by the risk in the other group).

Now a note on epidemiological terminology which can be incredibly confusing. A ratio can be calculated from both the measures of risk defined above. If we use the ratio between the proportions it is known as the *Relative Risk*; if we use the ratio between the odds it is called the *Odds Ratio*. Both the Relative Risk and the Odds Ratio are measures of relative risk in a general sense. Reading epidemiological texts, you will come across the term 'risk ratio' – used as a synonym for the Relative Risk or with reference to both the Relative Risk and Odds Ratio. In this book we use 'relative risk' as an overarching term referring to the ratio of either two risks or two odds, Relative Risk (note capitals) to mean the ratio of two risks and Odds Ratio to mean the ratio of two odds.

Example: In a trial of nicotine gum, a group of smokers were given gum and a control group were not. Out of 6328 smokers who were given nicotine gum, 1149 stopped smoking. Out of 8380 smokers in the control group, 893 stopped. So the numbers who did not give up smoking are 6328 – 1149 = 5179 and 8380 – 893 = 7487, respectively.

These figures can be shown on a 2 × 2 table, which often helps to support calculating relative risks.

	Given nicotine gum	No nicotine gum
Gave up smoking	1149	893
Did not give up	5179	7487
Total	6328	8380

The Relative Risk = risk of stopping smoking in nicotine-gum group/risk of stopping smoking in the control group. The Odds Ratio = odds of stopping smoking in the nicotine-gum group/odds of stopping smoking in the control group. NB We can see here that the word 'risk' can be applied to an outcome which we want (i.e. stopping smoking) as well as to an outcome we want to avoid such as death. Therefore:

Relative Risk = (1149/6328)/(893/8380) = 1.70
Odds Ratio = (1149/5179)/(893/7487) = 1.86.

This can be put into words such that we can say someone who uses nicotine gum is 1.7 times more likely to give up smoking as someone who does not. Or the odds of someone stopping smoking if they use nicotine gum are 1.86 times greater than if they don't.

Relative Risks can be used as a measure of the *strength of association* between a risk factor and an outcome (e.g. smoking and lung cancer) or a measure of the effectiveness of an intervention in causing an outcome (e.g. nicotine gum and stopping smoking). Odds Ratios are calculated in case–control studies (see page 64) because in case–control studies we can only derive the odds of exposure among cases (those with the condition of interest) and the odds of exposure in controls (those without the condition of interest). In instances when the condition under study is rare, Odds Ratio approximates to the Relative Risk. This approximation is useful as it helps us interpret studies simply and assumes that an Odds Ratio quoted is an approximation of a Relative Risk, but it must be remembered that this only holds for rare conditions. The following example illustrates this point.

Example: In the nicotine-gum example from earlier the Relative Risk and the Odds Ratio are similar (1.70 and 1.86), but imagine that the prevalence of stopping smoking was much higher:

	Given nicotine gum	No nicotine gum
Gave up smoking	3000	2000
Did not give up	3328	6380
Total	6328	8380

Calculating the Relative Risk and Odds Ratio now we find:

Relative Risk = (3000/6328)/(2000/8380) = 1.99
Odds Ratio = (3000/3328)/(2000/6380) = 2.87

The Relative Risk is now much smaller than the Odds Ratio and we cannot assume that an Odds Ratio quoted in a study for a very common outcome would be the same as a Relative Risk.

Relative Risks are also useful in epidemiology as they provide a single summary statistic where no difference (i.e. no association between a risk factor and an outcome or no effect of an intervention) will give a Relative Risk of 1. A Relative Risk greater than 1 suggests there is an association between the risk factor or intervention and the outcome. So if the outcome is something we want (such as cure or reduced mortality) a Relative Risk greater than 1 is good but if we want less of the outcome (such as death) then a Relative Risk below 1 is good.

Exercise 3.6   Relative Risk

The Relative Risk of death due to lung cancer among smokers is 15.34 compared to non-smokers. The same study found that the Relative Risk in smokers for coronary heart disease (CHD) was 1.45. What is your interpretation of these findings?

Smokers are 15.34 more likely to die of lung cancer compared to non-smokers. This risk is very high and there is a strong association between smoking and lung cancer. However, for CHD the risk is much smaller as smokers are at only 1.45 times higher risk of dying due to CHD compared to non-smokers.

Absolute risk reduction

The *absolute risk reduction* (ARR) is the difference in the rate of adverse events between study and control populations:

Absolute risk reduction (ARR)

$\quad$ = experimental event rate (EER) − control event rate (CER) $\qquad$ (3.8)

The ARR is a measure of the absolute effect of exposure and is a guide to individual needs and benefits. It may be estimated in cohort studies but not in case–control studies (see below).

When to use relative risk and when to use absolute risk reduction

In general, relative risks are more useful for expressing the population impact of a risk factor or intervention and absolute risks are more useful when considering individual needs and benefits. For example, if the risk of recurrence of a cancer goes from an absolute risk of 5% down to 2.5% after treatment with a new drug, the relative risk reduction is 50% (50% of 5% is 2.5%) but the absolute risk reduction is only 2.5% (5% minus 2.5% = 2.5%). So, any one individual, with a small risk to begin with, reduces their risk by a small absolute amount. However, across a population this may be a significant risk reduction.

Exercise 3.7   Relative risk and absolute risk reduction

In a clinical trial the event rate in the control group is 40 per 100 patients, and the event rate in the treatment group is 30 per 100 patients. Calculate the Relative Risk and ARR in this trial.

Relative Risk = (40/100) ÷ (30/100) = 1.33, ARR = (40% – 30%) = 10%.

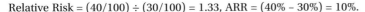

Number needed to treat

The *number needed to treat* (NNT) is another summary measure that is helpful in making decisions over which interventions are effective. The NNT is the number of people who (on average) need to receive a treatment to produce one additional successful outcome. If, for example, the NNT for a treatment is 10, the practitioner would have to give the treatment to 10 patients to prevent one patient from having the adverse outcome over the defined period, and each patient who received the treatment would have a 1 in 10 chance of being a beneficiary.

For example, if the NNT for the use of nicotine chewing gum in helping people stop smoking for at least 1 year is 14, we need to treat 14 smokers by giving them nicotine gum, for one extra person to stop smoking.

Calculation of NNT

If a disease has a death rate of 100% without treatment and treatment reduces that mortality rate to 50%, the ARR is 100/100–50/100 = 0.5. How many people would we need to treat to prevent one death? In this example treating 100 patients with the otherwise fatal disease results in 50 survivors. This is equivalent to one out of every two treated, an NNT of 2.

Alternatively, the NNT to prevent one adverse outcome equals the inverse of the absolute risk reduction, i.e. NNT = 1/ARR.

Example: Using data from the example on page 55 we can calculate the NNT for nicotine gum. Out of 6328 smokers who were given nicotine gum, 1149 stopped smoking.
Out of 8380 smokers in the control group, 893 stopped smoking.
NNT = 1/ARR = 1/[(1149/6328) – (893/8380)] = 1/(0.182 – 0.107) = 1/0.075 = 13.3.
The NNT is always rounded up and in this case it will be 14. The NNT gives more information than relative risk because it takes into account the baseline frequency of the outcome. Exercise 3.8 illustrates this.

Exercise 3.8   NNT

A drug reduces the risk of dying from a heart attack by 40% (Relative Risk = 0.60). In terms of relative risk, this drug has the same 'clinical effectiveness' for everyone. Calculate the NNT if it is given to people with a 1 in 10 annual risk of dying from a heart attack and to people with a 1 in 100 risk.
For a risk of 1/10:
The original risk is 1/10 (0.1) and with the drug 0.6 × 1/10 = 0.06
So the ARR is 0.1 – 0.06 = 0.04
And the NNT = 1/0.04 = 25
For a risk of 1/100:
The original risk is 1/100 (0.01) and with the drug 0.6 × 1/100 = 0.006
So the ARR is 0.01 – 0.006 = 0.004
And the NNT = 1/0.004 = 250

So we can see that the NNT is much higher when the risk of the condition (incidence rate) is lower. If the drug causes serious side effects in 1 in 100 people then we would probably not use it for people with a low risk but it would still be an effective treatment for people with high baseline risk. So the NNT helps us estimate how likely the treatment is to help an individual patient.

Measures of population impact

So far we have considered how we measure the rates of disease or risk factors in populations and how we measure the effects of risk factors or interventions in populations exposed to them compared to unexposed populations. Another useful measure when looking at the health of populations or individuals is a measure of what proportion of death or disease can be attributed to specific causes. For individuals, the *attributable risk* (AR) is the difference between the event rates in the exposed and unexposed populations and is usually expressed as an attributable fraction (AF).

$$AF = \frac{(\text{event rate in exposed population} - \text{event rate in unexposed}) \times 100}{\text{event rate in exposed population}} \quad (3.9)$$

For example, in deciding whether or not to indulge in a dangerous sport such as rock climbing, the attributable risk of injury (i.e. the risk due solely to the rock climbing and not other causes) must be weighed against the pleasures of participation.

For populations, the *population attributable risk* is the reduction in the risk (incidence) for a population if the population were to be entirely unexposed to the factor under study (such as smoking). Like AR this is often expressed as a fraction, the population attributable fraction (PAF).

PAF = attributable risk × prevalence of exposure to risk factor in population; or
Population attributable risk = Rate in population − Rate in unexposed   (3.10)

The population attributable risk tells us what proportion of a population's disease or death experience is due to a particular cause and can indicate the potential impact of control measures in a population (i.e. what proportion of disease would be eliminated in a population if its disease rate were reduced to that of unexposed persons). Population attributable risk is, therefore, particularly relevant to decisions in public health. The following exercises examine the risks attributable to smoking at a population level.

A classic study of smoking and mortality [5, 6]

Exercise 3.9   Attributable risks

The British Doctors' Study [5, 6] was set up in 1951 to investigate the relationship between smoking habits and mortality. A total of 59,600 members of the medical profession in the United Kingdom were asked to fill in a simple questionnaire on smoking habits. Complete replies were received from 34,440 men – that is, about 69% of the male doctors who were alive when the questionnaire was sent. Further inquiries about changes in smoking habit were made in 1957, 1966, 1971 and 1991; i.e. after 6, 15, 20 and 40 years. Of the initial respondents in 1951, 17% were classified as non-smokers. In the first 20 years of follow-up (1951–71) a total of 10,000 deaths occurred in the 34,440 men, 441 of which were from lung cancer and 3191 from ischaemic heart disease (IHD); see Table 3.2.

From Table 3.2
a. **Calculate relative risks (as Relative Risks) and attributable fractions for the data in Table 3.2 relative to non-smokers?**

LIVERPOOL JOHN MOORES UNIVERSITY
LEARNING SERVICES

Table 3.2 The British Doctors Study [6]. Death rate for men by cause of death and cigarette smoking habit

Cause of death	Death rate per 1000	
	Smokers	Non-smokers
Lung cancer	0.9	0.07
IHD	4.87	4.22

Table 3.3 Annual death rate by smoking status [6]

	Annual death rates per 100,000 from lung disease
Heavy smokers	224
Non-smokers	10
Total population	74

b. (i) Which disease is most strongly related to cigarette smoking?
   (ii) Which disease has the largest number of deaths statistically attributable to cigarette smoking?

a. The Relative Risks are 12.86 (0.9/0.07) for lung cancer and 1.15 (4.87/4.22) for IHD. The attributable fraction is 92% ([(0.9–0.07) /0.9] × 100) for lung cancer and 13.3% ([(4.87–4.22) /4.87] × 100) for CHD.

b. (i) The data shows that 92% of lung cancer is attributable to smoking and 13.3% of CHD. In CHD both Relative Risk and AR are not very high suggesting not much of the disease could be prevented by stopping smoking as compared to lung cancer.

   (ii) Ischaemic heart disease. The death rates from IHD in the population as a whole is high: 4.87/1000 in smokers and 4.22/1000 in non-smokers. Smoking is one of several causes of IHD mortality.

Annual death rates from lung cancer are given in Table 3.3.

From Table 3.3, calculate the Relative Risk and population attributable risk of lung disease associated with smoking.

Relative Risk for heavy smokers is 224/10 = 22.4 compared to non-smokers.
   Population attributable risk is 74–10 = 64 deaths per 100,000 person years

Summary

Table 3.4 summarises the concepts explained so far in the epidemiological description of disease (or risk factors) by time, place and person.

Table 3.4 Summary of concepts

Concept	Definition	Comment
Dynamic population	Population in which person–time experience can accumulate from a changing group of individuals	Ideal in cohort studies as everyone contributes to the denominator
Static population	Fixed population with no loss to follow up	Difficult to achieve as people tend to drop out of studies
Period prevalence	The number of existing cases of an illness during a period or interval, divided by the average population	A problem may arise with calculating period prevalence rates because of the difficulty of defining the most appropriate denominator
Point prevalence	The prevalence of a condition in a population at a given point in time	Prevalence data provide an indication of the extent of a condition and may have implications for the provision of services needed in a community
Incidence	Number of new cases in a defined period of time	Used in cohort studies
Risk	Risk can be thought of as a probability of developing disease	Preventive measures try and address risk factors
Incidence rate	The proportion of new cases of the target disorder in the population at risk during a specified time interval. It is usual to define the disorder, the population, and the time, and is reported as a rate	Can be calculated in cohort studies
Relative Risk	Incidence among exposed/incidence among unexposed	Important in aetiological enquiries
Risk ratio	Another term for relative risk	Important in aetiological enquiries
Odds Ratio	Ratio of odds of exposure in cases and controls	Used for studying associations
	In cohort studies, it is the odds of outcome in exposed and unexposed	Can be used in cohort studies
Absolute risk reduction	The absolute arithmetic difference in rates of unwanted outcomes between experimental and control participants in a trial, calculated as the experimental event rate (EER) minus the control event rate (CER)	Inverse of this provides numbers needed to treat (see below)
Number needed to treat (NNT)	The inverse of the absolute risk reduction or increase and the number of patients that need to be treated for one to benefit compared with a control NNT = 1/ARR	The ideal NNT is 1, where everyone has improved with treatment and no-one has with control. Broadly, the higher the NNT, the less effective is the intervention
Attributable fraction	The risk of disease occurrence or death ('risk') in a group that is exposed to a particular factor, which can be attributed to that factor attributable risk = (incidence in exposed – incidence in unexposed) × 100/incidence in exposed	This suggests the amount of disease that might be eliminated if the factor under study could be controlled or eliminated
Population attributable risk or risk fraction	The difference between event rates in populations exposed or unexposed to a risk factor Population attributable risk = rate in population – rate in non-exposed Or Population attributable fraction = attributable risk × prevalence of exposure to risk factor in population	This provides an estimate of the amount by which the disease could be reduced in the population if the suspected factor is eliminated or modified

Types of epidemiological study

We now move on to consider how various epidemiological study designs help answer questions about health and health-care. Epidemiologists often adopt what Rudyard Kipling stated decades ago 'I keep six honest serving men; they taught me all I know. Their names are what, why, when, how, where and who'.

Epidemiologists seek answers to the following questions:

- **Description**. What is the extent of disease or risk factors in this population?
- **Prognosis**. How does this disease progress, what is its natural history?
- **Aetiology**. What are the causes of disease? What risk factors increase the chance of becoming diseased?
- **Prevention/treatment**. How well does an intervention work to prevent or treat a condition?

Different types of study will help us answer the different questions above. Epidemiological studies can be divided into descriptive and analytical studies and they can be further subdivided.

Hennekens and Buring [1] classified epidemiological design strategies as shown in Box 3.2.

Descriptive studies help us to describe the health status of populations whereas *analytical* studies, some of which are observational in nature, are employed to study associations – test hypotheses or establish aetiology. Interventional studies, which are part of analytical study design, provide us with information on what works to prevent or treat a disease.

Box 3.2 Epidemiological study designs

Descriptive studies

Population (correlation or ecological studies)

Individual

    Case reports

    Case series

    Cross-sectional surveys

Analytical studies

Observational studies

    Case–control studies

    Cohort studies

Interventional studies

    Clinical trials

    Community trials

Descriptive studies

These studies attempt to describe patterns of diseases within and between populations. They seek to answer the question 'What is the extent of disease or risk factors in this population?' They often use routinely collected data to identify relationships between the prevalence of disease and other variables such as time, place and personal characteristics. Data collection can take place at the level of the population or individual.

Population studies

Here, variables are measured at population or group level. These are also called correlation or ecological studies. In these studies the unit of analysis is an aggregate of individuals and information is collected on this group rather than on individual members. The statistical relationship between exposure and outcome is calculated using the correlation coefficient. The correlation between exposure and outcome can be positive or negative. An example of a population study would be an analysis of the childhood immunisation coverage at ward level using the Index of Multiple Deprivation. Here, both deprivation (exposure) and immunisation coverage (outcome) are measured at community level. However, there are two problems with this approach. Firstly, the observed association may be due to confounding factors (see below). Secondly, beware of the so-called '*ecological fallacy*'. Observations made at population or aggregate levels may not be true at an individual level. For example, it may not be true that all children living in deprived communities are unvaccinated and all those living in affluent areas are fully vaccinated. Ecological studies generate hypotheses but cannot be used to test them.

Individual studies

These are *case reports*, *case series* and *cross-sectional studies*. A case report describes the medical details of one case of disease. For example, this is helpful in the post-marketing surveillance of licensed drugs when rare adverse outcomes not found in original studies may be seen. Case series (descriptions of several patients) can also be useful in generating hypotheses for further testing.

In cross-sectional studies both exposure and outcome are measured at individual and population level at the same point in time. Classical examples are the health and lifestyle surveys undertaken in various populations. In the Health Survey for England various health determinants and health-status indicators are measured on a sample of the English population (see Chapter 4). The major disadvantage of this design is that it cannot determine whether the outcome preceded the exposure or was due to the exposure as both are measured simultaneously. Hence this design is not suitable to test hypotheses but can help planning the services needed.

Analytical studies

A better way to assess the strength of an association between a suspected risk factor and a disease is to perform a study which tries to analyse the effect of the proposed risk factor, while minimising interference from other variables such as age and sex, which might have an independent effect on the development of disease. Such variables are called confounding variables and are discussed in more detail later in this chapter. Analytical studies can be grouped into *observational* studies and *interventional* studies.

Observational studies describe the distribution of diseases in human populations and investigate possible aetiological factors to explain that distribution. The investigators have no control over who is or is not exposed to the factor under study. In interventional studies, the investigator decides who is exposed and who is not. Observational studies can be subdivided into *case-control* and *cohort* studies. Interventional studies can be subdivided into *clinical* trials and *community* trials.

Observational studies

(a) Case-control studies

In this type of study, people who have been identified as having the disease (the *cases*) are compared with people who do not have the disease (the *controls*) (Figure 3.6). Allocation to groups is on the basis of the presence or absence of disease. The investigator looks back (retrospectively) to discover if in the past the cases had more or less exposure to the proposed risk factor than the controls. Should this be the case then the investigator might conclude that there was, indeed, a relationship between exposure to the risk factor and development of disease (generally by calculating an Odds Ratio). It is important that the cases and the controls be as similar as possible (except for the presence of the disease) in order to reduce the effects of confounding variables. Failure to do this adequately leads to the introduction of *bias* into the results and may invalidate the study. Bias is discussed further later in the chapter.

Figure 3.6   A case–control study design.

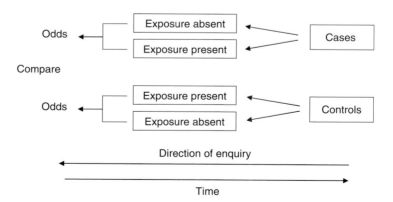

A classic case–control study – oral contraceptives and pulmonary embolism [7]
In the late 1960s, Vessey and Doll interviewed women who had been admitted to hospital with venous thrombosis or pulmonary embolism without medical causes (cases). The controls were women who had been admitted to the same hospital with other diseases and who were matched for age, marital status and parity. The investigators found that those who had pulmonary embolism were six times more likely to have used oral contraceptives compared to women who did not have the condition.

(b) Cohort studies
In a cohort study, a comparison is made between subjects allocated to groups on the basis of their *exposure* to the proposed risk factor. The aim is to compare the development of the disease in an exposed group with that in an unexposed group. If the exposure occurred before the study started then the allocation to groups is done at the beginning of the study and the exposed group compared with a selected, unexposed, control group. If, however, the exposure occurs during the study period then allocation is done at the end of the study and those subjects who were not exposed act as the controls for those who were.

   All subjects are followed up to record the development of the disease and at the end of the study the incidence of the disease in the exposed group is compared with the incidence in the unexposed group (usually calculated as a Relative Risk) (Figure 3.7). Any difference between the two groups is likely to be due to the difference in their exposure to the risk factor, provided that the groups are similar in regard to other factors such as age and sex. The evidence obtained from a cohort study is felt to be better than that from a case–control study because of the danger in the latter of introducing bias through inadequate selection of controls and the problems of reliable retrieval of historic information. Often a case–control study is followed by a cohort study when more evidence of an association is needed (Figure 3.7). However, cohort studies tend to be more time-consuming and expensive to perform.

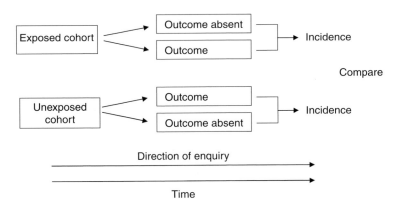

Figure 3.7   A cohort study design.

A classic cohort study – the Whitehall studies [8]

The Whitehall studies of civil servants were set up in 1967 and included 18,000 men in the UK Civil Service. The first Whitehall study showed that men in the lowest employment grades were much more likely to die prematurely than men in the highest grades. The second Whitehall study that followed was set up to determine what underlies the social gradient in death and disease, and to include women. In 1985, all non-industrial civil servants aged between 35 and 55, in 20 departments in central London, were invited to a cardiovascular medical examination at their workplace. The authors recruited 10,308 civil servants. This study found an inverse relationship between socio-economic position and the occurrence of coronary heart disease, diabetes and metabolic syndrome. A steep gradient in the incidence of coronary events with socio-economic status was observed in the study such that people of lowest socio-economic status were between two and three times more likely than the wealthiest to suffer coronary events.

 Can you think of some of the possible reasons for the differences in health status observed among the civil servants?

Many differences between the civil servants could influence health status. These include their income and socio-economic status, access to and pattern of utilisation of health services, and lifestyle. For example, levels of smoking, obesity and physical activity could differ leading to increased risk of diabetes and heart disease.

Interventional studies

In interventional (sometimes called experimental) studies, the investigators have control over who is and who is not exposed to the factor under investigation. Such interventional studies look at the effect of changing the exposure of the population to a factor. This is usually done by either removing a harmful factor or adding a beneficial or protective factor, and interventional studies provide information on prevention or treatment.

The whole population (termed the reference population) cannot be practically studied so two groups are chosen from the population to be representative. The reference group might be the whole population or those with a certain disease or condition. The desired intervention is administered to the intervention group while a placebo is administered to the control group.

Wherever possible it is important that the participants in the study have the same chance of being allocated to the intervention or control groups. The process of allocation is termed *randomisation*. A study where randomisation occurs between an intervention and control group is called a *randomised controlled trial* (RCT). It is regarded as the best form of evidence of association as the randomisation process should ensure that the two groups are similar except in terms of exposure to the intervention under study.

Both intervention and control groups are followed up and the development of disease in each group recorded. A significant difference in disease incidence between the groups may indicate that this was the result of the intervention and that the factor added or removed has a real effect on the development of the disease. Sometimes it is not possible to identify a control group and it may then be necessary to use the whole population before the intervention as an historical control against which the whole population after the intervention may be compared. These studies can be considered as cohort studies as they follow two groups of people over time to determine the outcome. The major difference is that the investigator has control over who is exposed and who is not. Interventional studies can be subdivided into clinical trials and community trials.

What measure of association do you expect to be used in interventional studies? (Hint – remember these are similar to cohort studies)
Relative Risk.

(a) Clinical trials
These are studies of the effect of a specific treatment on patients who already have a particular disease, in comparison with another treatment (or a placebo) on a similar group of people, also with the disease (see Figure 3.8 overleaf). These are normally only ethical when it is not known which of the treatments is more effective and the term used to denote this is *equipoise*.

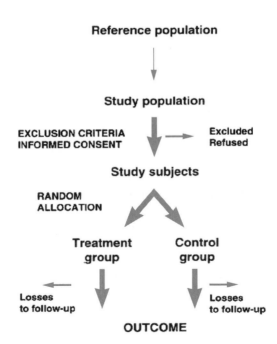

Figure 3.8   Design of a clinical trial.

A classic clinical trial – diabetes control [9]

In the Diabetes Control and Complications Trial (DCCT) a group of investigators from many centres tested whether intensive control of blood glucose in patients with insulin-dependent diabetes (IDDM) decreases long-term micro-vascular and neuro-logical complications. Intensive control consisted of administration of insulin by external insulin pump or by three or more daily insulin injections and was guided by frequent blood-glucose monitoring. The control group received conventional therapy with one or two daily insulin injections. The researchers concluded that intensive therapy effectively delays the onset and slows the progression of diabetic retinopathy, nephropathy and neuropathy in patients with IDDM as the rate of neuro-pathy was around four times higher in the control group.

Exercise 3.10   Intervention studies

Think through the following questions.
a. What do you understand by the term randomisation?
b. What do investigators attempt to achieve by randomisation?
c. What is the reference population?
d. Why are interventional studies regarded as providing better evidence than observational studies?

a. The aim behind randomisation, where study subjects are randomly allocated to the two groups (often termed as 'arms') in a trial, is to produce comparable treatment and control groups.

b. If it is effective, both known and unknown factors that could influence the outcome will be equally distributed between the two groups. This is the reason why the randomised controlled trial is such a powerful study design. Other epidemiological studies have to make statistical adjustments for known confounders.

c. The reference population is the population from which the study population is drawn and to which the results of the trial are to be extrapolated. If the study population is dissimilar to the reference population in some way (e.g. contains more people of one age group or sex or is generally sicker) then the results of the study may not be reliably applied to the rest of the population. This is called external validity and is discussed further later in the chapter.

d. Interventional studies are regarded as providing better evidence as they provide the best control for confounding factors so that we are able, with more certainty, to regard the results as truth.

(b) Community trials

These trials are undertaken in community settings and the unit of intervention could be individuals, families or communities, or geographical areas.

A classical community trial – perinatal and maternal mortality in rural Pakistan [10]

This RCT involved randomising communities to the intervention and control groups. Seven sub-districts (talukas) of a rural district in Pakistan were randomised: three were assigned to the intervention group where traditional birth attendants were trained and issued disposable delivery kits; female health workers linked traditional birth attendants with established services and documented processes and outcomes; and obstetric teams provided outreach clinics for antenatal care. Women in the four control talukas received usual care and there was no additional input from the research team. The authors concluded that training traditional birth attendants and integrating them into an improved health-care system were achievable and effective in reducing perinatal mortality as the Odds Ratio for perinatal death was 0.7 and that for maternal mortality was 0.74 in the study group.

Summary

Table 3.5 summarises the main features of the different types of epidemiological study.

Interpreting results of epidemiological studies

Before we conclude that the results of studies are valid (true), we need to consider the factors that might fully or partly explain the observed results. They include *chance* and *error* (random or systematic).

Table 3.5 Main features of the different types of epidemiological study

Design	Descriptive/ Observational/ Interventional	Retrospective/ Prospective	Aim	Specific comparison group/No such group
Case-series (clinical and population)	Descriptive	Retrospective	Describes diseases in individuals	No
Cross-sectional	Descriptive	Retrospective	Describes disease or risk factors in populations	Usually not
Case–control	Observational	Retrospective	Examines association	Yes
Cohort (prospective and retrospective)	Observational	Prospective and retrospective	Examines associations of disease and/or outcomes with risk factors exposed to	Usually yes (though it may be integral to the study population)
Trial	Interventional	Prospective	Tests effectiveness of interventions to prevent or treat disease	Yes, with exceptions

Chance

The observed results of a study could be due to chance. The effects of chance are quantified using statistical techniques and the two common measures employed are probability (*P value*) and *confidence interval* (CI). These are explained here but readers are advised to refer to statistical texts to expand further their knowledge in this area [11, 12].

The *P* value is the probability (ranging from zero to one) that the results observed in a study (or results more extreme) could have occurred by chance. Convention is that we accept a *P* value of 0.05 or below as being statistically significant and we call this the significance level. This means that when a *P* value of less than 0.05 is quoted it suggests that the association is real and not due just to chance. Because this means that 5% of the time (1 time in 20) we would find an association purely by chance, when we are making many comparisons we often use a *P* value of 0.01, so that *P* values of 0.01 or below are deemed statistically significant and signify a real association.

The confidence interval (CI) quantifies the uncertainty in measurement. It is defined as 'a range of values for a variable of interest constructed so that this range has a specified probability of including the true value of the variable.' The range of values is called the confidence interval, and the end points of the confidence interval are called confidence limits. It is conventional to create confidence intervals at the 95% level – this means that 95% of the time properly constructed confidence intervals should contain the true variable of interest. One useful feature of confidence intervals is that one can easily tell whether or not statistical significance has been reached, just as when using the *P* value. If the confidence interval spans the value reflecting 'no effect' (e.g. the value 1 for a relative risk), this represents a difference that is not statistically significant. If the confidence interval does not enclose the value reflecting 'no effect' this represents a difference that is statistically significant. Apart from statistical inference, confidence intervals show the largest and smallest effects that are likely, given the observed data.

Error

Estimates of measures of associations such as Relative Risk and Odds Ratio may differ from their true value. This may be a result of random error or of systematic error. Random error results in an estimate being equally likely to be above or below the true value. Systematic error, which is caused by a consistent discrepancy in the measurement, results in an estimate being above or below the true value, depending on the direction of the discrepancy. For example, while measuring blood pressure, random error could occur due to the time of measurement, the status of the person whose blood pressure is measured and random fluctuations. However, the causes of systematic error are different: for example, use of the wrong cuff size and deafness in the person making the measurement. In observational studies there is a greater potential for various biases to be introduced that need to be addressed.

Random error

The major cause of random error in epidemiological studies is *sampling error* caused simply by the random nature of the sample.

Random error means that we might conclude that there is no association when there is one. This is called a *type II* or beta error and is harmful as we do not become aware of risk factors for disease or effective treatments. A study must be designed with sufficient *power* to detect an association if one exists. Power is often increased by increasing the sample size in the study or by optimising the ratio of cases to controls, or exposed to unexposed.

Random error might also lead us to conclude that there is an association where none exists. This is potentially more harmful as we may decide to intervene in an ineffective way based on these results (e.g. to give an ineffective drug with potentially adverse effects). This is named *type I* or alpha error. Setting a significance level of 0.05 means that there will be a 5% chance of making an alpha error and, if the potential harms are great, we might set a lower alpha level (significant *P* value) such as 0.01.

Sampling error cannot be eliminated, but one of the aims of good study design is to reduce it to an acceptable level within the constraints imposed by the availability of finite resources. Ways to reduce random error include taking multiple readings and training those taking measurements to ensure standardisation.

Systematic error

Systematic error may take one of three main forms, selection bias, information bias or confounding.

Selection bias: This is a major problem in case–control studies where it gives rise to non-comparability between cases and controls. It is found when cases (or controls) are chosen to be included in (or excluded from) a study by using criteria that are related to exposure to the risk factor under investigation. In cohort studies, selection bias can appear as participants are lost during follow up.

Example: In a case–control study of the aetiology of lung cancer, controls were selected from people who were suffering from non-malignant respiratory disease. Smoking is a cause of chronic bronchitis and thus the controls would have a higher prevalence of smoking than the population from which the people with lung cancer was drawn. As a consequence, the strength of the association between smoking and lung cancer would be underestimated. The controls should have been selected from the general population, which would have avoided this bias.

Much of the effort that goes into the design of good case–control studies is spent on the careful selection of controls in order to eliminate selection bias.

Information bias: This involves study subjects being misclassified either according to their disease status, their exposure status, or both. Differential misclassification occurs when errors in classification of disease status are dependent upon exposure status or vice versa. For example, in a case–control study, a case's recall of his or her past 'exposure' to risk factors may differ from the recall of a control because the process of having the disease will have caused the person to think much more about possible exposures than is the case for the controls.

Example: In a case–control study investigating the association between congenital defects in new-born babies and maternal exposure to X-rays, women with babies with congenital defects are more likely to recall their X-rays due to apparent association. The effect of this would be to over-estimate the strength of association, as the cases would appear to have a higher exposure to the risk factor.

Confounding: This occurs when an estimate of the association between an exposure and a disease is confused because another exposure, linked to both, has not been taken into account. For a variable to be a confounder, it must be associated with the exposure under study and it must also be independently associated with disease risk in its own right (see Figure 3.9). Both these criteria are met in the two examples which follow:

Example 1: Consider a study of the association between work in a particular occupation and the risk of lung cancer. A comparison of death rates due to lung cancer in the occupational group and in the general population may appear to show that the occupational group has an increased risk of lung cancer. If this still persists after taking into account the different age structures of the two groups, it is necessary to consider whether people in the occupational group smoke more (or less) heavily than people in the general population. If this is not taken into account, the inference is invalid.

Example 2: Age at menopause may confound estimates of the association between replacement oestrogens (taken for relief of menopausal symptoms) and breast-cancer risk. This is because an early age at menopause is associated with both a reduced risk of breast cancer and a greater use of replacement oestrogens.

Figure 3.9   Confounding.

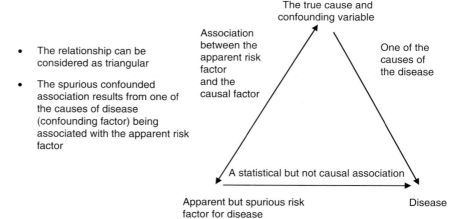

- The relationship can be considered as triangular

- The spurious confounded association results from one of the causes of disease (confounding factor) being associated with the apparent risk factor

Confounding may be avoided by appropriate study design, as could be achieved in Example 2 by only studying women who had their menopause at a particular range of ages. However, it may also be controlled for in the analysis, provided that the confounding factors have been identified and information on them has been collected. The control of confounding at analysis is a widely used strategy, much of the statistical methodology in epidemiology being concerned with this issue.

Exercise 3.11 Confounding

For each of the examples 1–3 consider the following questions:
a. What is the apparent association?
b. What else might cause the outcome and could it also be related to the apparent cause?
c. Therefore, what is the confounded factor and what is the confounding (causal) factor?
d. How can we check whether the possible confounder is having an effect?
(1) People who drink alcohol have a raised risk of lung cancer.
(2) People living in an affluent seaside resort have a higher mortality rate than the country as a whole.
(3) African Americans are heavier users of crack cocaine than 'white' Americans.
See Table 3.6.

Table 3.6 Confounding questions answered

The confounded association	One possible explanation	The confounded factor	The confounding (causal) factor	To check the assumption
a. People who drink alcohol have a raised risk of lung cancer	Alcohol drinking and smoking are behaviours which go together	Alcohol, which is a marker for, on average, smoking more cigarettes	Tobacco, which is associated with both alcohol and with the disease	See if the alcohol–lung cancer relationship holds in people not exposed to tobacco: if it does, tobacco is not a confounder
b. People living in an affluent seaside resort have a higher mortality rate than the country as a whole	A holiday town attracts the elderly, so has a comparatively old population	Living in a resort is a marker for being, on average, older	Age, which is associated with both living in a resort and with death	Look at each age group specifically, or use age standardisation to take into account age differences
c. African Americans are heavier users of crack cocaine than 'white' Americans	Poor people living in the American inner city are particularly likely to become dependent on illicit drugs	Belonging to the racial category 'African American'	Poverty and the pressures of inner-city living, including the easy availability of drugs	Use statistical techniques to adjust for the influence of a number of complex socio-economic factors

As can be seen from the exercise above, we need to consider the potential confounders before we conclude that the association is causal. In case (b), although we observe higher mortality in coastal towns this is not due to the geographical area but the different age structure between resort towns and other areas of the country. Resort towns tend to have a higher proportion of elderly as people tend to settle in these areas after retirement. Here, age is a potential confounder because it is a surrogate for age-related causal factors. There are various ways of tackling confounders including advanced statistical techniques such as multivariate analysis.

Validity (truth)

Once we have established that the results from the epidemiological studies are not due to chance or error (including confounding) we need to determine if our results are *valid* and if any association seen is causal. Validity is the extent to which a variable or intervention measures what it is supposed to measure, or accomplishes what it is supposed to accomplish.

In the context of epidemiological studies, validity has two components, internal and external validity. The *internal validity* of a study refers to the integrity of the experimental design and relates to inferences about the study population itself. The *external validity* of a study refers to the appropriateness by which its results can be applied to non-study patients or populations. This will depend upon the similarities or otherwise between the study population and the population to which the results are extrapolated. This is often termed the generalisability of a study.

When we are assured that the results of a study are valid we can consider, where relevant, the issue of *causality*. Much of epidemiology seeks to relate causes to the effects they produce, that is, to determine aetiology. Epidemiological evidence by itself is rarely sufficient to establish causality, but it can provide powerful circumstantial evidence. A statistical association between two or more events or other variables may be produced under various circumstances. The presence of an association does not necessarily imply a causal relationship.

To learn more about aetiology, associations between the disease and the hypothesised cause resulting from natural experiments must be observed. According to Hill [13], causality is more likely if the association can be shown to be:

1. Strong (e.g. is statistically significant and has a large relative risk).
2. Dose-related (i.e. the greater the risk factor the greater the effects).
3. In the right time sequence (cohort studies show that exposure precedes outcome).
4. Independent of recognised confounding factors.
5. Consistent between different studies. (We are more likely to believe an association which has been demonstrated several times and we now look for systematic reviews and meta-analyses to increase our confidence in associations.)
6. Plausible. However, we need to be aware that this may not always be necessary because medical science advances all the time and some of the biological

mechanisms will evolve in future years. In the 1980s, HIV/AIDS research was in its earliest stages. A relationship was discovered between the incidence of AIDS-like symptoms in homosexual men (the largest portion of the population displaying these symptoms at the time), and the use of alkyl nitrites, more commonly called 'poppers'. As science stood at that time the biological agent had not been identified and various mechanisms were put forward including the 'poppers' hypothesis [14]'. However, with the discovery of the causative agent, all these theories disappeared and a biological mechanism was established.

7. Reversible (removing the exposure should remove the risk). Two kinds of cause are sometimes distinguished. A necessary cause is one whose presence is required for the occurrence of the effect. A sufficient cause is one which can cause the effect alone. In practice, most causal factors are neither necessary nor sufficient, but contributory.

Conclusion

In this chapter we have described the ways in which we measure the extent of health problems within and between populations and the scientific basis for conclusions we reach on disease causality, prevention and treatment. Without this knowledge we cannot know where best to concentrate our efforts to have the greatest effect on population health. We recommend the accompanying book in this series which provides a more detailed coverage of the field of epidemiology [15]. Chapter 5 continues this theme and looks at how the strength of evidence on which we base healthcare decisions is judged.

REFERENCES

1. C. Hennekens and J. Buring, *Epidemiology in Medicine*, Boston, MA, Little, Brown and Company, 1987.

2. Hippocrates, *The Genuine Works of Hippocrates*, transl. Frances Adams, Baltimore, MD, Williams & Wilkins, 1939.

3. Committee on Assessing Interactions Among Social, Behavioral, and Genetic Factors in Health, M. L. Hernandez and D. G. Blazer (eds.) *Genes, Behavior, and the Social Environment: Moving Beyond the Nature/Nurture Debate*, Washington, DC, National Academic Press, 2006.

4. G. Rose, Sick individuals and sick populations. *International Journal of Epidemiology* **30** (3), 2001, 427–32.

5. R. Doll and A. B. Hill, The mortality of doctors in relation to their smoking habits; a preliminary report. *British Medical Journal* **228**, 1954, 1451–5.

6. R. Doll and R. Peto, Mortality in relation to smoking: 20 years' observations on male British doctors. *British Medical Journal* **273**, 1976, 1525–36.

7. M. P. Vessey and R. Doll, Investigation of relation between use of oral contraceptives and thromboembolic disease. *British Medical Journal* **2**, 1968, 199–205.

8. J. E. Ferrie, P. Martikainen, M. J. Shipley and M. G. Marmot, Self-reported economic difficulties and coronary events in men: evidence from the Whitehall II study. *International Journal of Epidemiology* **34** (3), 2005, 640–8.

9. The Diabetes Control and Complications Trial Research Group, The effect of intensive treatment of diabetes on the development and progression of long-term complications in insulin-dependent diabetes mellitus. *New England Journal of Medicine* **329** (14), 1993, 977–86.

10. A. H. Jokhio, H. R. Winter and K. K. Cheng, An intervention involving traditional birth attendants and perinatal and maternal mortality in Pakistan. *New England Journal of Medicine* **352** (20), 2005, 2091–9.

11. D. G. Altman, *Practical Statistics for Medical Research*, London, Chapman & Hall/CRC, 1991.

12. B. R. Kirkwood and J. A. C. Sterne, *Essential Medical Statistics*, 2nd edn., Oxford, Blackwell Science, 2003.

13. A. B. Hill, The environment and disease: association or causation? *Proceedings of the Royal Society of Medicine* **58**, 1965, 295–300. (online at www.edwardtufte.com/tufte/hill)

14. J. P. Vandenbroucke and V. P. Pardoel, An autopsy of epidemiologic methods: the case of "poppers" in the early epidemic of the acquired immunodeficiency syndrome (AIDS). *American Journal of Epidemiology* **129** (3), 455–7.

15. P. Webb, C. Bain and S. Pirozzo, *Essential Epidemiology. An Introduction for Students and Health Professionals*, 2nd edn., Cambridge, Cambridge University Press, 2011.

4

The health status of the population

Padmanabhan Badrinath and Jan Yates

Key points

- Determining the health status of a population is essential before planning effective interventions to improve health and to prevent disease.
- Measures used to compile such a health profile include:
  - mortality (for example, all deaths, deaths from specific causes, in specific subsets of the population standardised to account for different population structures, deaths in and around childbirth, years of life lost);
  - objectively measured morbidity (for example, infectious disease rates, hospital activity, primary care data, registered diseases);
  - data on determinants of health and well-being (for example smoking, unemployment, social status);
  - analysis of health inequalities;
  - data collated at regional or national level by statistical organisations or public health observatories.

Introduction

Public health practitioners are frequently called upon to determine the health status of a population. This is central to understanding the health experiences of the people within the population and to planning effective interventions to improve their health. Public health surveillance ensures that relevant data are used to inform public health decision making.

It is important to consider both health and disease and their determinants, what contributes to well-being as well as what conditions we must address. Both qualitative and quantitative measures are important as not every outcome can be measured or

Essential Public Health, Second Edition, ed. Stephen Gillam, Jan Yates and Padmanabhan Badrinath.
Published by Cambridge University Press. © Cambridge University Press 2012.

> **Box 4.1 Finagle's law**
>
> The information you have is not the information you want. The information you want is not the information you need. The information you need is not what you can get or is not known. The information that is known can't be found in time.

counted easily. We can count deaths, numbers of operations or measure blood pressure but people's perceptions of their care or feelings of well-being can only be measured qualitatively. In addition it is important to consider both self-reported (subjective) and measured (objectively verified) elements so that interventions can be carefully planned and monitored and shown to meet the needs of patients and the public. As well as absolute counts it is useful to have information on trends to help predict the need for interventions in the future. Lastly, the information must be related to knowledge of health and other service structures (e.g. numbers of doctors, social workers), processes (e.g. admission rates, unemployment registrations), and outcomes (e.g. death) so that action can be taken. This chapter outlines some of the key indicators of health status which are typically included within a health profile. Therefore this chapter links to many of the other public health tools – it is integral to the understanding of needs (Chapter 6), it requires skills in epidemiology (Chapter 3), it is necessary to evaluate services (Chapter 11) and it informs prioritisation decisions (Chapter 7). We see once more that public health skills are not used in isolation but must be integrated in practice (see Part 2).

Note that the data described in this chapter come with a 'health warning' (Box 4.1). Data are not without flaws and should never be used without first considering their completeness, accuracy and relevance. Data can be difficult to collect, collate and analyse and it is worth considering carefully the use to which the data will be put and whether they are fit for purpose (Box 4.2).

Measuring mortality

One of the most commonly used epidemiological measurements is the incidence of death. It is generally the starting point for a health profile but does not contain information on the extent of ill health within a population or other factors which determine well-being. Many countries require physicians to record cause of death and these mandatory reports form the basis of mortality files, which can inform health profiling. Although many countries have vital registration systems it is important to remember that there may be many reasons why these are not completely accurate, such as limited recording of multiple pathologies in old age or non-statutory birth and death registration systems (see Chapter 2).

Box 4.2 Are the data you have fit for purpose?

You should ask the following questions of any data obtained:

1. Are the data related clearly to specific ages and sexes? If the disease or determinant you are interested in may vary by age or sex you may need to standardise rates to allow comparisons.
2. Are the data clearly related to a specific time period? Time trends are helpful in supporting the planning of health-care or other public health interventions. Data often take time to collate and it is important to use the most up-to-date information available.
3. Are the data clearly related to specific geographical locations? You need to ensure that the data you have are related to your population and take care in extrapolating information from other populations to your own.
4. Are the data complete? Are there any population groups missing? Will whoever inputs the data have included every case? Some causes of death may be more easily identified and recorded more frequently than others and some may carry stigma (for example HIV) and be less well recorded. Population surveys of self-reported health have variable uptake rates and may not be representative of the whole population. Are the same data collected across geographical areas? – Data coverage in rural areas may be less complete than urban ones.
5. Are the data accurate? What do the definitions of data fields mean? For example, what clinical indications would a field called 'CHD' include? Has it been transcribed from original data allowing the introduction of errors? Are the data coded and are the codes used in the same way by everyone? Have the definitions changed over time if you are looking at time trends?
6. Are the data relevant to the question you have? It is often tempting to use readily available routine data without real thought as to whether they are right for the job!

For comparative purposes, it is usual to express the number of deaths as a rate. The crude death rate is the average number of deaths in a given population and time period, usually expressed per hundred thousand population over one year, e.g. 967/100,000 for all causes in England and Wales in 2009.

1. **2100 deaths occurred in an area of 250,000 population in 2011. What is the crude death rate?**
2. **200 of these were deaths due to cancer. What is the cancer death rate?**

1. 2100 deaths per 250,000 people means $(2100 / 250,000) \times 100,000 = 840$ deaths per 100,000 population.
2. 200 deaths per 250,000 people means $(200 / 250,000) \times 1000 = 80$ deaths per 100,000 population.

Differences in the age structure of populations affect crude rates and for most epidemiological purposes it is usual for them to be refined. This enables us to compare the mortality of our population with other similar populations. One way is to compare age- and sex-specific death rates. These are routinely published in the UK by the Office of National Statistics, for 5- and 10-year age groups. In order to have a single summary figure which allows for different age or sex distributions, standardised death rates are used. These make use of a standard (or reference) population, e.g. the population of England and Wales in 2009.

The directly standardised death rate (DSR) is the death rate that would have occurred in the reference population if it had had the age- and sex-specific death rate of the population being studied (the study population). However, the age-specific death rates of every group must be known, making calculations tedious if more than one population is being studied, and age-specific death rates may not be available.

Indirect standardisation leads to a standardised mortality ratio (SMR), which is the ratio of the deaths observed in the study population to the number of deaths that would have occurred if it had the age- and sex-specific death rates of the reference population, multiplied by 100. This is the most common type of standardisation in the UK and is used to compare populations differentiated by such variables as age, sex, geographical region, time and social class. The appropriate reference population varies, e.g. with occupation or socio-economic class it is the national population aged 15–64 years. When an SMR is used to show trends in mortality, the reference population is the study population at one particular point in time. The SMRs can be misleading if the populations being studied differ widely, from each other or from the reference population, in age and sex structure.

3. **The crude death rates for two towns, A and B, are 10.4 per 1000 and 20.1 per 1000 respectively. The directly standardised death rate (DSR) for A and B are 14.5 per 1000 for A and 15.7 for B. What does this mean?**
4. **The coronary heart disease (CHD) SMR for your population is 130. What does this mean?**

3. More people die in town B per year but, after accounting for age and sex, the two towns have roughly similar death rates. This may indicate that the age and/or sex structure of the two towns differs. It may be that town B has larger numbers of older people and a higher death rate would be expected. When the standardised death rates are compared this age structure difference is accounted for and the death rates look more similar. This demonstrates that differences in crude rates generally need more investigation.

4. An SMR of 130 means that there are 30% more deaths from coronary heart disease in this population than would be expected if the age and sex structure were the same as the reference population. An SMR of 100 is the baseline, higher SMRs indicate worse health and SMRs lower than 100 indicate better health than

Box 4.3 Proportional mortality

Proportional mortality =

$$\frac{\text{Deaths assigned to the disease in a year}}{\text{Total deaths in the same population in the same year}} \times 100$$

expected. An SMR this high would suggest that interventions to prevent CHD are needed for this population and that it is likely that more services for CHD will be needed by this population than the average.

Sometimes it is helpful to demonstrate the proportion of the overall mortality that may be ascribed to a specific cause and emphasise the importance of a particular cause of death. Here we use proportional mortality (also known as the attributable mortality rate, see Box 4.3).

5. What is the proportional mortality for cancer in the example in questions 1 and 2 above?

5. Cancer deaths = 200, Total deaths = 2100. Proportional mortality = (200/2100) × 100 = 9.5%

Since the 1850s there have been attempts to aid epidemiological analysis and health planning by standardising the classification of death statistics. This allows comparisons between countries and supports international collaboration by providing a common language. The international classification has been overseen by the World Health Organization since 1948 and is called the International Classification of Diseases (10th revision) or ICD-10. Since 1948 the classification has also included causes of morbidity (see later).

Deaths around the time of childbirth or in infancy are helpful indicators in many countries of the scale of infectious disease or malnutrition and point to the need for public health interventions such as childhood vaccination programmes or improved breast feeding. Indicators used here are perinatal mortality, neonatal mortality, post-neonatal mortality, maternal mortality, stillbirth rate and infant mortality rates (actually ratios). The definitions of these are:

- Perinatal mortality rate: Stillbirths + deaths in the first week ÷ total births.
- Neonatal mortality rate: Deaths in the first 28 days per 1000 live births (early neonatal death – first week, and late neonatal death – subsequent 3 weeks).
- Post-neonatal mortality rate: Post 28 days to first-year deaths ÷ live births.
- Maternal mortality rate: Deaths due to complications of pregnancy, childbirth or from puerperal causes within 42 days ÷ live births.
- Stillbirth rate (synonym, foetal death rate): Stillbirths per 1000 total births.
- Infant mortality rate: Deaths at <1 year ÷ live births.

6. High rates of perinatal mortality are observed in UK-born Pakistani and Caribbean babies. What might be the reasons for this?

6. Reasons can include late booking for care, deprivation, consanguinity, reluctance to terminate a foetus which is known to be seriously malformed and lack of social support. These suggest that interventions to improve perinatal mortality include both those aimed at specific causes of death and those aimed at broader lifestyle factors.

There are many causes of perinatal death, including congenital abnormalities, immaturity and low birth weight, maternal diseases in pregnancy and obstetric problems. Factors associated with increasing perinatal death are higher maternal age, higher parity, lower socio-economic class and ethnicity [1, 2].

Another indicator of child health is the under-5 mortality rate: the number of deaths of children less than 5 years old divided by the number of live births in a year multiplied by 1000. This indicator measures child survival. It also reflects the social, economic and environmental conditions in which children (and others in society) live, including their health-care. Although under-5 mortality is decreasing globally the rate in some areas is still significantly higher than others (129/1000 births in sub-Saharan Africa in 2009 compared with 22/1000 in Oceania and a global average of 33/1000 [3].

Life expectancy and years of life lost (YLL)

Mortality rates alone give only a partial picture of the public health impact of diseases. The significance of common causes of death (e.g. pneumonia at the end of life) may eclipse rarer but devastating causes of death earlier in life (e.g. road traffic fatalities). Life expectancy provides an estimate of the average expected life span of a population based on current patterns of mortality. Years of potential life relate to the average age at which deaths occur and the expected life span of the population so provides a measure of the relative importance of conditions in causing mortality.

Years of life lost are calculated for each person who died before age 75. For example, a person who died at age 30 would contribute 45 potential years of life lost. (Deaths in individuals aged 75 or older are not included in the calculation). Years of life lost are the sum of the YLL contributed for each individual. They can be expressed as a rate where the total years of life lost by the total population less than 75 years of age are divided by the population count.

Figure 4.1 illustrates that using YLL (in this case standardised to account for population differences) shows a much higher burden of disease than mortality (here directly standardised – DSR – to allow comparison).

In addition to the use of years of life lost, the use of life expectancy as a measure of a population's health status can be modified by using adjustments such as those used in developing quality-adjusted life years (QALYs; see Chapter 7). Health or quality-adjusted life expectancies give an indication of the quality of life expected rather than just the extent.

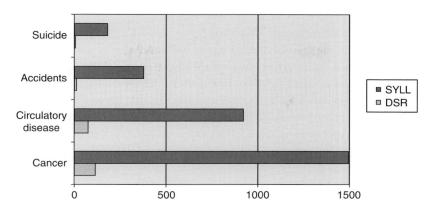

Figure 4.1 Directly standardised death rates (DSR) and standardised years of life lost (SYLL) (2006) in persons under 75 for selected causes, England. Data source www.nchod.nhs.uk.

Measuring morbidity

Morbidity is defined as 'any departure, subjective or objective, from a state of physiological or psychological well-being. In this sense, sickness, illness and disease are similarly defined and synonymous' [4]. Morbidity statistics will be described (with the UK as an example) under the following headings:

1. infectious diseases;
2. hospital data;
3. primary care data;
4. disease registers.

Infectious diseases

In the UK and many other countries certain communicable diseases are notifiable by law. This system provides a rich source of information on one aspect of the health of a population. Other data are available from alternative surveillance systems (see Chapter 10) and are helpful in determining public health policy such as vaccination requirements, sexual health service needs and likely sources of communicable disease outbreaks for a population.

However, these notification and reporting systems may be incomplete. Despite this they have been shown to provide valid information that is relatively consistent and can be used as a crude indicator of change in prevalence of diseases in the community.

Hospital data

The origins of concern for recording hospital activity can be traced to the eighteenth century and an early proponent in the UK was Florence Nightingale. However, it was not until after the founding of the NHS in 1948 that a system for collecting these data was introduced. Today, hospital episode statistics (HES) data are collected on patient administration systems (PAS) and diagnostic/operation coding is added at hospital trust level. The following data are recorded:

- demographic, e.g. age, sex, marital status, residence, ethnic codes;
- administrative, e.g. length of stay, waiting list and source of admission;
- clinical speciality, main condition and operation details.

Hospital activity data are only a proxy measure of morbidity and represent process data on those treated by the hospital system (see Chapter 11). However, data about utilisation by speciality, principal diagnosis and operation can provide indices of morbidity. Accident-and-emergency and out-patient data are also available. Coding of the clinical elements of HES allows linkage to ICD-10 coding and international comparisons.

Primary care data

The main focus for medical care outside hospitals in the UK is general medical practice. Some 90% of illness episodes are dealt with in the context of primary care. Data can be collected via relatively infrequent patient surveys or through routine patient data collection such as disease registers to support the management of chronic conditions (e.g. coronary heart disease, diabetes, epilepsy). This source of data is useful as, although not always complete, it is available at very small population levels and can be used effectively to engage local clinicians in health improvement or health-care quality initiatives. For example, an audit of statin prescribing to those people identified in a practice register as having coronary heart disease might be used to encourage greater rates of prescribing in women (which tend to be lower). Incentive systems may operate to encourage general practitioners to increase the amount of data collected, which can be used for audit and monitoring as well as for one-to-one patient care during consultations.

Specialist disease registers

It is possible to establish special data collection systems for some diseases. They provide richer sources of information than routine data but are costly to establish and maintain. A good example of a disease register is that for cancer. Cancer registration is established in many countries including the UK, many European countries and the USA. In the UK, the Ministry of Health set up a system in 1923 through the Radium Commission to follow up patients treated with radium. This was the origin of the regional cancer registries, which collect details of age, sex, place of birth, occupation, site of primary tumour, type of tumour and date of initial diagnosis. Information about survival and incidence are obtained through linking this clinical data on individuals to the national death registration system. As with the other data sources there are concerns about completeness of registration, accuracy of particulars and effectiveness of follow-up. However, cancer registration has proved an invaluable source of cancer morbidity and survival data.

Self-reported health status, risk factors and determinants of health

Not all ill health is reported and details of the determinants of health, such as diet, smoking, housing and physical-activity levels cannot be collected solely through health systems. Thus we need to consider other data sources when aiming for a complete profile of the health of our population.

Population surveys

Many countries administer regular health surveys. Typically, they sample a population and ask a standard series of questions repeatedly over time, for example annually or decennially. Whilst these surveys tend to cover a range of topics such as employment, housing tenure and family nature they often have a health component (see Box 4.4 for UK examples).

Some health information may be available from full descriptive population surveys (see Chapter 3). These are also carried out in many countries, often less frequently than smaller, sampled surveys. Data from UK censuses are available at a local level and can help define the self-reported health of small populations. However, as the census takes place only every 10 years, the data become increasingly inaccurate as the next census approaches.

Box 4.4 Examples of UK surveys

In the UK in 1971 the General Household Survey was developed as an instrument to examine the interaction between different education, employment, social security and health departmental policies. The sampling frame was obtained through the electoral registers from which households were identified. Approximately 12,000 households were approached annually to undertake a detailed interview questionnaire, which resulted in a response rate of about 70%.

The health section included data about how activity was limited by acute or chronic illness, contacts with health and social services, consultations with GPs, hospital outpatients or admissions, smoking and alcohol consumption and other specific topics such as sight or hearing. The time period for recall varied from 2 weeks for acute illness and GP consultation to 1 year for inpatient care. One advantage of this system was the ability to cross-tabulate health data with other social variables such as housing, employment, income etc. In the UK, National Statistics published the findings annually until 2011.

In addition, the Health Survey for England is administered annually and produces data on health status and related activities (e.g. smoking, obesity, diet, mental health, physical activity).

Local health surveys

It is also possible to carry out local health surveys to obtain a picture of the population's perception of important health issues. These are time-consuming and must be carried out with rigorous methodology to be valid but can provide information not obtainable in any other way.

As well as quantifying the mortality and morbidity experience of a population directly, quantifying the degree of health risk experienced provides useful intelligence on which to assess likely future health and well-being status and care needs as well as plan current public health or preventive interventions.

A wide range of data may be used for this purpose, some examples are given here:

- Data on prevalence of risky behaviours such as smoking, hazardous drinking, being overweight or obese. This can be collected as part of routine health-care and the creation of registers such as those maintained by UK general practitioners or through the use of population surveys.
- Social statistics, including data on care needs, sickness and injury benefit payments, and absences from work resulting from illness.
- Registers such as disabled, blind and partially sighted registers held by local government authorities or organisations.
- Accident reports for road accidents and accidents at home.
- School health reports including dental surveys.
- Educational attainment statistics and workforce information including worklessness and occupational types.
- Income and poverty data collected by national or local government agencies.
- National food surveys, which collect data on food consumption and expenditure.
- Indices of deprivation. These combine different deprivation-related domains and produce measures with which to compare different geographical areas. An example in England is the Index of Multiple Deprivation 2010, which incorporates domains relating to health and disability, employment, income, education, skills, crime, living environment and barriers to housing and services.
- Commercially available geodemographic data, which classify the population into types based on their socio-economic status and preferences and is used to target interventions to small population areas in ways which are meaningful to that 'type' (Chapter 8). Examples used in the UK provide information on which newspapers and other forms of media communication are most likely to appeal to people living in certain geographic areas, which can then be used to target prevention and other messages.

Measures of inequality

The aim of profiling a population is to guide the delivery of interventions such that the best outcomes, tailored for a specific population, are achieved. A primary aim of such intervention is frequently the narrowing of health inequalities, so a population profile would not be fit for purpose without the inclusion of measures of health inequality.

Chapter 15 looks at the topic of health inequality in detail but the inclusion of measures of inequality within a population health profile is so fundamental that it is worth an additional mention here.

Various methods are used to measure inequalities. In the simplest form, any data such as rates of disease, mortality or access to services can be compared across populations to give an indication of inequality. These can be shown numerically or, increasingly, as pictorial atlases that are visually easy to interpret. Increasing in complexity, a range of data can be combined to provide aggregate indices such as those used to measure deprivation. Attempts are also now made to combine data to provide summative measures of inequality with the intention of providing a more direct indicator of the degree of inequality present within and across populations. An example is the slope index of inequality (SII), a single score which represents the gap between the best-off and worst-off deprivation deciles within a district for a chosen indicator such as all-cause mortality. Care must be taken, as with measures of risk, to be clear whether relative or absolute inequality is being discussed. An area which is twice as deprived as another may be little different if both levels of deprivation are very low. Further information on measuring inequalities can be found in the Internet Companion.

Conclusion

The collation of the information described in this chapter to form succinct health profiles, which can be updated and utilised effectively, requires considerable skill – and effort. Observatories have been founded in some countries, and globally, to facilitate access to the data (such as the World Health Organization's Global Health Observatory, which brings together health data at a country level). However, much of the data can only be found at small population levels and must be obtained through bespoke collection systems. Local interpretation is required of all data to enable appropriate public health action to be taken in the context of more anecdotal and qualitative information.

In the UK, local government agencies are required to develop Joint Strategic Needs Assessments (Chapter 6), which collate this local public health intelligence and drive the development of local strategy and services to meet the needs of the population (Chapter 1).

Public health practitioners must be familiar with the indicators that are established to monitor the health status of our communities. These indicators also help us to understand and evaluate the effects of current interventions and programmes (Chapter 11). For some indicators, new research will be required to generate the information needed.

Summary exercise

Use the information in this chapter, your own knowledge and some additional research if necessary to complete the following table.

Type of data	Advantages in health profiling	Disadvantages in health profiling
Mortality statistics		
Notifiable infectious disease rates		
Hospital episode data		
General practice (primary care) data		
National surveys		
Disease registers		

Possible answers:

Type of data	Advantages in health profiling	Disadvantages in health profiling
Mortality statistics	Provide an indicator of a clear outcome Generally easy to count Often available at small population levels	Cause of death may be inaccurately recorded May be incomplete if no mandatory death registration system Does not give an indicator of the burden of long-term health conditions or of loss of potential life
Notifiable infectious disease rates	Good population coverage Mandatory Regularly updated Clinician and laboratory based so local Provides trends over time	Not all infectious diseases are notifiable Time-consuming to collect and analyse so timeliness may be an issue
Hospital episode data	Contains a patient identifier so can be linked to other person-based datasets Coded by disease categories Collected by hospital so local Covers the majority of major diseases Relatively complete	Process (rather than outcome) based There may be inconsistencies in coding across areas or over time Data are recorded twice (by clinicians and then entered onto a database by coders) and errors may be introduced
General practice (primary care) data	Local Provides a source of data that cannot be obtained elsewhere (for example, prevalence of heart failure)	May not be very complete There may be inconsistencies in coding across areas or over time There are usually incentives for completion which may skew what is collected It is time-consuming to collect, collate and analyse

Type of data	Advantages in health profiling	Disadvantages in health profiling
National surveys	Random sampling should ensure the results are applicable to the whole population	Those which do not have complete population coverage need care with extrapolation to a local population
	Can provide information not obtainable elsewhere (for example subjective health status)	Response rates may be low (some groups tend to respond worse than others, for example young men)
	Generally they have a core set of questions which can be used to determine trends over time	May not be very frequent so data become out of date
		Do not necessarily cover all population groups such as travellers and migrant workers
Disease registers	Rich source of disease-specific data which can be linked to other data sources	Not all diseases are recorded in this way
	Provides trends over time	Time-consuming and expensive to maintain
	Local	

REFERENCES

1. S. Bundey, H. Alam, A. Kaur, S. Mir and R. Lancashire, Why do UK-born Pakistani babies have high perinatal and neonatal mortality rates? *Paediatric Perinatal Epidemiology* **5**(1), 1991, 101–14.

2. A. Hobbiss, Are perinatal and infant mortality rates improved for second generation Pakistani mothers? *Research Findings Register* (H1060R), 2002.

3. The Inter-agency Group for Child Mortality Estimation, Levels & Trends in Child Mortality Report, New York, NY, UNICEF, 2010. See: http://www.unicef.org/media/files/UNICEF_Child_mortality_for_web_0831.pdf.

4. J. M. Last, *A Dictionary of Epidemiology*, 4th edn, Oxford, Oxford University Press, 2004.

5

Evidence-based health-care

Padmanabhan Badrinath and Stephen Gillam

Key points

- Evidence-based practice integrates the individual practitioner's experience, patient preferences and the best available research information.
- Incorporating the best available research evidence in decision making involves five steps: *asking* answerable questions; *accessing* the best information; *appraising* the information for validity and relevance; *applying* the information to care of patients and populations; and *evaluating* the impact for evidence of change and expected outcomes.
- Although practitioners need basic skills in finding evidence, a health librarian is an invaluable asset.
- There are specific checklists available to appraise research papers critically, and every practitioner should possess the skills to appraise the published literature.
- The major barriers to implementing evidence-based practice include the impression among practitioners that their professional freedom is being taken away, lack of access to appropriate training, tools and resource constraints.
- Various incentives including financial ones are used to encourage evidence-based practice.

Introduction – what is evidence-based health-care?

How much of what health and other professionals do is based soundly in science? Answers to the question 'is our practice evidence based?' depend on what we mean by practice and what we mean by evidence. Some studies have estimated that less than 20% of all health-care interventions are underpinned by robust research [1]. This varies from discipline to discipline. For example, studies examining clinical decisions

Essential Public Health, Second Edition, ed. Stephen Gillam, Jan Yates and Padmanabhan Badrinath.
Published by Cambridge University Press. © Cambridge University Press 2012.

in the field of internal medicine found that most primary therapeutic clinical decisions are based on evidence from randomised controlled trials [2].

Sackett *et al.* defined evidence-based medicine (EBM) as 'the conscientious, explicit, and judicious use of current best evidence in making decisions about the care of individual patients. The practice of evidence-based medicine means integrating individual clinical expertise with the best available external clinical evidence from systematic research' [3]. The expansion of EBM has been a major influence on clinical practice over the last 15 years. The demands of purchasers of health-care keen to optimise value for money have been one driver. A growing awareness among health professionals and their patients of medicine's potential to cause harm has been another. Since the early 1990s, EBM has steadily embraced other disciplines and public health is no exception. Public health practitioners with limited resources need to target these efficiently. Public health interventions are often costly and policy makers need evidence to invest appropriately. In this chapter we examine the nature of what is nowadays more broadly referred to as evidence-based health-care (EBHC) and discuss its limitations. It is worth noting that in the UK this field continues to expand, particularly into the arena of social care, which often goes hand in hand with the provision of health-care. Increasingly, the term 'evidence-based practice (EBP)' is used as a catch-all. Whilst this chapter focuses on health-care, the principles of EBP we describe apply equally to other disciplines.

The tools necessary for EBHC

The tools needed to practice in an evidence-based way are common across disciplines. Doctors, public health practitioners, nurses and allied health professionals all need the skills to ensure that the work they do, whether with individual clients or patients, or in the development of programmes and policies, is based on sound knowledge of what is likely to work.

Of the following five essential steps, the first is probably the most important:

1. convert information needs into answerable questions, i.e. by asking a focused question;
2. track down best available evidence;
3. appraise evidence critically;
4. change practice in the light of evidence;
5. evaluate your performance.

Step 1. Asking a focused question

Before seeking the best evidence, you need to convert your information needs into a tightly focused question. For example, it is not enough to ask 'Is alcohol-based gel more effective than soap and water in a hospital setting?' We need to convert this into an answerable question: 'For persons entering a hospital, is hand rubbing with a waterless, alcohol-based solution, as effective as standard hand washing with anti-septic soap for reducing hand contamination [4]?

The PICO approach can be used as a framework to focus a question by considering the necessary elements. It contains four components (shown below with our alcohol-based question from above as an example):

Patient or the population (those entering a hospital);

Intervention (use of alcohol-based hand solution);

Comparison intervention (use of antiseptic soap and water);

Outcome (reduction in the contamination of hands).

Some practitioners add a fifth element to the question – time. It may be important to determine the time-frame, for example when using an alcohol-based solution we may only be interested in contamination-free hands in the subsequent few hours, but when considering the effectiveness of cancer treatment we might want to know about mortality rates after 5 years.

Form a focused clinical question using the PICO format to find the evidence for the effectiveness of smoking cessation interventions in adult smokers who have had a heart attack.

P   Adult smokers who have had a heart attack.

I   Providing smoking cessation intervention.

C   Providing usual care.

O   Mortality and quit rates.

This gives us the question 'In smokers who have had a heart attack does a smoking cessation intervention in comparison with usual care reduce mortality and improve the quit rate?' [5]

Step 2. Tracking down the evidence

The second step in the practice of evidence-based health-care is to track down the best evidence.

Doctors may all too easily assess outcomes in terms of surrogate pathological end points rather than commonplace changes in quality of life or the ability to perform routine activities ('the operation was a success but the patient died'). Traditionally, doctors making decisions about what works have attached much weight to personal experience or the views of respected colleagues. Over time, doctors' knowledge of up-to-date care diminishes [6, 7] so there is a constant need for the latest evidence and simple ways to access and use it. A study of North American physicians has shown that up-to-date clinical information is needed twice for every three patients seen but they only receive 30% of this due to lack of time, dated textbooks and disorganised journals [8].

So, rather than rely on colleagues or textbooks, EBHC encourages the use of research evidence in a systematic way. Once a question has been formulated, the research base is then searched to find articles of relevance.

Table 5.1 Levels of evidence (Scottish Intercollegiate Guidelines Network)

1++ High-quality meta-analyses, systematic reviews of RCTs, or RCTs with a very low risk of bias

1+ Well-conducted meta-analyses, systematic reviews, or RCTs with a low risk of bias

1– Meta-analyses, systematic reviews, or RCTs with a high risk of bias

2++ High-quality systematic reviews of case–control or cohort studies. High-quality case–control or cohort studies with a very low risk of confounding or bias and a high probability that the relationship is causal

2+ Well-conducted case–control or cohort studies with a low risk of confounding or bias and a moderate probability that the relationship is causal

2– Case–control or cohort studies with a high risk of confounding or bias and a significant risk that the relationship is not causal

3 Non-analytic studies, e.g. case reports, case series

4 Expert opinion

So what do we look for? What is evidence? Care needs to be taken in relying on published articles. Many reviews reflect the prejudices of their authors and are anything but systematic. Even mainstream journals have a propensity to accept papers yielding positive rather than negative findings, e.g. in assessing treatments, so-called 'publication bias' [9,10]. Most books date rapidly. Hence the prominence nowadays accorded to properly conducted systematic reviews at the top of the hierarchy of evidence. A widely used ranking of the strength of evidence is shown in Table 5.1 [11]. Another popular hierarchy of evidence is the one developed by the Centre for Evidence Based Medicine in 1998, which was revised in 2011 [12].

Table 5.1 reminds us of the three main types of epidemiological study designs: descriptive, observational and interventional, which were considered in Chapter 3. When searching for evidence we should look for the highest level suitable to our question. A question relating to the effectiveness of an intervention will most appropriately be answered by a randomised controlled trial (RCT) or a systematic review of RCTs. The RCT is the gold standard as robust randomisation ensures that study and control groups differ only in terms of their exposure to the factor under study; the observed results are due only to the intervention and not to confounding variables. The Scottish Intercollegiate Guidelines Network (SIGN) takes into account the potential biases in its hierarchy of evidence. We can find answers to questions about the causes of a disease from case–control or cohort studies. However, questions beginning 'Why?' are often not answered by these kinds of study. What factors, after all, go to make a 'good nurse' or a 'good public health practitioner' and how easily are they measured? It is not possible to answer the question 'Why do women refuse an offer of breast screening?' with any of the study types mentioned so far. Another example would be: 'What leads to inappropriate use of medicines in elderly inpatients?' In these cases one looks for a qualitative study. Qualitative studies use methods such as interviews, diaries and direct observation to provide detailed information to describe the experiences of participants. Qualitative data are then analysed rigorously to lead to conclusions. Detailed coverage of qualitative methodology is beyond the scope of this book (see Pope and Mays' book [13] for an introduction to this topic) but it is important to remember that not every question can be answered using the classical hierarchy above. Qualitative methods can generate a wealth of knowledge to contextualise many of the decisions health professionals must make.

Consider the questions below. What studies would be most appropriately conducted to answer them: RCT, cohort, case–control, cross-sectional, qualitative?
   a. For what conditions do patients call their GP out of hours?
   b. What are the barriers to hand washing in a hospital setting?
   c. Does paternal exposure to ionising radiation before conception cause childhood leukaemia?
   d. What is the most sensitive and specific method of screening for genital chlamydial infection in women attending general practice?
   e. Does laparoscopic cholecystectomy cause less morbidity and a swifter return to work than a small-incision cholecystectomy?
   f. Do clinicians change their practice as a result of education?
   g. For a given patient with asthma, does beclamethasone give better symptomatic control than fluticasone?
   h. How do patients and carers view the service provided by a mental health team?
   i. How does smoking cessation affect the risk of stroke in middle-aged men?
   j. Is this new vaccine against avian flu effective?
   k. Do cooking sessions and information provision improve people's diet in deprived community settings?
   a. Cross-sectional study.
   b. Qualitative study.
   c. Case–control study.
   d. Cross-sectional study.
   e. Randomised controlled trial.
   f. Cohort study.
   g. Randomised controlled trial.
   h. Qualitative study
   i. Cohort study.
   j. Randomised controlled trial.
   k. Cohort study.

There are various sources of evidence. These include primary and secondary sources of literature. Primary sources are the thousands of original papers published every year in research journals. However, to deal with the vast amount of information available, more and more people now turn to secondary sources of evidence and the single most important source of systematic reviews is the Cochrane Database (www.cochrane.org). The Cochrane Collaboration (named after Archie Cochrane, an early pioneer of EBM) is an international endeavour to summarise high-quality evidence in all fields of medical practice. It has slowly transformed many areas of clinical practice. In this textbook's Internet Companion you will find more information about the Cochrane Library and relevant internet links.

So it is important to have basic skills in searching the literature, although the help of expert librarians may be needed. Research papers are catalogued in a variety of databases searchable on the internet. For many medical or public health queries the database Medline is a good starting place. Other databases are available for specialist queries such as those in the fields of mental health and nursing. Using the PICO format here is helpful as it can be used to generate search terms with which to query the databases. Databases may have tools to support the user in this such as the 'Clinical Queries' tool in PubMed, which is a US National Library of Medicine's service to search the biomedical research literature [14].

We can use our example question from earlier to demonstrate how a search might work. Our focused question was 'In smokers who have had a heart attack does a smoking cessation intervention in comparison with usual care reduce mortality and improve quit rate?'

What study type would be appropriate for answering this question?
Randomised controlled trials are possible, where smokers who have had
a heart attack are randomised to receive smoking cessation intervention or usual
care, to give a measure of the relative effectiveness of the smoking cessation
intervention.

Using the PICO format, list the key words we need to use to search databases through a search function such as PubMed's Clinical Queries.
Smokers, heart attack, cessation, counselling, mortality. In Clinical Queries, as we select an option to indicate our interest is in therapy (i.e. intervention studies) the term 'randomised controlled trial' is automatically added to the key words. In other search systems or databases this may need to be added manually.

The journal articles found using this strategy are:

1. N. A. Rigotti, A. N. Thorndike, S. Regan *et al*. Bupropion for smokers hospitalised with acute cardiovascular disease. *American Journal of Medicine* **119**(12), 2006, 1080–7.
2. E. A. Dornelas, R. A. Sampson, J. F. Gray, D. Waters and P. D. Thompson. A randomised controlled trial of smoking cessation counseling after myocardial infarction. *Preventive Medicine* **30**(4), 2000, 261–8.

Look at these results. Are these articles relevant?

Yes. Bupropion is used to help smokers quit their habit. The second study is an RCT testing the effectiveness of smoking cessation counselling in patients who have had a heart attack.

In the search for evidence it should be remembered that not every piece of information which might help us answer our question may be published. Studies may be in progress which could inform our action; negative studies, which could help tell us what NOT to do, may not have made it as far as a publication; many pharmaceutical companies have unpublished information; conference reports might provide helpful information. As we move down the hierarchy it becomes more difficult to find this kind of evidence (called 'grey' literature) from readily available sources but some databases and repositories are available. This is a good time to seek the help of an expert librarian!

Refer to the Internet Companion for more exercises to develop your skills in searching the literature to answer your questions.

Step 3. Appraising the evidence

To be able to determine whether we should act on the results of the studies found in the search we must be able critically to appraise a range of study types. It is important to have an understanding of the basic epidemiological concepts outlined in Chapter 3, to be able to understand the results presented and to have a systematic approach to the appraisal. In brief, we are looking to determine whether we believe the results sufficiently to act on them and change our practice. In order to do this we ask a series of questions about the study which include:

- Did the research ask a clearly focused question and carry out the right sort of study to answer it?
- Were the study methods robust?
- Do the conclusions made match the results of the study?
- Can we use these results in our practice? This might include an assessment of whether the results are due to chance, 'big' enough to make a real difference and whether the same results are likely to occur in our own situation.

There are standard checklists available to support systematic appraisal of different types of study designs. We can use these to help determine how valid the findings of the study are, and whether the findings can be generalised to our own population.

Table 5.2 shows a checklist for appraising a randomised controlled trial, the most appropriate primary design to generate evidence of effective interventions. This checklist is taken from the UK Critical Appraisal Skills Programme (CASP) in Oxford [15].

It is important to be able to analyse critically the results of all study types but, as the volume of scientific literature increases, it is perhaps most important to be able to use systematic reviews effectively to guide practice. It has been estimated that a general physician needs to read for 119 hours a week to keep up to date; medical students are alleged to spend 1–2 hours reading clinical material per week – and that's more than

Table 5.2 The CASP critical appraisal tool for systematic reviews

Screening questions

1. Did the review ask a clearly focused question? Yes / Can't tell / No

    Consider if the question is 'focused' in terms of:

    the population studied

    the intervention given or exposure

    the outcomes considered

2. Did the review include the right type of study? Yes / Can't tell / No

    Consider if the included studies:

    address the review's question

    have an appropriate study design

Is it worth continuing?

Detailed questions

3. Did the reviewers try to identify all relevant studies? Yes / Can't tell / No

    Consider:

    which bibliographic databases were used

    if there was follow-up from reference lists

    if there was personal contact with experts

    if the reviewers searched for unpublished studies

    if the reviewers searched for non-English-language studies

4. Did the reviewers assess the quality of the included studies? Yes / Can't tell / No

    Consider:

    if a clear, pre-determined strategy was used to determine which studies were included.

    Look for:

    a scoring system

    more than one assessor

5. If the results of the studies have been combined, was it reasonable to do so? Yes / Can't tell / No

    Consider whether:

    the results of each study are clearly displayed

    the results were similar from study to study (look for tests of heterogeneity)

    the reasons for any variations in results are discussed

6. How are the results presented and what is the main result?

    Consider:

    how the results are expressed (e.g. Odds Ratio, Relative Risk, etc.)

    how large this size of result is and how meaningful it is

    how you would sum up the bottom-line result of the review in one sentence

7. How precise are these results?

    Consider:

    if a confidence interval were reported. Would your decision about whether or not to use this intervention be the same at the upper confidence limit as at the lower confidence limit?

    if a P value is reported where confidence intervals are unavailable

8. Can the results be applied to the local population? Yes / Can't tell / No

    Consider whether:

    the population sample covered by the review could be different from your population in ways that would produce different results

    your local setting differs much from that of the review

    you can provide the same intervention in your setting

Table 5.2 (*cont.*)

Screening questions

9. Were all important outcomes considered? Yes / Can't tell / No
   Consider outcomes from the point of view of the:
   > individual
   > policy makers and professionals
   > family/carers
   > wider community
10. Should policy or practice change as a result of the evidence contained in this review? Yes / Can't tell / No
   Consider:
   > whether any benefit reported outweighs any harm and/or cost. If this information is not reported can it be filled in from elsewhere?

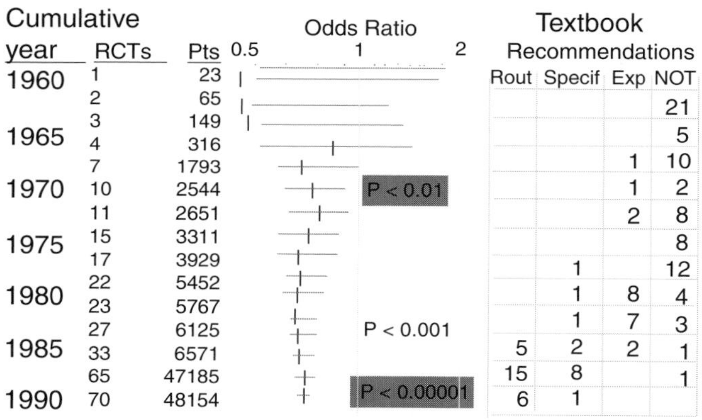

Figure 5.1   Results of meta-analyses of thrombolysis for myocardial infarction (MI), according to when they could have been carried out, and the textbook recommendations at the time (Pts = patients): routine, in specified circumstances, as experimental treatment, or not recommended.

Cumulative year	RCTs	Pts	Odds Ratio	Textbook Recommendations

the doctors who teach them [16]. Also, a single study of insufficient sample size or of otherwise poor quality may yield misleading results. The right answer to a specific question is more likely to come from a systematic review. This is a review of all the literature on a particular topic, which has been methodically identified, appraised and presented. The statistical combination of all the results from included studies to provide a summary estimate or definitive result is called meta-analysis.

Antman *et al.*'s classic study of research into the effectiveness of thrombolysis demonstrates the importance of systematic review and meta-analysis for proponents of EBM [17]. The first study, showing that streptokinase reduced mortality following myocardial infarction, was published in 1960. The results of this meta-analysis are shown in Figure 5.1. Whilst early RCTs showed a treatment effect (Odds Ratio below 1), the confidence intervals around these effect–size estimates were wide, showing imprecision, and went above 1, which indicates the possibility of no effect.

The power of meta-analysis is clearly demonstrated by the narrowing of these confidence intervals as the number of RCTs increased. From around 1970, the beneficial effect of thrombolysis seems clearly apparent but some 30 years after the first RCT and nearly 20 years after meta-analysis might have decided the question, thrombolytics were still not being routinely recommended in clinical practice. Because reviews have not always used scientific methods, advice on some life-saving therapies has often been delayed. Other treatments have been recommended long after controlled trials have shown them to be harmful.

Step 4. Changing practice in light of evidence

Actually following through on the results of your appraisal of new evidence – implementation – is the most difficult of the five steps. Some change can be self-initiated; other circumstances require change in those around you. The implementation of effective public health interventions often requires change in others, and public health practitioners often act as advocates for EBHC, encouraging other professionals to act on results of an assessment of the evidence base. The management of people and an understanding of how they will react are invaluable. Chapter 1 has already covered the theoretical models of change in some detail and we can use evidence-based practice to determine how to implement change (see Box 5.1).

There is no magic bullet (see Chapter 11). Most interventions are effective under some circumstances; none is effective under all circumstances. A diagnostic analysis

---

Box 5.1 Evidence of effectiveness of interventions to change professional behaviour [18]

There is good evidence to support:

Multifaceted interventions. By targeting different barriers to change, these are more likely to be effective than single interventions.

Educational outreach. This can change prescribing behaviour.

Reminder systems. These are generally effective for a range of behaviours.

There are mixed effects in the following:

Audit and feedback. These need to be used selectively.

Opinion leaders. These need to be used selectively.

There is little evidence to support:

Passive dissemination of guidelines. However, there is some evidence to support use of guidelines if tailored to local needs and associated with reminders.

of the individual and the context must be performed before selecting a method for altering individual practitioner behaviour. Interventions based on assessment of potential barriers are more likely to be effective.

Step 5. Evaluating the effects of changes in practice

Commonly, this step will involve a clinical audit (see Chapter 11). Depending on how frequently the intervention or activity under scrutiny is performed, a review of behaviour will be undertaken some months after instigation of the change.

If we go back to the example of use of alcohol-based gel from Step 1 how would we know that practice has changed?
There are various ways of ascertaining whether practice has changed. We could observe those entering the hospital. Once we identify people who are not using the alcohol-based gel we need to identify the barriers. These could include sheer callousness or lack of knowledge of the risks associated with contaminated hands and these could be addressed by awareness-raising initiatives and training.

Limitations to EBHC

Evidence is only one influence on our practice. Education alone may not change deeply ingrained habits, e.g. patterns of prescribing. Knowledge does not necessarily change practice. This is true for practitioners and patients or the public. An example is the continued use by patients of complementary therapies, which professionals consider to be ineffective. Doctors are sceptical of their benefits and attempt to restrict their use on the basis of scientific evaluations, which show either that most such therapies are not effective or that there is no evidence that they are [19]. The public continue to use them and research has shown that 26% of adults have taken a herbal medicine in the previous 2 years [20], possibly because they meet personal needs that conventional treatments do not.

Hence we need to consider employing other incentives to change. Financial incentives are used to promote interventions known to be effective (e.g. target payments to increase immunisation uptake). In the NHS the Quality and Outcomes Framework (QOF) payment system has been introduced to improve the quality of clinical care and promote evidence-based practice [21]. Evidence suggests that financial incentives might improve provider performance in preventive interventions such as offering a smoking cessation service [22]. Chapter 11 looks in more detail at quality improvement in health-care.

The most strident criticisms of EBHC have come from those physicians who resent intrusions into their clinical freedom. The use of evidence-based protocols has been demeaned [23] as 'cookbook medicine'. A more powerful philosophical argument is mounted by those arguing that a rigid fixation on randomised controlled trials risks ignoring important qualitative sources of evidence [24].

In addition, there may be times when high-quality evidence from the upper echelons of the hierarchy simply does not exist. This should not prevent action! The lack of RCTs does not mean an intervention is ineffective, it means that there is no evidence that it is effective, a clear distinction. In these cases, one looks further down the hierarchy and uses the best level of evidence available. When no research evidence exists there is nothing wrong with asking colleagues for their opinions; the practice of EBHC simply means we should at least carry out the search.

Conclusion

The terms 'evidence-based medicine' and 'evidence-based health-care' were developed to encourage practitioners and patients to pay due respect – no more, no less – to current evidence in making decisions. Evidence should enhance health-care decision making, not rigidly dictate it [25]. Public health practitioners need to consider their population's health- and social-care needs and what effective interventions are available to meet them. Finally, the practitioner must consider society's and individuals' preferences. The art of EBHC lies in bringing all these considerations together. Use the following example to practice putting all the steps together for a specific issue.

Evidence-based practice is not solely the province of the health sector. Here is an example of EBHC in the community setting.

Your community is concerned about the high rates of road traffic accidents locally and local councillors have asked you for help. Keeping in mind the principles of EBHC list the steps you would take and how you would proceed.

1. You need to frame an answerable question. This might be 'What community-based interventions are successful at reducing road traffic accidents and deaths in children aged up to 16 years?'
2. Identify the evidence for the specific intervention. A simple search in PubMed using the key words reducing, road traffic accidents, yields several studies including articles on road-safety training programmes, speed cameras and penalty points for drivers.
3. Critically appraise the evidence. A closer look at the papers may show that some are not relevant to the local situation (e.g. as they are not RCTs or were undertaken in non-UK settings). There may be promising studies, the results of which could be applied locally [26].
4. Develop ways of implementing the evidence if found to be appropriate. One option might be to explore the possibility of installing speed cameras after appropriate consultation with the local community.

5. Undertake an evaluation to determine if the intervention has produced the intended outcome. The introduction of a new intervention should always be accompanied by an explicit evaluation strategy, which identifies the objectives of the intervention and plans to measure success in a robust way.

REFERENCES

1. R. Smith, Where is the wisdom ...? *British Medical Journal* **303**, 1991, 798–9.
2. G. Michaud, J. L. McGowan, R. van der Jagt, G. Wells and P. Tugwell, Are therapeutic decisions supported by evidence from health care research? *Archives of Internal Medicine* **158**(15), 1998, 1665–8.
3. D. L. Sackett, W. M. Rosenberg, J. A. Gray, R. B. Haynes and W. S. Richardson, Evidence based medicine: what it is and what it isn't. *British Medical Journal*, **312**, 1996, 71–2.
4. A. DiCenso, G. Guyatt and D. Ciliska, *Evidence-Based Nursing: A Guide to Clinical Practice*, St. Louis, MO, Mosby, 2005.
5. K. Korenstein and T. McGinn, The impact of an intensive smoking cessation intervention. *Mount Sinai Journal of Medicine* **75**, 2008, 552–5.
6. N. K. Choudry, R. H. Fletcher and S. B. Soumerai, Systematic review: the relationship between clinical experience and quality of health care. *Annals of Internal Medicine* **142**, 2005, 260–73.
7. P. G. Ramsey, J. D. Carline, T. S. Inui *et al.*, Changes over time in the knowledge base of practicing internists. *Journal of the American Medical Association* **266**, 1991, 1103–7.
8. D. G. Covell, G. C. Uman and P. R. Manning, Information needs in office practice: Are they being met? *Annals of Internal Medicine* **103**, 1985, 596–9.
9. P. J. Easterbrook, J. A. Berlin, R. Gopalan and D. R. Matthews, Publication bias in clinical research. *Lancet* **337**(8746), 199, 867–72.
10. K. Dickersin, The existence of publication bias and risk factors for its occurrence. *Journal of the American Medical Association* **263**, 1990, 1385–9.
11. Scottish Intercollegiate Guidelines Network, SIGN 50: A guideline developer's handbook, Annex B. Edinburgh, SIGN. See: http://www.sign.ac.uk/guidelines/fulltext/50/annexb.html.
12. M. Dawes, Putting evidence into practice. Revised level of evidence helps to find the best evidence in real time. *British Medical Journal* **342**, 2011, 885–6.
13. C. Pope and N. Mays (eds.), *Qualitative Research in Health Care*, 3rd edn., Oxford, Blackwell Publishing/BMJ Books, 2006.
14. PubMed Clinical Queries. See: http://www.ncbi.nlm.nih.gov/pubmed/clinical.
15. Critical Appraisal Skills Programme. Making sense of evidence. See http://www.casp-uk.net.
16. D. L. Sackett, W. S. Richardson, W. Rosenberg and R. B. Haynes, *Evidence-based Medicine: How to Practise and Teach EBM*. Edinburgh, Churchill Livingstone, 1997, pp. 8–9.
17. E. M. Antman, J. Lau, B. Kupelnick, F. Mosteller and T. C. Chalmers, A comparison of results of meta-analyses of randomized control trials and recommendations of clinical experts. *Journal of the American Medical Association* **268**, 1992, 240–8.
18. University of York, NHS Centre for Reviews and Dissemination, Getting evidence into practice. *Effective Health Care Bulletin* **5**, 1999. See http://www.york.ac.uk/inst/crd/EHC/ehc51.pdf.

19. E. Ernst, A systematic review of systematic reviews of homeopathy. *British Journal of Clinical Pharmacology* **50**, 2000, 577–82.

20. Medicines and Healthcare products Regulatory Agency (MHRA), *Public perception of herbal medicine*. Drug Safety Update, March 2009. See http://www.mhra.gov.uk/Safetyinformat ion/DrugSafetyUpdate/CON088122.

21. T. Doran, C. Fullwood, H. Gravelle *et al.*, Pay-for-performance programs in family practices in the United Kingdom. *New England Journal of Medicine* **355**(4), 2006, 375–84.

22. J. Roski, R. Jeddeloh, L. An *et al.*, The impact of financial incentives and a patient registry on preventive care quality: increasing provider adherence to evidence-based smoking cessation practice guidelines. *Preventative Medicine* **36**(3), 2003, 291–9.

23. B. G. Charlton and A. Miles, The rise and fall of EBM. *Quarterly Journal of Medicine* **12**, 1998, 371–4.

24. J. Popay and G. Williams, Qualitative research and evidence-based healthcare. *Journal of the Royal Society of Medicine*, **91**(Suppl. 35), 1998, 32–7.

25. S. E. Straus and F. A. McAlister, Evidence-based medicine: a commentary on common criticisms. *Canadian Medical Association Journal* **163**, 2000, 837–41.

26. C. Wilson, C. Willis, J. K. Hendrikz, R. Le Brocque and N. Bellamy, Speed cameras for the prevention of road traffic injuries and deaths. *Cochrane Database of Systematic Reviews* **10**(11), 2010, CD004607.

6

Health needs assessment

Stephen Gillam, Jan Yates and Padmanabhan Badrinath

Key points

- Health needs should be distinguished from the need for health-care, which is nowadays defined in terms of ability to benefit.
- Health-care needs assessment is central to the planning process.
- There are three commonly contrasted approaches to needs assessment: corporate, comparative and epidemiological.
- Many toolkits and other resources have been developed to assist those undertaking health-care needs assessments.

Theoretical perspectives

Health professionals spend much time learning to assess the needs of individuals; many know less about defining the needs of a population. The need for health underlies but does not wholly determine the need for health-care. Health-care needs are often measured in terms of demand, but demand is to a great extent 'supply-induced' (see Chapter 7). For example, variations in general practice referral or consultation rates have less to do with the health status of the populations served than with differences between doctors, such as their skills or referral thresholds [1].

There is no generally accepted definition of 'need'. Last's notion of the 'clinical iceberg' of disease [2] (see Chapter 3) has been supported by various community studies indicating much illness is unknown to health professionals. Needs can be classified in terms of diseases, priority groups, geographical areas, services or using a lifecycle approach (children/teenagers/adults/elderly). Bradshaw's often-quoted taxonomy highlighted four types of need [3]:

- expressed needs (needs expressed by action, for instance visiting a doctor);
- normative needs (defined by experts);

Essential Public Health, Second Edition, ed. Stephen Gillam, Jan Yates and Padmanabhan Badrinath.
Published by Cambridge University Press. © Cambridge University Press 2012.

- comparative needs (comparing one group of people with another);
- felt needs (those needs people say they have).

Health or health-care?

Health is famously difficult to define. The World Health Organization's definition of health embraces the physical, social, and emotional well-being of an individual, group or community and emphasises health as a positive resource of life, not just the absence of disease [4]. Health needs accordingly encompass education, social services, housing, the environment and social policy.

The need for health-care is the population's ability to benefit from health-care, which is in turn the sum of many individuals' ability to benefit [4]. As well as treatment, health-care includes prevention, diagnosis, continuing care, rehabilitation and palliative care. The ability to benefit does not mean that all outcomes will be favourable but implies outcomes that will, on average, be effective. Some benefits may be manifested in changes of clinical status; others, such as the benefits of reassurance or the support of carers, are difficult to measure. Diagnosis and reassurance form an important part of primary care when many people may require no more than a negative diagnosis. Health needs assessment thus requires knowledge of the incidence of the health problem (risk factor, disease, disability), its prevalence, and the effectiveness of services to address it.

Individual or population?

Clinicians focus on the individual and need is defined in terms of what can be done for the patients they see. However, this may neglect the health needs of people not receiving care, e.g. attending surgery or outpatients departments. Traditionally, the clinical view enshrined in such notions as 'clinical freedom' has taken little account of treatment cost. Services of doubtful efficacy are provided if they may be even remotely beneficial to patients. In contrast, the view of public health professionals who adopt a population approach seeks to prioritise within finite budgets. Individual clinical decisions may be made without considering the opportunity costs of treatment, while at a population level such opportunity costs must be minimised if the health of the population is to be maximised.

The ethical conflicts raised are not easily resolved. Health professionals will only reluctantly withhold interventions of minor benefit for the greater good of potential patients. Tension between what is best for the individual and what may be best for society will always present a dilemma for clinicians. In reality, a complex range of considerations of which cost-effectiveness is but one will always determine both clinical and strategic decision making (see Chapter 7).

Need, supply or demand?

Health-care is never organised as a 'pure' market. Its products are heavily subsidised and regulated in all countries. The main reason for this is asymmetry of information whereby patients lack knowledge of their own treatment needs and depend on health-care providers to make appropriate decisions. The clinician acts as the patient's 'agent' to translate demands into needs. However, the literature on variation in referrals, prescribing and other activity rates reveals that this agency relationship is complex.

Professional perceptions of need may differ from those of consumers [5]. The latter are more likely to be influenced by external factors such as media coverage and the opinions of relatives and friends. Consumers' priorities vary with age, health status and previous experience of health-service use.

The health problems considered to constitute need may change over time. Much universal screening activity, for example in the field of child health surveillance, is no longer supported by research evidence. New needs accrue with the development of new technology. There is usually a time lag before lay demand (for health) reflects scientific evidence of need (for health-care). Unfortunately, an even longer time lag distorts the provision of health services. Their supply is affected by historical factors, and by public and political pressures. The closure of hospital beds is ever politically charged. Health services tend to be regarded as untouchable even when their useful-ness has been outlived, while medical innovations are generally implemented before they have been fully evaluated. The pharmaceutical industry, the professions them-selves and the media are among interested parties that can manipulate demand. (How would you assess the need for treatments for Pre-diabetes or Hypoactive Sexual Desire Disorder?)

The relationship between need, demand and supply is illustrated in Figure 6.1. It shows seven fields of services divided into those for which there is a need but no demand or supply (segment 1), those for which there is a demand but no need or supply (segment 2), those for which there is a supply but no need or demand (segment 3), and various other degrees of overlap. Any intervention can be fitted into one of these fields. Rehabilitation after myocardial infarction may be needed but not supplied or demanded. Antibiotics for upper-respiratory-tract infection may be demanded but not needed or supplied, and so on. Much effort is required on behalf of patients, providers and purchasers to make the three cycles more confluent. Something is known about how to change professional behaviour through financial incentives, protocols, education, audit and even contracts (see Chapter 11): the factors influencing patient preferences are less well understood.

From Figure 6.1, seven types of service can be identified. See if you can provide examples of services in each segment.

1. Services where there is a need but no demand or supply. Family-planning and contraceptive services are needed in many parts of the developing world to improve women's reproductive health. They are frequently neither *demanded* nor *supplied*.

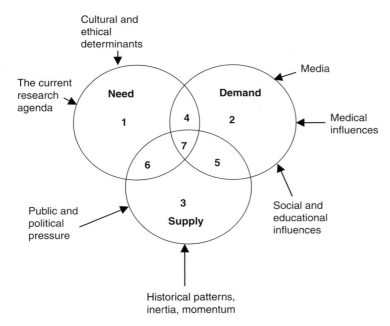

Figure 6.1 Need, demand and supply.

2. Services for which there is a demand but no need or supply. Patients may ask for (*demand*) expectorants for coughs and colds. However, cough mixtures are ineffective (no *need*) and seldom prescribed (no *supply*).

3. Services for which there is a supply but no need or demand. The provision of routine health checks in people over 75 years. Most people do not request these (no *demand*), but in some practices they are provided (*supply*). Research suggests that the benefits of such checks do not outweigh the costs (no *need*).

4. Services for which there is a need and demand but no supply. Substance misuse is a common and dangerous affliction. Methadone maintenance programmes can reduce the physical risks of heroin addiction (*demand*) and may increase the chances of drug misusers giving up (*need*), but are not always available (no *supply*).

5. Services for which there is a demand and supply but no need. People may request (*demand*) and be prescribed (*supply*) long-acting benzodiazepines for insomnia. In the long term, this is not effective (no *need*).

6. Services for which there is a need and supply but no demand. Even when it is offered, not all health-care staff take up the opportunity of Hepatitis B immunisation (*supply* but no *demand*). Yet they are at risk of Hepatitis B infection and immunisation is effective at preventing it (*need*).

7. Services for which there is a need, demand and supply. People with insulin-dependent diabetes ask for (*demand*) insulin, it is effective at maintaining their health (*need*) and the UK National Health Service, unlike many others, can afford to provide it (*supply*).

Health needs assessment (HNA) in practice

In the UK, after the so-called 'internal market' between health-care purchasers and providers was introduced in the early 1990s, purchasing decisions based on the needs of the population to achieve 'health gain' came into focus. Commissioning organisations with the responsibility to purchase care have been required to assess the needs of their population and to use these needs to set priorities and improve health. Public health practitioners, with their training and origins in epidemiology, disease control and health promotion, developed a number of techniques to assess population needs. At the same time, there was greater interest in involving the general public in shaping services and a number of techniques have been developed to assess health needs from the user's perspective.

Why is assessing needs and priorities important?

The majority of health-care is currently commissioned by primary care trust 'clusters' of practices, which place contracts with providers of care (such as acute hospital trusts). The commissioning of much health-care transfers to clinically led groups in 2013 under the current plans of the Coalition government. Central to current and future commissioning in the UK are the 'Joint Strategic Needs Assessments', undertaken jointly between health and social care in local government [6]. These and other needs assessments should specify:

- the quantity of health-care activity required (e.g. numbers of operations, admissions, attendances at emergency departments, in/out-patients, etc.);
- the quality of care required, by specifying and monitoring standards (with measures such as infections, rates of venous thrombo-embolism, or readmissions within 30 days of discharge).

The aim of a health needs assessment is therefore to describe health problems in a population and detect differences within and between different groups in order to determine health priorities and unmet need (see Box 6.1). It should identify where people are able to benefit either from health-service care or from wider social and environmental change and balance any potential change against clinical, ethical and economic considerations: that is, what should be done, what can be done and what can be afforded [7].

Health needs assessment is thus a method that:

- is objective, valid and takes a systematic approach;
- involves a number of professionals and the general public;
- involves using different sources and methods of collecting and analysing information (including epidemiological, qualitative and comparative methods);
- seeks to identify needs and recommends changes to optimise the delivery of health services.

> **Box 6.1 Five objectives of a health-care needs assessment [8]**
>
> 1. **Planning**. This is the central objective of needs assessment; to help decide what services are required; for how many people; the effectiveness of these services; the benefits that will be expected; and at what cost.
> 2. **Intelligence**. Gathering information to get an overview and an increased understanding of the existing health-care service, the population it serves and the population's health needs.
> 3. **Equity**. Improving the spatial allocation of resources between and within different groups.
> 4. **Target efficiency**. Having assessed needs, measuring whether or not resources have been appropriately directed: i.e. Do those who need a service get it? Do those who get a service need it? This is related to audit.
> 5. **Involvement of stakeholders**. Carrying out a health needs assessment can stimulate the involvement and ownership of the various players in the process.

The NHS and health systems across the world face similar pressures. These include the rising cost of health-care due to continuing scientific advances, increasing life expectancy and rising public expectations. At the same time, most countries face similar dilemmas: health-service resources are limited and people face inequitable access to existing care. People whose health needs are greatest are least likely to have access to health-care (the 'inverse care law' referred to several times throughout this book). Finally, there are concerns about the appropriateness, effectiveness and quality of that care. The challenge is to make decisions that maximise the benefit for the population, taking into account the resources available. Needs assessment helps this decision making and involves at least three steps.

Step 1. Identifying health priorities by defining the population under scrutiny and collecting and analysing routine data – comparative needs assessment

Routine data indicate what it is that people are dying from and why they consult general practices, hospitals and social services. This will help to prioritise topics for local discussion (Step 2) with a range of other local agencies and professionals. These data allow comparisons to be drawn between local services and those available in other geographical areas. It is also possible to compare these data with previously set standards. For example, one might compare hospital rates of health-care-acquired infections with government standards.

Many data are already available and provide information to 'start the ball rolling'. Chapter 4 gives an indication of routinely available information, which may be accessed from health-care organisations. Discussions about the data will help lead to a consensus on what areas are priorities. It can also be a starting point to involve the public.

There are some disadvantages. The data may be quite old (it often takes up to two years for routine data to become available), diseases may have been mis-diagnosed or not reported, and hospital data may reflect different admission policies for the same condition. Nevertheless, data collection does help to start the process and is a means to approaching others who have a contribution to make.

Step 2. Agreeing local priorities by involving other agencies, users and the public – corporate needs assessment

There are a confusing number of terms for this process, including community appraisals, rapid appraisals and community surveys. Many of the techniques have been pioneered in developing countries by researchers using qualitative methods [9] – semi-structured interviews, for example. These approaches to understanding behaviours and beliefs may reduce the distorting effect of measuring needs through the eyes of health professionals.

Professionals from other agencies, including local government and the voluntary sector, may have differing ideas from health professionals and it is important to take these ideas into account. It is also important to consider the ideas of users and carers about what improves their health. These factors may include having a job, adequate housing, better choice of food or a bus route. It is important to be aware of the limitations of professional knowledge. There are a number of ways of getting the public involved including:

- Citizens' juries – representatives of the public or local opinion leaders are selected. Experts give evidence and jurors have an opportunity to ask questions and debate.
- User consultation panels – local people are selected as representatives of the locality. Typically, members are rotated to include a broad range of views. Topics are considered in advance and members are presented with relevant information. A moderator facilitates the meeting.
- Focus groups – semi-structured discussion groups of six to eight people led by a moderator.
- Questionnaire surveys – these can be postal, distributed by hand or electronically. This is often most appropriate when the issues behind questions are well known.
- Panels – these are large sociologically representative samples (around 100) of a population in a primary care trust, a clinical commissioning group, or a health board, which are surveyed at intervals.
- Interviews – for example, with patients after a clinic visit on the quality of care, or with health workers on what they know of people's perceptions of local needs.
- Rapid appraisal – involves the public directly in the assessment and definition of local needs through a series of face-to-face interviews with local informants who have a knowledge of the community [9]. From these interviews and from appraisal

of local documents about the neighbourhood or community, a list of priorities is drawn up. This is then assessed collectively by means of a public meeting. Working groups develop action plans. The approach is 'bottom-up' and the key philosophy is not only of public involvement but of a collective response to health needs.

Step 3. Undertaking an epidemiological needs assessment

This stage involves examining specific priorities in more detail (Box 6.2). It looks carefully at matters such as the size of the problem, what is currently being provided and what interventions may help. Recommendations can then be made on what changes are needed.

An epidemiological approach to assessing health needs involves three kinds of measurement. It measures:

1. The size of the problem. It looks at how much illness or ill health there is in the community by assessing the incidence and prevalence.
2. The current services that exist to meet this burden. It examines how local provision compares with other areas, whether the services meet the needs or whether they are over- or under-provided.
3. Whether the services are effective. If new services are required to meet unmet need it looks at what is known about what works or will make a difference.

Resources for health-care are always finite so the purpose of this type of needs assessment is to identify health improvements which can be achieved by reallocating resources to remedy over-provision (sometimes) and unmet need. Toolkits are available to help undertake needs assessment at a local level [7].

Policy, planning, and strategy development

The cycle of planning for health-care delivery should originate in an assessment of needs: where are we now and where do we want to get to? The rest of the process is mostly concerned with how to get there (Figure 6.2). Comprehensive needs assessment will generate a bewildering array of possible needs. There are many ways of identifying priorities and this issue is discussed in Chapter 7.

Box 6.2 Priorities for the purposes of HNA may comprise:

A whole speciality such as mental health

A disease such as coronary heart disease

A client group such as substance misusers

Groups waiting for interventions such as those waiting for hip operations

Vulnerable groups such as ethnic minorities

Socially deprived groups such as tenants of particular housing estates

Figure 6.2   The planning cycle.

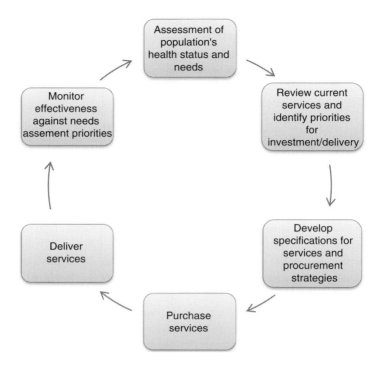

At whatever level in the system priorities are being agreed, the process should involve as many of the people who will be affected by the choice as reasonably possible. Teams need to take careful stock of their current work when making a decision. In many important areas work may already be on-going (for example, heart disease prevention). Few health professionals are not already overloaded. There is little point in setting grandiose objectives that cannot realistically be attained.

Audit and evaluation (to see whether we have got to where we want to go) is therefore integrally related to needs assessment (Chapter 11). Indeed, the selection of audit topics should be framed by systematic assessment of priority needs. It can too often be governed by ad hoc medical choices.

A description of the planning process may falsely imply an orderly sequence. Few practitioners with experience of planning and policy-making will subscribe to this myth of rational planning (Chapters 1 and Chapters 16). In real life, it is rarely possible to maintain forward progress around the cycle for long. The process is iterative rather than cyclical. The commonest causes of disruption, other than shortage of finance, are vague objectives, lack of information and changing circumstances, people and politics. An understanding of the contingent nature of much planning is important in effecting change. However, consideration of both the planning process and policy-making process as a cycle is helpful when working at a local level within the NHS or partner organisations such as local authorities or voluntary sector organisations.

Table 6.1 An example of local policy and planning

Stage	Possible local actions
Assessment of health status and need	Local needs assessment is carried out and identifies high levels of adolescent drinking and local 'hot spots' such as town-centre venues. Police enforcement activity levels are high in specific locations and public perception of street safety has been worsening. Local emergency departments report disorder issues and levels of alcohol-related admissions are higher than the national average. General practitioners are surveyed and low levels of awareness of the effectiveness of brief interventions to address excess alcohol use are found.
Review current services and prioritise	Stakeholder engagement takes account of the local context (e.g. local consumption levels, the ease of availability, views of local health professionals, views of local schools, the level of enforcements, local political imperatives, local commercial interests, and the views of the public) and identifies a need to share information between health and the police, to provide additional capacity in emergency departments, to provide brief intervention training to GPs and to adjust policing policies in certain locations.
Develop service specifications and procurement plans	A specification is drawn up for an alcohol specialist nurse to be based in the emergency department, an information system to enable data sharing and the provision of brief intervention training in general practice. A business case for an additional community safety officer capacity is drawn up. Key decision-making forums approve additional resources based on a cost-effectiveness analysis.
Purchase services	Local procurement guidance is followed and potential service providers assessed to determine which are the most appropriate.
Deliver services	Funding is provided, staff are employed, services commence delivery.
Monitor and evaluate services	Key performance indicators on which to assess outcomes have been specified to enable service monitoring and evaluation. These are collected on an on-going basis and any issues they highlight are reviewed.

Devising services to reduce the harm caused by alcohol can be used as an example to consider how the planning cycle would work in practice. Alcohol-harm reduction has been a UK government priority for several years and the local translation of this into action will depend on local needs. Use the stages in Figure 6.2 to consider how a local alcohol policy might be developed.
Table 6.1 provides some suggestions.

Conclusion

Health needs assessment is the first and, arguably, most important step in planning and evaluating the delivery of care. It is not possible to tell how good the care is, how efficient or how cost-effective it is if we do not know what our population needs, i.e. what services they will benefit from. Certainly in UK health policy this is increasingly recognised and assessment of both health needs (for example, the needs of a specific minority population, not restricted simply to the need for NHS services) and health-care needs (for example, the needs of a locality for mental health-care) are pre-requisites for the assignment of resources. See the Internet Companion for a further example of a health-care needs assessment with the needs of prisoners as the focus.

REFERENCES

1. M. Roland and A. Coulter, *Hospital Referrals*, Oxford, Oxford University Press, 1993.
2. J. M. Last, The iceberg: completing the clinical picture in general practice. *Lancet* **2**, 1963, 28–31.
3. J. S. Bradshaw, A taxonomy of social need. In G. McLachlan (ed.), *Problems and Progress in Medical Care: Essays on Current Research, 7th series*, London, Oxford University Press, 1972.
4. A. Stevens and J. Raftery, *Health Care Needs Assessment: The Epidemiologically Based Needs Assessment Reviews*, Oxford, Radcliffe Medical Press, 1994, vols. 1 and 2.
5. J. Wright and D. Kyle, Assessing health needs. In D. Pencheon, C. Guest, D. Melzer and J. A. Muir Gray (eds.), *Oxford Handbook of Public Health Practice*, 2nd edn., Oxford, Oxford University Press, 2006, ch. 1.3, pp. 20–31.
6. Joint Strategic Needs Assessment (SNA): A spring board for action. See: http://www.idea.gov.uk/idk/aio/27014541.
7. J. Pallant, *Health needs assessment toolkit*. Mid Hampshire PCT, 2002. See: http://courses.essex.ac.uk/hs/hs915/Mid%20Hampshire%20PCT%20HNA%20Toolkit.pdf.
8. H. Annett and S. Rifkin, Guidelines for rapid participatory appraisal to assess community health needs: a focus on health improvements for low income urban and rural areas. Geneva, World Health Organization, 1995.
9. Health Care Needs Assessment, University of Birmingham. See: http://www.hcna.bham.ac.uk/index.shtml.

7

Decision making in the health-care sector – the role of public health

Jan Yates and Stephen Gillam

Key points

- In the UK, funding decisions are made at three main levels: nationally at the Department of Health and the NHS Commissioning Board; locally within commissioning organisations, and at the front line between clinicians and patients in hospitals and general practices.
- In order to make funding decisions it is necessary to determine the priority status of different options and to make decisions between them.
- Priority setting should be a transparent process based on a clear set of criteria, for example:
  - Is there a need for the service?
  - Is there an intervention or service which is proven to be effective and which will meet this need?
  - Is the intervention acceptable and appropriate for the health-care system?
  - Is the service cost-effective?
- Priority setting needs to take place within a clear ethical framework.

Introduction

Health-care systems within most countries are resource-limited – budgets are finite and not every service one would like to provide can be funded. In publicly funded health systems, those responsible for procuring health-care need to be able to explain how taxpayers' money has been spent. Decisions are made at both an individual patient and a population level. At an individual level, the decision might be: should this patient get a prescription for a statin to lower her blood cholesterol and, if so, which statin should it be? At a population level, the decision might be: will a commissioning organisation purchase a heart-failure specialist nurse or an additional sexual health clinic? In the UK,

Essential Public Health, Second Edition, ed. Stephen Gillam, Jan Yates and Padmanabhan Badrinath.
Published by Cambridge University Press. © Cambridge University Press 2012.

funding decisions are made at various levels. Individual clinicians, managers within commissioning organisations and hospitals, local politicians and civil servants in the Department of Health all make decisions which affect what public health and treatment services are available to populations. Some decisions are more appropriately made by individuals at a local level but the need for some specialised services may be very low for small populations. For example, less than 20 liver transplants are needed for every million people and decisions over funding liver-transplant services are taken at larger population levels by specially configured service commissioning groups. In the UK, a National Specialist Commissioning Advisory Group decides on very specialised services for rare conditions such as liver transplantation.

How these kinds of decisions are made is the focus of this chapter. We will look briefly at one framework for priority setting and consider what factors should be taken into account when comparing options. This will include an examination of basic health economic concepts. While this chapter primarily takes examples from health-care, the same principles can be applied to decision making in other sectors relevant to the public's health such as local government (e.g. social care, transport, leisure facilities).

A framework for setting priorities

In order to plan services which are effective and can be adequately resourced it is important to consider the need for each service within a clear public health framework. A series of questions need to be considered before a service is funded and these are shown in Figure 7.1.

Identifying the proposed service

This may sound easy but is frequently very difficult. Many services continue to be funded based on historical actions, the activity (say hip replacements) we saw last year is provided and funded again this year plus a little bit extra to account for population increasing and ageing. New interventions and service options are always potentially available but very rarely do we make decisions which lead to disinvestment in services rather than investment in new ones. Why might this be the case?

In reality, those funding and delivering health-care are making decisions within defined resource limits and choosing between different options. The same is true for making decisions about individuals so we focus in the remainder of this chapter primarily on how you might make these kinds of choices.

Assessing need

The assessment of needs is discussed in detail in Chapter 6. The use of needs assessment is crucial to determining which interventions for which health and health-care issues are likely to benefit the population most and so become priorities. Populations

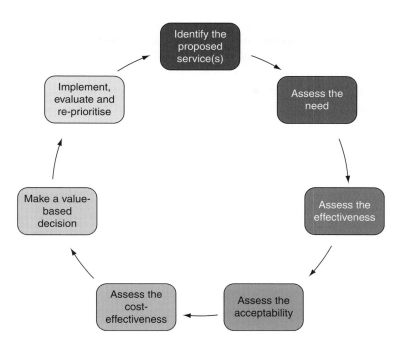

Figure 7.1   A framework for setting priorities.

vary according to age, sex, ethnicity and many other determinants of health and the need for health services will vary accordingly. Public health specialists' role here is to ensure that services are targeted to those who most need them. One major way in which this will be done in the future within the UK is via local-authority-level Joint Strategic Needs Assessments. These will compile local-level epidemiological information with knowledge of local service delivery and therefore drive health and well-being service commissioning across a locality.

At an individual level, this assessment of need takes the form of a robust examination, which determines the nature of the condition needing treatment. As mentioned in the introduction to this book, the processes of individual and community needs assessment are analogous.

Assessing evidence of effectiveness

If an intervention doesn't work it shouldn't be provided by a publicly funded health-care organisation. Repositories of evidence such as the Cochrane Library are valuable. Critical appraisal skills ensure the best possible assessment of the effectiveness of potential services or interventions (see Chapter 5).

However, evidence can be difficult to obtain. There are many interventions for which the quality and quantity of evidence are limited. Public health interventions often fall into this category as they may be multifaceted. Outcomes are only partly due to the intervention we are interested in (for example, how much of a reduction in lung cancer mortality in men can be attributed to smoking cessation services and how much is to treatment services or tobacco taxation?). Pragmatic solutions are often needed and the best available evidence is used to inform decisions.

The evidence base changes over time and interventions previously thought to be effective may prove not to be in the light of further research. It can be difficult to reduce a service already in place and decisions such as these need careful implementation. For example, the evidence to support use of grommets in children with glue ear is limited. However, parents, and sometimes clinicians, need to be reassured that a useful service is not being withheld.

Assessing acceptability

Services that are not acceptable to patients or the public will be less well used and potentially inefficient. When introducing new treatments, services or public health interventions the views of patients and the public on what services are needed should be taken into consideration.

When introducing public health interventions which rely on people to change their behaviours, the people being targeted should be involved in the planning stages.

We discussed some ways that patients, the public and local communities can be involved in health needs assessment in Chapter 6. The same methodologies can be used to involve people in setting priorities.

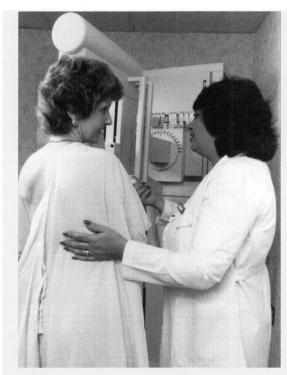

Mammography – an acceptable intervention?

Assessing cost-effectiveness

Costs must be factored into decision making. However, money is not the only cost and saving lives is not the only benefit. Costs and benefits should be measured accurately and compared between different interventions and outcomes. How do we determine whether £1m spent on coronary care to improve cardiac outcomes is more useful than £1m spent on cancer prevention?

Health economics applies traditional economic theory to consider problems in health-care. Economic evaluation helps decision making by considering the outputs of competing interventions in relation to the resources that they consume. Relevant outputs must be defined, costs measured, and studies relating outputs to their costs undertaken.

Economic evaluation

Economic evaluation can be defined as '...the comparative analysis of alternative courses of action in terms of both their costs and consequences' [1]. For a smoking cessation service we would be comparing the costs (i.e. the resources consumed) and the consequences (outputs or benefits) of having a smoking cessation service against the costs and consequences of not having one.

Costs are generally divided into direct and indirect costs. Direct costs can be easily identified as the expenditure associated with the activity (for example, the cost of 10 minutes of a general practitioner's time and the cost of a prescription). Indirect costs are more difficult to measure and might include items such as a share of the overheads (such as heating and lighting) for the building in which a doctor works. Opportunity costs should also be considered (see Box 7.1).

Box 7.1 Opportunity cost

An opportunity cost is 'the amount lost by not using the resource (labour, capital) in its best alternative use'. For example, the financial cost of admitting an elderly patient with influenza and respiratory problems to a surgical ward (due to lack of beds) is relatively low (cost of bed, nursing etc.). However, the opportunity cost of the admission may be much higher (for example, cancelled operations, increased waiting lists).

What might be some of the direct, indirect and opportunity costs of providing pneumococcal vaccine to an elderly population? How does this differ from the perspective of the health-care provider and the patient?

You may have thought of:

- Direct costs: to provider – cost of immuniser time, cost of vaccine; to patient – bus fare or fuel costs of travel for vaccination.
- Indirect costs: to provider – share of venue costs, share of administrator time to book clinic slots and respond to queries, time costs of e.g. lost work.
- Opportunity costs: for example, the nurse could have been training other nurses or doing a baby clinic instead. There may be increased waiting times for other clinics. The patient may have missed an opportunity to visit family or attend a social event.

Options are rarely straightforward and the concept of *marginal or incremental* costs is helpful. Increasingly, health-care interventions make small, additional gains to health. Decisions are generally not whether to have a service or not but whether to improve our service in certain ways.

Thus, while we could compare, for example, a smoking cessation service with none, we are more likely to compare the current service (say, one nurse-led clinic per month) with an improved service (say, two clinics per month). In this case we would compare the number of people who quit smoking from our original service with the number we predict for our improved service. We can then quote the benefits in terms of additional quitters per pound spent on the additional clinic. This is a marginal cost and tells us how much we could gain from our service improvement. The alternative is to focus on *programme budgets*: funding for different types of care such as cancer, diabetes or mental health. Expenditure can be analysed against outcome to identify priorities [2].

Table 7.1 illustrates the different types of economic evaluation.

Table 7.1 Types of economic evaluation

Type of evaluation	Costs measured in:	Benefits measured in:	Smoking cessation example:
Cost minimisation	Money	Not measured	Cost of one clinic compared to cost of two
Cost-effectiveness	Money	Natural units – units relevant to the intervention	Costs per additional quitter
Cost utility	Money	Comparable units – often QALYs	Cost per additional QALY* gained for the quitters
Cost-benefit	Money	Money	Here you would need to value the benefits in terms of how much they were worth in financial terms – difficult to do

*see Box 7.2.

Cost minimisation does not count what we gain but assumes the benefits of each option are the same. This type of analysis is often used in medicines management when alternative drugs having the same clinical indication and effects are compared according to price and the cheapest prescribed. However, it is rarely the case that all consequences are equal. Within a *cost-effectiveness analyses* we measure the two sets of costs and compare the outcomes in units of relevance for the intervention. This may be lives saved or life years gained. From Table 7.1, with smoking cessation we might count the number of additional people who quit smoking. However, this does not allow us to say whether we should invest in smoking cessation in preference to exercise classes or weight-management clinics as the outcomes are not comparable.

This is where *cost-utility analyses* are useful as they measure all outcomes in terms of an index of benefit, which is comparable across different types of service. The quality-adjusted life year is the most commonly used index of benefit. This allocates a quality of life value (between 1 (perfect health) and 0 (death)) and combines quantity and quality of life to derive the quality adjusted life year (QALY). Although the cost-utility method has the advantage that different interventions can be compared across a broad range of choices in resource allocation, a number of methodological problems remain (see Boxes 7.2a and 7.2b).

A new drug enables patients to live for 5 years rather than dying within 2 years. However, they live with a minor disability and a quality of life equal to 80% of a full healthy life year. But, if they do not receive the drug, their quality of life for the 2 years they live is only 60% of a full healthy life year. How many QALYs are generated by the intervention?

5 years of life at 80% quality:

$$\text{QALYs} = 5 \times 0.8$$
$$= 4$$

or

2 years of life at 60% quality:

$$\text{QALYs} = 2 \times 0.6$$
$$= 1.2$$

So QALYs generated

$$= 4 - 1.2$$
$$= 2.8$$

From question 3 below we can see that whilst programme b is the more cost-effective it does cost a lot more! Consider how you might persuade a health-care organisation that programme b is a preferable investment. While useful, this model does not reflect the complexities of measuring the impact of interventions on multiple outcomes.

Box 7.2a How a QALY is constructed

A quality-adjusted life year (QALY) combines the quantity and quality of life. It is the arithmetic product of life expectancy and a measure of the quality of the remaining life years.

It takes 1 year of perfect-health life expectancy to be worth 1 and regards 1 year of less-than-perfect life expectancy as < 1.

Patients, the public and professionals are asked to judge the quality value (utility) for one year of life lived with the relevant condition and these values are then used multiplicatively with the number of years lived in this state to give the QALY.

E.g. an intervention which results in a patient living for an additional 4 years rather than dying within 1 year, and where quality of life for both treated and untreated patients is 0.6 will generate:

4 years extra life @ 0.6 QoL values = 2.4

less 1 year @ reduced quality = 0.6

generates 2.4–0.6 = 1.8 QALYs

QALYs can therefore provide an indication of the benefits gained from a variety of medical procedures in terms of quality of life and additional years for the patient.

Box 7.2b Disadvantages of QALYs

- It is argued that seeking to compare the incomparable (different treatments, different states) with crude tools is methodologically flawed and that their use oversimplifies complex health-care issues by reducing what should be a multifaceted assessment of options to simple quantitative values.
- QALYs are not based on an individual's assessment of value and the values determined by others may not reflect those of every patient.
- QALYs are controversial. They can be seen as 'ageist': reduced life expectancy results in lower QALY values so that interventions for elderly patients may compare poorly with those for young patients. Conversely, QALYs can be seen as 'insufficiently ageist' if one considers that the elderly have already had a 'fair innings' and the young are more deserving of treatment.
- QALYs may disadvantage those already disabled as their quality of life is already lower; interventions for the disabled may yield fewer QALYs than those for healthier people.
- QALYs may lack sensitivity within a disease area as not every subdivision within or level of complex conditions will have been valued and one value may be applied to subdivisions with varying health states (for example, the quality of life with a condition like depression might vary considerably depending upon the severity of the depression).

Consider the following two health improvement programmes. Which is the most cost-effective?

(a) Provision of home safety equipment for the elderly. This increases quality of life by 0.1 and the benefit lasts for 10 years. The extra cost is £1500 per life year.

(b) Intensive post-natal care for low-birth-weight babies. This improves quality of life by 0.8 and the benefits last for 35 years. The care costs £125,000.

(a) QALYs gained $= 10 \times 0.1$

$\qquad = 1$

Cost $= 10 \times £1500$

$\qquad = £15,000$

Cost per QALY gained

$\qquad = £15,000/1$

$\qquad = £15,000$ per QALY

(b) QALYs gained $= 35 \times 0.8$

$\qquad = 28$

Cost $= £125,000$

Cost per QALY gained

$\qquad = £125,000/28$

$\qquad = £4464$ per QALY

Programme b is more cost-effective.

The most useful health economic analyses for public health tend to be *cost-utility* studies. Ideally, analyses should be carried out alongside the original effectiveness studies but this adds to the cost of the study and is not always possible. It is important to understand from whose perspective the evaluation is being carried out as the costs and benefits will vary if considered from a health-care-provider perspective, that of a patient or that of society. For example, in a recent study of nine alternative treatments for alcohol dependence, only three were found to be cost-effective when considered from the perspective of the patient who has to give time and money to attend the treatment [3]. See the Internet Companion for further information.

Making value-based decisions

There will always be competing needs to consider. Once we have assured ourselves that the proposed services are needed, effective, acceptable and cost-effective, we must still decide whether to fund them. This isn't as simple as asking 'Is there enough money to pay for this?' Frequently, funding one initiative means something else cannot be funded – there is an opportunity cost. Increasingly, there may be an additional requirement to ensure the overall expenditure on an intervention is cost-neutral or even cost-saving, i.e. that over time the ill health prevented saves the health system money. For example, identifying alcohol overuse in primary care and providing a brief intervention is estimated to be able to save the NHS in England £18m per year in treatment costs (as well as saving 240 lives).

These kinds of judgements are ultimately also value-based. We weigh up options using ethical frameworks, implicitly or explicitly, to judge worth. Different ethical approaches upon which people base decisions, both in health-care and in daily life, are summarised in Table 7.2.

Table 7.2 Ethical approaches

Decisions are based on:	Explanation
The view that there is a right and a wrong	This approach is often seen in the popular press and media. Media headlines highlighting emotive issues around cancer treatments can make a dramatic impact on the public consciousness and influence the way in which decisions are made.
What powerful professionals think	There is a strong tradition, rapidly shifting now, of paternalism within health services. In a paternalistic system, decisions over treatment were pre-eminently the right of (mostly male) clinicians. There remain strong political preferences for or against imposing interventions on the population.
The greater good	Public health decisions may use a utilitarian framework, which aims to maximise the good consequences for a population. This does not mean that everyone gets the same service but that each receives health-care based on his or her need. This is equity rather than equality and attempts to bring the greatest good to the greatest number.
What we have always done	Health-care decisions about what services to fund are often made on the basis of what was bought last year. In these circumstances, services change very little and costs generally go up in line with inflation.
Standards	We also tend to believe that everyone has the right to a minimum standard of service and many decisions are made based on guidance or targets set by experts (such as NICE). In England, interventions recommended in NICE technology appraisals must be funded by the health-care system.
Need in an emergency	Another way of making decisions is by applying the 'rule of rescue' [4]. Why do we mount a rescue for the survivors of a disaster when their chances of survival are slim? Why do we spend resources on critical care for patients where the effectiveness is limited? If we feel shocked by the circumstances of an individual and offer intervention based on this psychological imperative without thought for the opportunity costs, we are operating under the rule of rescue. For whole populations this kind of decision making may take place in large-scale emergencies such as an influenza pandemic (see Chapter 10) when funds are diverted to controlling an immediate threat.

Box 7.3 Beauchamp and Childress principles (and rules) of biomedical ethics

Beauchamp and Childress posit four major principles of biomedical ethics and four minor rules:

Principles:

- **Respect for autonomy**. This important principle is implicit in the requirement for consent for procedures. It can be difficult to apply this principle to those who are unable to make informed decisions such as minors or those with learning difficulties.
- **Non-maleficence**. Avoid harm. The need to avoid harm must frequently be weighed against the next principle when considering treatments with potential benefits and with some side effects.
- **Beneficence**. Do good. Too much beneficence can be paternalistic! For example, our need to prevent the harm caused by obesity might lead us to coerce overweight people into lifestyle changes.
- **Justice**. This principle reiterates the public health concept of equity in that a regard for fairness is important.

Rules:

- **Veracity**. The truth. It is difficult to make decisions based on falsehood but the ability to be able to identify one common truth is debatable.
- **Privacy**. The right of patients to withhold information is seen to be important but may hinder the diagnostic process.
- **Confidentiality**. This is of increasing importance in modern health-care and the need to handle patient-identifiable data sensibly is plain throughout many health-care systems.
- **Fidelity**. Trust. The relationship between clinician and patient requires trust; public health decisions which restrict treatments may jeopardise that trust.

An ethical framework commonly used to guide clinical judgements is that of Beauchamp and Childress [5] (see Box 7.3). This can be adapted to form the basis of prioritisation decisions made in health-care settings. The principles may conflict with each other. For example, the decision to offer an expensive treatment to one patient from a limited budget permits them autonomy and enables the health carer to do good for that individual. However, the treatment may have side effects, which must be weighed against the benefits, and there may be insufficient funds left to treat others – thus unjustly restricting their right to treatment. Decisions around individual patient needs may conflict with the needs of populations and public health professionals are often involved in mediating over complex decisions.

Use the Beauchamp and Childress principles to decide whether you think funding stop-smoking services with specialist advisors to help individuals and groups quit through the use of motivational therapies and drugs would be ethically justified.

You may have considered some of the following points:

Autonomy:

- Smoker's right to choose when to stop or not to stop.
- Addictive nature of nicotine reduces smoker's autonomy.
- Advertising and peer pressure may reduce autonomy.

Non-maleficence:

- Need to ensure non-smokers are not exposed to harmful tobacco smoke.
- Cessation may increase harm transiently (e.g. operative risk increases 4 weeks post-cessation).
- Adverse effects of cessation therapies.

Beneficence:

- Harms of smoking well documented so cessation is doing good.
- Smokers' friends and families are benefited by cessation.

Justice:

- Should we spend on this if we consider it self-inflicted?
- Should we fund one or several courses of treatment?

There are also legal imperatives on those making decisions. In the UK, NHS organisations are required to abide by a variety of laws as they make decisions which impact on patients, including those around equality and meeting the needs of patients as well as remaining in financial balance. These duties, as within the Beauchamp and Childress principles, can conflict with each other and a robust process not only serves the needs of patients and the public but also enables organisations to assure their stakeholders that their decisions are fair and defend them, in a court of law, if necessary. Priority-setting committees are frequently used, which have explicit frameworks to advise organisations on the use of funds.

Conclusion

The aim overall is to provide a more robust decision than would be achieved through a less systematic approach, to ensure that resources are used cost-effectively and to enable improvement in the health of individuals and populations. Having made such decisions, the last stage of the framework proposes implementing the decision followed by evaluation and re-starting the cycle. More on the quality of health-care and evaluation can be found in Chapter 11.

REFERENCES

1. M. F. Drummond, *Methods for the Economic Evaluation of Health Care Programmes*. Oxford, Oxford University Press, 1997.
2. Department of Health. *Program budgeting tools and data*. See: http://www.dh.gov.uk/en/Managingyourorganisation/Financeandplanning/Programmebudgeting/DH_075743.
3. L. J. Dunlap, G. A. Zarkin, J. W. Bray, *et al.*, Revisiting the cost-effectiveness of the COMBINE study for alcohol dependent patients: the patient perspective. *Medical Care*, **48**(4), 2010, 306–13.
4. A. R. Johnsen, Bentham in a box: technology assessment and health care allocation. *Law, Medicine and Health Care* **14**(3–4), 1986, 172–4.
5. T. L. Beauchamp and J. F. Childress, *Principles of Biomedical Ethics*, 3rd edn., New York, NY, Oxford University Press, 1989.

Improving population health

Stephen Gillam and Jan Yates

Key points

- Health promotion focuses on the social, economic and environmental determinants of health and aims to help people increase control over their own health.
- Many different groups and organisations are involved in health promotion within and without the NHS for it encompasses health policy, education, legislative action and community development.
- Disease prevention at the level of the high-risk individual is increasingly effective but population-wide approaches have greater potential to improve population health.
- Psychological models of behaviour change can support both individuals and organisations to improve health.

Disease prevention

Cervical cancer is 20 times more common in Columbia than in Israel. Twenty percent of Afghan children die before the age of 5, compared with 0.5% of children in the UK. Ischaemic heart disease death rates vary by a factor of two in different wards in Luton. In other words, diseases that are common in one place will usually prove to be rare somewhere else. Such variations suggest that common diseases – with their roots in lifestyle, social factors and the environment – are preventable but there are several misconceptions about prevention.

Prevention and cure are not alternative ways of dealing with illness. Much that we consider 'cure' in the classical medical sense is, in reality, prevention. (Consider, for example, the treatment of high blood pressure or hypothyroidism). Although some

Essential Public Health, Second Edition, ed. Stephen Gillam, Jan Yates and Padmanabhan Badrinath.
Published by Cambridge University Press. © Cambridge University Press 2012.

treatments do effect a permanent 'cure', most merely prevent or retard the development of pain, handicap or more serious consequences.

It is often held that 'prevention is cheaper than cure'. Successful reduction of incidence
rates of common diseases ought, in theory, to reduce health-care costs. In practice, this
hope has been frustrated and the costs of health services have generally risen in inverse
proportion to disease rates (consider how cardiology services have expanded as death
rates from heart disease have declined). Preventive medicine such as screening can be
very expensive. For example, the annual cost of the NHS cervical screening programme is
approximately £160 million – but it saves around 4500 lives each year [1].

Preventive medicine is but one small part of the wider field of health promotion. In
Chapter 8 we listed three main approaches to improving the population's health. How
health-care can be made more effective is examined in Chapter 11 but most of the
activities that promote health occur beyond the world of clinical medicine. How we
change unhealthy behaviours and alter social determinants of health is the subject of
this chapter.

Natural history of disease

We need to begin by looking at the progression of disease in the community (represented simply in Figure 8.1).

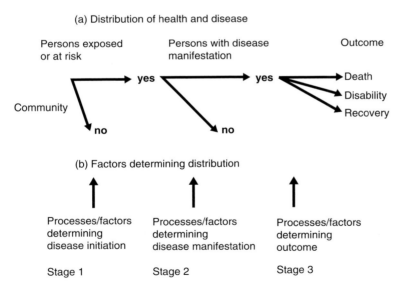

Figure 8.1   Natural history of
disease in the community.

The first stage in the development of a disease is exposure to risk. A risk factor is an
aspect of personal behaviour or lifestyle, an environmental exposure or an inherited
characteristic, which is known to be associated with a particular health-related outcome (see Chapter 3).

What behavioural and other risk factors do you associate with the onset of cardiovascular disease?

Your list might include: tobacco smoking, high fat diet and abnormal lipid profiles, raised blood pressure, diabetes mellitus and raised blood glucose, lack of exercise, haemostatic factors – e.g. raised fibrinogen, inflammatory markers such as C reactive protein, homocysteine, stress (though the evidence is highly contested).

The next step is to consider factors and processes that determine whether or not a disease is manifest. Pathological processes may ensure a disease progresses to be symptomatic but many other factors will determine whether or not a person with symptomatic disease seeks or gains access to health services. These include increasing awareness of the meaning of symptoms (influenced by education and cultural factors) or whether or not appropriate care is available. A further set of factors determine the outcome of any episode of care. Outcomes can broadly be classified into three: death, disability and recovery.

What processes or factors might determine the outcomes for someone diagnosed with diabetes mellitus?

Age, severity of disease, level of education or health awareness which might influence adherence to dietary and treatment regimes, socio-economic status which may have a bearing on dietary and other relevant lifestyle choices (e.g. exercising to reduce obesity), ethnicity if written material to assist self-care is inappropriate, quality of care in general practice, access to specialist hospital care or services in the community (e.g. retinal screening), availability of funding to provide optimal drug therapy, level of support from carers or others.

At any one time, all three stages of a disease exist in the community. The processes and factors working at each stage may overlap. Medical care, however, has tended to concentrate on treating outcomes but these are the end-stage of a complex process. To reduce the burden of disease at stage 3, we need to tackle stages 1 and 2 as well. The community's health needs are the totality of what is required to interrupt the natural history at all three stages.

Levels of prevention

Preventive activities are commonly categorised at one of three levels:

- Primary prevention – these are actions designed to prevent the occurrence of the problem, e.g.:

    health education;
    genetic counselling;
    immunisation;
    protection from carcinogens.

- Secondary prevention – these are actions designed to detect and treat the occurrence of a problem before symptoms have developed, e.g.:
    screening;
    early diagnosis.
- Tertiary prevention – these are actions designed to limit disability once a condition is manifest, e.g.:
    limitation of disability;
    rehabilitation;
    prevention of relapse.

Illustrate the different levels of prevention by considering ischaemic heart disease.

Primary prevention	Encourage healthy lifestyles: not smoking, healthy diet, exercise.
Secondary prevention	Detection of risk factors, e.g. high blood pressure, raised cholesterol levels, hyperglycaemia etc. and action to reduce these.
Tertiary prevention	Cardiac rehabilitation and patient education after ischaemic events such as myocardial infarction to reduce risk factors.

The stages of the natural history can be seen to correspond to the three levels of prevention. Simplistically, the aim of public health practice can be described as shifting the problem to the left in terms of its natural history and shifting the problem upwards in terms of the level of prevention.

Approaches to prevention

Strategies for prevention

The epidemiologist Geoffrey Rose described two broad approaches to prevention (Figure 8.2):
- The high-risk strategy aims to protect those individuals at the high end of the risk distribution. They are usually a small proportion of that distribution.
- The population strategy aims to reduce the underlying causes. It is concerned with factors that affect the whole population [2].

The high-risk strategy avoids interference with those who are not at special risk. Interventions are appropriate to the individuals targeted and this strategy is regularly accommodated within the ethos and organisation of medical care. Appropriate targeting improves its cost-effectiveness. Genomic science may further segment populations in terms of their responsiveness to preventive interventions [3].

Figure 8.2   High-risk individual
and population-based strategies
for prevention.

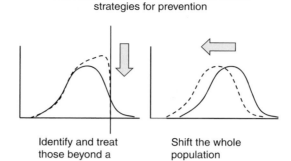

High-risk individual and population-based
strategies for prevention

Identify and treat
those beyond a
threshold for risk
factor

Shift the whole
population
distribution of risk
factor

Figure 8.2   High-risk individual and population-based strategies for prevention.

However, the high-risk strategy has a limited impact on the behaviour of populations and has hitherto been limited by our ability to predict individuals' futures. Population strategies, on the other hand, by tackling behaviours and other risk factors en masse, offer large benefits for populations. Taking strokes as an example, a 5-mm lowering of blood pressure across the population might achieve a 33% reduction in strokes (approximately 75,000 in the UK each year). This compares with a 15% reduction in the number of strokes if all cases of hypertension (defined as those people with blood pressure higher than a set threshold) were detected and treated [4].

However, with a population strategy, the benefits to the individuals may be small and both subjects and health professionals may be poorly motivated to implement mass strategies. This is the so-called *prevention paradox:* where preventive measures bringing large benefits to the community offer little to each participating individual. However, recent evidence affirms that countries able to implement strategies targeted at individuals on the basis of baseline risks will also see major health gains [5]. In other words, Rose's famous dichotomy is less clear cut. Thus, preventive medicine must embrace both approaches but – at least in low- to middle-income countries yet to introduce simple policy changes aimed at smoking and dietary change – the power resides with population strategies.

It is important in passing to distinguish two kinds of mass preventive measures. The first consists of removing or reducing an unnatural exposure, e.g. stopping smoking, reducing dietary intake of saturated fat and salts. The second type of mass preventive measure consists of adding some unnatural factor in the hope of conferring protection (e.g. folic acid to prevent neural-tube defects, fluoridation of water supplies to prevent dental caries, even statins to reduce blood lipid levels and prevent excess risk of heart disease). For such measures there can be no prior presumption of safety and the required evidence of benefit must be stringent.

The public health approach to disease screening presents a further ethical dilemma with its focus on maximising participation in screening rather than on informed participation. For example, current recommendations for the primary prevention of coronary heart disease in groups at high risk depend on screening through primary care and provision of risk-related advice or treatment. However, we lack evidence for the cost-effectiveness of multiple risk factor interventions delivered through primary care [6]. Presenting the uncertainties associated with the assessment and reduction of cardiovascular risk to individuals may actually be more cost-effective than screening conducted in a traditional, public health paradigm if it results in participants who are more motivated to reduce their risks [7].

Prevention in clinical practice

A sharp distinction between health and disease is a medical artefact for which nature provides no support. Not so long ago, this proposal was regarded as revolutionary. A spectrum of disease is now seen to be the norm rather than the exception; even infectious diseases come in all sizes from obvious clinical cases to symptomless infections.

Physiological variables such as blood pressure, serum cholesterol, body mass index, and bone mineral density are important in the aetiology of common diseases. They are not direct causes of disease, like smoking, but are intermediates between those external factors and disease itself. Risk can be reduced by lowering high levels of these variables by drug treatment or lifestyle change. However, terminology that regards extreme values as indicating a disease state (such as hypertension, hypercholester-olaemia, osteoporosis and obesity) and average values as being 'normal' (normoten-sive, normocholesterolaemia) is misleading. Clinical guidelines specify risk-factor thresholds; these have been set at successively lower levels over time and redefined as 'action levels' but they still deny treatment below specified values.

The notion that we intervene only when an individual risk factor reaches a threshold is misguided. Meta-analyses of cohort studies have been used to plot the relationships between risk factors and diseases [8]. Far from demonstrating risk-factor thresholds, these plots yield reasonably straight lines, and this is so whether the level of the risk factor on the horizontal axis is plotted using an arithmetical or proportional scale (Figure 8.3). In other words, there is a constant proportional change in risk for a given change in the risk factor from any starting level. These continuous dose–response relationships have a crucially important implication: anyone at high risk should be 'treated'.

For example, blood-pressure-lowering drugs should not be limited to people with high blood pressure, nor cholesterol-lowering drugs to people with high serum cholesterol concentrations. The constant proportional relations indicate that the absolute reduction in risk from changing the risk factor will be large in people who are at high risk for any reason (existing disease, smoking status or older age, for example), regardless of the starting value of the risk factor.

The major determinant of risk is existing disease. Without preventive treatment, mortality from heart disease in people who have had a myocardial infarction in the

Figure 8.3 Incidence of ischaemic heart disease (with 95% confidence intervals) according to diastolic blood pressure, serum cholesterol and body mass index – data from cohort studies.

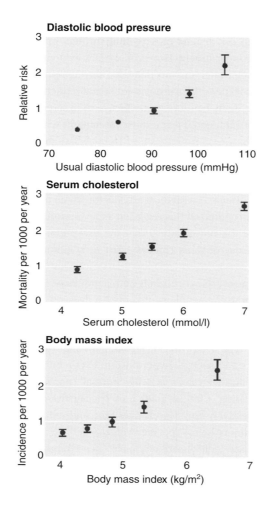

past is about 5% per year for the rest of their life. Mortality from stroke in people who have had a stroke is similar. Both rates are much higher than in people with no history of cardiovascular disease; coronary mortality is 0.3% per year in men aged 60, for example, or about 0.5% per year in men with high cholesterol or blood pressure [8]. Anyone with existing disease (a previous myocardial infarction or stroke, for example) should be treated irrespective of the level of the risk factors being modified.

Another problem with the notion of intervening only above a threshold level is illustrated in the case of cardiovascular disease and age. In people without known cardiovascular disease, age is the most important determinant of risk. Mortality from ischaemic heart disease and from stroke doubles with about every 8 years of increasing age [9]. In England and Wales, 95% of deaths from heart disease occur in the quartile of the population at oldest age (men over 55 and women over 60). Offering preventive treatment only to people with relatively high values of a variable means that only a small proportion of those destined to have disease events will be targeted. People of a given age with relatively high values of the physiological variables are at similar risk as people a few years older with average levels; it is illogical to offer preventive treatment to the former but not the latter. In people without cardiovascular disease, intervention to change risk factors should be introduced when a person's risk of a disease event over the next few years exceeds a specified value (e.g. using the Framingham or Q-risk scoring systems). Because there is substantial benefit from lowering these physiological variables from any starting value in persons at high risk, all the reversible risk factors should be changed, not just those judged 'abnormal'. Reducing only variables with high values loses most of the potential benefit.

Behaviour change

Behaviour change in theory

Some public health programmes can impose benefits on people without them having to change their own behaviour (e.g. the provision of clean water). However, many preventive projects require some behaviour change on the part of the public/patient. Unless frontline health professionals have the skills to assist in that behaviour change, the goals of the programme may be thwarted. This subsection looks at ways of changing behaviour.

Much of human disease is due in whole or in part to the attitudes and behaviour of individuals. Cholera, typhoid, poliomyelitis and infectious hepatitis are all transmitted faeco-orally, so their spread depends upon personal habits, as well as policies for public sanitation, and the way food is prepared. The most important single cause of lung cancer is the habit of smoking cigarettes; the causes of coronary heart disease include a diet high in fat and salt and low in fruit and vegetables, physical inactivity and the use of tobacco. Cleanliness, smoking, diet and physical activity are all personal matters. However, the behaviour underlying each is, to a large extent, determined by the values of society and resultant attitudes. By changing knowledge and attitudes, one hopes to change behaviour, prevent many of these diseases and thus promote health. In reality, the link between these three is less straightforward [10].

Knowledge does not always lead to 'correct' behaviour. For example, many drivers who do not wear seat belts know what happens to an unrestrained driver in an accident. Knowledge and behaviour can be out of step for many reasons:

- There is a perception of no personal threat from the behaviour.
- There are rewards from the present behaviour.
- The benefits of change are too long-term.
- There is social pressure.
- There is a belief that change will have no effect or that there is no value or benefit in the outcome of the change.
- There is a belief that "I cannot change".

Simply telling people what is good for them is not an effective health change strategy. Four pre-conditions are necessary for behaviour change to take place. You must:

- want to change;
- believe you can change;
- believe change will have the desired effect;
- know how to change.

Self-efficacy is the belief in your own ability to effect change. Patients with low self-efficacy will find it hard to make changes because they lack confidence in their capacity to determine what happens to them. Self-efficacy is closely related to self-confidence and self-esteem. Where patients have low self-efficacy, it may be raised in various ways, for example, by helping the patient to remember or recognise someone else who made the change ("If they did it, then so can I."). Action-efficacy is the belief that the change will remove the threat caused by the original behaviour. Achieving early successes breeds confidence, thus reinforcing both self- and action-efficacy. It is particularly important that a person with low self-efficacy does not have further experiences that will reinforce his/her poor self-image. Setting realistic, measurable goals is more likely to ensure successful practice. Physical feedback that tells you that you are doing something right increases self-efficacy (e.g. the 'feel good' factor in exercise, which fuels the desire for more exercise).

The theory of reasoned action suggests that a person's behavioural intention depends on the person's attitude about the behaviour and subjective norms (BI = A + SN). If a person intends to adopt a behaviour then it is likely that the person will do it. Behavioural intention measures a person's relative strength of intention to perform a behaviour. Attitude consists of beliefs about the consequences of performing the behaviour multiplied by his or her valuation of these consequences. Subjective norms are seen as a combination of perceived expectations from relevant individuals or groups along with intentions to comply with these expectations. In other words, a person's voluntary behaviour is predicted by his/her attitude toward that behaviour and how he/she thinks other people would view them if they performed the behaviour [11].

Another well-known model identifies stages in behaviour change (Figure 8.4) [12]. Developed in the field of addictions, these stages can be illustrated by the example of someone giving up smoking

- **Pre-contemplation**. At this stage, the smoker does not perceive that he/she has a problem. Others, though, might be pointing out a problem.
- **Contemplation**. The smoker begins to recognise that he/she has a behaviour which is a problem for them. He/she thinks about the problem – is it bad enough to need action? What action might I take? Who could help? At this stage, the smoker might discuss his/her problems with others, including those who have previously been smokers.
- **Action**. This is when the attempt to change behaviour takes place. It can include seeking advice; joining a support group; using a nicotine patch; keeping charts of progress.

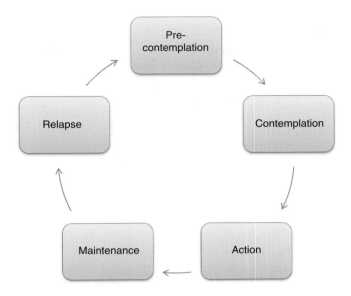

Figure 8.4   Stages in behaviour change.

- **Maintenance**. Once the smoker has reached the desired level of performance (say, abstinence), he/she has to keep to that level. This may involve special strategies for recognising a high-risk situation (e.g. "When I go to the pub with the bowls team, there's always a lot of smoking") and designing strategies for dealing with them (e.g. "When the game is finished, I will remind the team that they must not let me have a cigarette even if I ask for one in the pub").
- **Relapse**. Despite a person's best efforts, relapses occur and s/he needs to be warned that this can happen. The commonest triggers of relapse are events that trigger a low emotional state, e.g. accidents, job loss, relationship difficulties or social pressure, especially when the pressure catches the person unawares. The role of the health professional is to accept the relapse as normal and not as an indication of weakness on the patient's part; to talk the relapse through and see what the patient can learn from it; and help the patient re-establish short-term targets.

Behaviour change in practice

Individual behaviour is generally easier to change than the social and environmental circumstances that influence health outcomes. Evidence for the effectiveness of brief interventions delivered to individuals, generally in primary care, is strongest for smoking cessation and reducing harmful alcohol consumption [13]. Their cost-effectiveness is greatest for brief interventions among high-risk drinkers. Smoking cessation can generate QALY gains at a relatively low cost (see Table 8.1). The average costs of an intervention depend on who is delivering it and how. The salary costs of doctors are roughly double those of nurses. Training for nurses and other health

Table 8.1 Summary table of the cost-effectiveness for brief interventions [13]

Intervention	Cost-effectiveness rating			
	Effectiveness rating	Public sector costs saved	Quality of life gained	Incremental cost per QALY
Preventing harmful alcohol use				
Brief interventions in primary care for high-risk drinkers	***	***	*	Dominant – £13,600
Brief intervention in emergency departments	*	*	*	£6,600–23,100
Smoking cessation				
Brief interventions in primary care	***	*	**	£600–1,400
Reducing STIs and teenage conceptions				
One-on-one interventions in primary care	**	*	*	£3,200–9,600
Promoting physical activity and healthy weight				
Counselling by primary care staff	**	*	*	£2,300

professionals to deliver brief interventions could, therefore, yield major cost savings assuming they are as effective.

It is important to stress that mass media campaigns can change health behaviour and should be key components of government policy [14]. However, recent governments have retreated from a paternalistic position to a greater emphasis on individual choice. In the face of failures to control modern epidemics such as obesity using traditional forms of public education, new approaches are needed. Social marketing is an approach to promoting health, which draws heavily on the experience of the commercial sector. It focuses on individuals as consumers for whom health is something they wish to invest in. A definition of health-related social marketing is:

A systematic process using marketing techniques and approaches to achieve behavioural goals, relevant to improving health and well-being [15].

The features of social marketing when compared to past approaches based on public campaigns are set out in Figure 8.5.

Social marketing has three characteristics: it aims to achieve a particular 'social good' (rather than commercial benefit) with specific behavioural goals clearly identified and targeted; it is a systematic process phased to address short-, medium- and long-term issues; it utilises a range of marketing techniques and approaches (a 'marketing mix').

Here the 'social good' can be articulated in terms of achieving specific, achievable and measurable behavioural goals, relevant to improving health and well-being. A useful guide to social marketing is available on the National Social Marketing Centre website (www.nsms.org.uk).

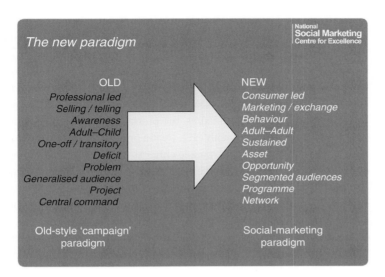

Figure 8.5 Social marketing compared to traditional campaigns.

Recent public health policy documents have made reference to the so-called 'nudge' approach to behaviour change. The theory of nudging assumes that most people make most decisions unconsciously and non-rationally and are influenced by contextual cues [16]. Their actions can thus be manipulated by changing the way choices are presented to them, for example making salad rather than chips a default side order in restaurants. Nudging is described as libertarian paternalism because no compulsion is involved. Nudging is often contrasted with 'nannying' and as working in voluntary partnership with, rather than regulating, business. However, the evidence for the effectiveness of nudging is weak [17]. Critics believe the government has misrepresented nudging as being in opposition to the use of regulation and legislation to promote health [18]. This obscures a failure to address upstream socio-economic determinants of disease. In reality, these approaches are not mutually exclusive. The challenges of tobacco and alcohol require more than just encouragement to change individual behaviours. Michael Marmot's review laid out much evidence for legislation, regulation, taxation and pricing policies in these areas (see Chapter 15).

Health promotion

Health has a wide variety of meanings ranging from an ideal state to the absence of medically defined disease. The former was encapsulated in the (in)famous World Health Organization definition of health as 'a state of complete physical, mental and social well-being and not merely the absence of disease or infirmity.' Unfortunately, health of this sort is more aspirational than obtainable. In the 1980s, the WHO promoted a more realistic definition of health in terms of the ability to function 'normally' in one's own society. Of more practical use is a definition of health that states the means by which its foundations can be achieved. These foundations include basic requirements such as adequate food, safe water, shelter, safety and security as well as education and information. The chosen definition of health itself has important implications for policy as it determines whether the emphasis is on multi-sectoral approaches or on technological solutions to tackling particular diseases.

Health promotion is identified as 'the process of enabling people to exert control over and to improve their health' [19]. Health promotion is not something that is done *on* or *to* people, it is done with people either as individuals or as groups. The purpose of this activity is to strengthen the skills and capabilities of individuals to take action, and the capacity of groups or communities to act collectively *to exert control* over determinants of their health. There are four main routes for health promotion (which are illustrated in the example in Box 8.1):

1. **Health education.** These are activities which are intended to lead to health-related learning. Typically, health education consists of interventions directed at

---

Box 8.1 Tobacco control as a health-promotion programme

- **Health education**. This is central and takes the form of major education campaigns such as television adverts and posters as well as interventions used to support those wanting to quit. Smoking cessation interventions have been funded and made widely available across the UK and several high-profile media campaigns have worked to increase the awareness of the public. Quit rates increase during times of these campaigns [20].

- **Legislation**. The increase in tax on tobacco products, age restrictions, smoking bans in public places and advertising restrictions have worked in several developed countries to bring the smoking rates down. Restrictions on smoking in public places have the knock-on effect of reducing smoking in homes [21]. Unfortunately, the tobacco companies have increased marketing in less-developed countries where the resources available for effective control are limited.

- **Community development**. This includes, for example, educational initiatives within schools, local policy development, working to understand and bridge cultural barriers to cessation, and work with teenage mothers on smoking in pregnancy.

- **Healthy public policy**. This is distinct from legislative action as it is often non-mandatory policy. The banning of smoking and provision of cessation advice in workplaces are policy initiatives, which provide supportive environments for those wanting to quit and triggers to those who may be at the pre-contemplation or contemplation stage.

individuals and led by professionals (for example, a community nurse or midwife encouraging a pregnant woman to stop smoking). Client-led interventions encourage individuals to make their own choices (for example, helping young people identify their own concerns and working with them to develop their own confidence and skills). Using a personal counselling approach to support behaviour change is preferable to crude 'health persuasion' ("You know, you really should eat less chips, Mrs Jones") which can appear authoritarian and may reinforce power differentials between 'professional' and 'patient'.

2. **Legislative action.** Interventions are led by professionals or experts but are intended to protect the health of the community (for example, lobbying for legislation for compulsory fluoridation by water companies). This approach also includes multi-agency working and can include health protection issues such as the compulsory notification of diseases (see Chapter 10).

3. **Community development.** Interventions take place within a defined community to identify local health issues and work with local people to take action on their concerns (for example, residents on a housing estate setting up a food co-operative). A community-empowerment model is often used, which aims to support members of communities to develop personally, form mutual support groups to tackle health-related issues identified by communities themselves and engage in collective political and social action to bring about change.

4. **Healthy public policy.** Tones and Tilford have defined health promotion as [22]: 'Health education × healthy public policy'. Healthy public policy focuses on the underlying determinants of good health and well-being. These can be summarised by the prerequisites of health as defined in the 1986 Ottawa Charter [23] – food, shelter, stable ecosystems, sustainable resources, peace, education, equity, income, and social justice. In many cases individuals can have little impact on their 'share' of these pre-requisites. In a time of war, your ability to access peace, shelter, food, indeed any of the prerequisites, is likely to be limited and beyond your control. If your income is low and you have no transport you may be unable to access cheaper, healthier food choices. Thus, healthy public policy covers the ways in which states can impact on the social, political, cultural and economic contexts in which we live and from there our ability to access resources that promote health. Policies which ensure fair taxation, reduce national debts, impose restrictions on sales and marketing, such as tobacco licensing and advertising legislation, would all come under the heading of healthy public policy.

The WHO's Bangkok Charter of 2005 [24] recognised the need to work in partnership with the corporate sector – hitherto demonised multinationals – to create healthier environments in which individuals can make choices. The values underpinning the charter are those of social justice, equity, human dignity, peace and security. The need to find constructive ways of working with the private sector is reflected in the WHO's *Framework Convention for Tobacco Control* [25], which includes an article helping tobacco growers to find economically viable alternative activities. However, critics of

LIVERPOOL JOHN MOORES UNIVERSITY
LEARNING SERVICES

recent UK public health policy point out that concordats with producers of tobacco, alcohol and fast food have frequently been flouted to the industries' advantage.

Who is responsible for health promotion?

The wide variety of influences on health means that health promotion is not the sole province of one professional group or organisation. The challenge for those working in the field and particularly for health-promotion specialists has always been to develop the skills and capacity of others so that they can then promote health as an integral part of their work.

An enduring role of public health is to champion the cause of disadvantaged groups in society. The underlying principle of advocacy – literally, to speak out – is to raise awareness of critical public health issues and mobilise communities and resources to promote better health. The process of advocacy uses data strategically, identifies and works with allies, deals with the opposition, works closely with the relevant community and uses the media strategically. Successful desired outcomes of advocacy are patient empowerment, less health-damaging behaviour, changes in policy, better services, better health and a better society. In addition to the tools of health education, epidemiological analysis and promoting community participation, social marketing is becoming an increasingly popular technique.

Advocacy action can take place at an individual level (for example, writing a letter to support a patient get better housing) or at an organisational level (for example, through discussions between practice collaborative and the local council to improve the play space for children on the local estate). Examples of advocacy actions at different levels are shown in Table 8.2. A dictionary of health promotion terms is included in the Internet Companion.

Conclusion

New knowledge has been used to protect and enhance health in a variety of ways and, in general, knowing what to do has been powerfully permissive of it being done [26]. The history of tobacco control through myriad means well illustrates this [27]. The diverse ways in which knowledge has been used extend well beyond processes we might describe as 'interventions'. The incremental gains from formal programmes may help but interventions that tell people what to do have often been ineffective. Decentralised approaches have also played important roles. For example, highly informal, horizontal channels transmitted knowledge about high-risk sexual practices and HIV among gay men in the 1980s. The example of HIV shows how, in highly literate and health-conscious populations, new knowledge may be disseminated through channels other than formal public health programmes. An informed public made their own good use of new knowledge, without the necessity of professional or administrative mediation.

Table 8.2 Advocacy action at various levels

Institutional	Government, UN agencies	National departments for health take various forms and provide the strategic framework for the health-care but other government departments are also crucial in creating change at a national level.
Organisational	National: NGOs e.g. Action on Smoking and Health, special interest groups; Local: practice, health-care commissioner	Local health-care organisations are often expected to take the lead on local action to promote health through partnerships in which local government has a crucial role to play. Within local authorities, health promotion may be traditionally associated with environmental health officers but departments of transport, housing, planning, leisure, education and social services are also taking a more active role with the increasing recognition of the wider determinants of health.
Community-based	Grass roots, local stakeholders, patients' group	Voluntary organisations are often commissioned to provide outreach services to community groups and set up community-based projects. Voluntary organisations can advocate on behalf of local people and are important partners in community development work.
Professional	Technical organisations, e.g. trade unions, educational bodies e.g. Royal Colleges	Health professionals and others who make up the primary health-care team have an essential role to play in health promotion. Moreover, health promotion is a core function for professional groups such as practice nurses, health visitors and school nurses. The relationships they establish with local people and communities mean they are all well placed to provide one-to-one support and advice.
Individual	Highly motivated individuals, either staff or patients or their carers	Health promotion specialists are core members of the multi-disciplinary and multi-organisational public health team. They are usually employed within health-care or local government with responsibility for developing strategy and stimulating and co-ordinating activities to promote health. They work in settings such as hospitals, schools and workplaces.

Health promotion at national and local level seeks to influence personal behaviour and policy making to secure change. In developed countries, increasing attention is being paid to the design and provision of environments which encourage healthy behaviours such as physical activity. In developing countries, health promotion still focuses on crucial interventions such as condom use, clean water and basic hygiene. Though politicians are inclined to retreat in the face of criticisms of the so-called 'nanny state', there is plenty of evidence that the electorate want governments to take a lead in developing healthy public policies [28]. The primary determinants of disease remain economic and social; remedies must therefore, in part, be economic and social. These are considered further in Chapters 15 and 16.

REFERENCES

1. UK National Screening Committee, The UK screening portal. See www.nsc.nhs.uk..
2. G. Rose, *The Strategy of Preventive Medicine*, Oxford University Press, Oxford, 1992.
3. R. Zimmern, Genomics and individuals in public health practice: are we buddies or can we meet the challenge? *Journal of Public Health* **33**, 2011, 477–82.
4. H. Arima, Effects of blood pressure lowering on major vascular events among patients with isolated diastolic hypertension: The Perindopril Protection Against Recurrent Stroke Study (PROGRESS) trial. *Stroke* **42**(8), 2011, 2339–41.
5. R. Jackson, J. Lynch and S. Harper, Preventing coronary heart disease. *British Medical Journal* **332**, 2006, 617–8.
6. S. Ebrahim and G. Davey Smith, Multiple risk factor interventions for primary prevention of coronary heart disease (Cochrane Review). *The Cochrane Library*, Issue 1, 2001. Update Software.
7. A.-L. Kinmonth and T. Marteau, Screening for cardiovascular risk: public health imperative or matter for individual informed choice? *British Medical Journal* **325**, 2002, 78–80.
8. M. R. Law and N. J. Wald, Risk factor thresholds: their existence under scrutiny. *British Medical Journal* **324**, 2002, 1570–6.
9. J. D. Neaton and D. Wentworth, Serum cholesterol, blood pressure, cigarette smoking, and death from coronary heart disease. *Archives of Internal Medicine* **152**, 1992, 56–64.
10. S. Rollnick, P. Mason and C. Butler, *Health Behaviour Change. A Guide for Practitioners.* Edinburgh, Churchill Livingstone, 2005.
11. M. Fishbein and I. Ajzen, *Belief, Attitude, Intention, and Behavior: An Introduction to Theory and Research*. Reading, MA, Addison-Wesley, 1975.
12. J. Prochaska and C. DiClemente, Stages and processes of self-change of smoking: towards an integrated model of change. *Journal of Consulting and Clinical Psychology* **51**, 1983, 390–5.
13. North West Public Health Observatory. Changing health choices. A review of the cost-effectiveness of individual-level behaviour change interventions. Liverpool, North West Public Health Observatory, February 2011.
14. M. Wakefield, B. Loken and R. Hornik, Use of mass media campaigns to change health behaviour. *Lancet* **376**, 2010, 1261–8.
15. National Social Marketing Centre for Excellence, *Social Marketing. Pocket Guide*, London, Department of Health, 2005.
16. R. Thaler and C. Sunstein, *Nudge: Improving Decisions About Health, Wealth and Happiness*, New Haven, CT, Yale University Press, 2009.
17. T. Marteau, D. Ogilvie, M. Roland, M. Suhrcke and M. Kelly, Judging nudging: can nudging improve population health? *British Medical Journal* **342**, 2011, d228.
18. C. Bonell, M. McKee, A. Fletcher, A. Haines and P. N. Wilkinson, Nudge smudge: UK Government misrepresents "nudge". *Lancet* **377**, 2011, 2158–9.
19. M. Lalonde, *A New Perspective on the Health of Canadians*, Ottawa, Government of Canada, 1974.

20. D. McVey and J. Stapleton, Can anti-smoking television advertising affect smoking behaviour? Controlled trial of the Health Education Authority for England's anti-smoking TV campaign. *Tobacco Control* **9**, 2000, 273–82.

21. R. Borland, H. H. Yong, K. M. Cummings, *et al.*, Determinants and consequences of smoke-free homes: findings from the International Tobacco Control (ITC) Four Country Survey. *Tobacco Control* **15** (suppl._3), 2006, iii42–iii50.

22. K. Tones and S. Tilford, *Health Promotion: Effectiveness, Efficiency and Equity*, 3rd edn, Cheltenham, Nelson Thornes, 2001.

23. World Health Organization, *Ottawa Charter for Health Promotion*, Geneva, WHO, 1986.

24. World Health Organization, *Bangkok Charter for Health Promotion in a Globalised World*, Bangkok, WHO, 2005.

25. World Health Organization, *Framework Convention for Tobacco Control*, Geneva, WHO, 2005.

26. J. Powles, Public health policy in developed countries. In R. Detels, R. Beaglehole, M. A. Lansang and M. Gulliford (eds.), *Oxford Textbook of Public Health*, 5th edn., Oxford, Oxford University Press, 2009, vol. **1**.

27. S. A. Glantz and E. D. Balbach, *Tobacco War: Inside the California Battles*. Berkeley, CA, University of California Press, 2000.

28. King'sFund, *Public Attitudes to Public Health Policy*, London, King's Fund, 2004.

9

Screening

Jan Yates and Stephen Gillam

Key points

- Screening is a tool to identify people at increased risk of a condition so that preventative action can be taken.
- Established criteria are used to judge when a screening programme should be introduced. These take account of the importance of the condition, the test, the treatment and the effectiveness of the programme as a whole.
- The performance of a screening test can be evaluated using calculations of sensitivity, specificity, predictive values and likelihood ratios.
- Screening will always identify so-called false negatives and false positives.
- Screening programmes are evaluated in the short and long term and potential sources of bias are considered in determining their effectiveness.
- Screening can incur harm and raises ethical questions. Health professionals and the public need to be aware of both the costs and benefits to society and individuals from screening as a public health activity.

Introduction

Screening is one of the most important preventive public health activities. This chapter provides some examples of effective screening programmes, considers what criteria are needed to demonstrate the effectiveness of a programme, how screening tests can be used to guide action and how screening programmes can be evaluated.

The UK National Screening Committee (see www.screening.nhs.uk) defines screening as:

a public health service in which members of a defined population, who do not necessarily perceive they are at risk of, or are already affected by a disease or its complications, are asked a

Essential Public Health, Second Edition, ed. Stephen Gillam, Jan Yates and Padmanabhan Badrinath.
Published by Cambridge University Press. © Cambridge University Press 2012.

question or offered a test, to identify those individuals who are more likely to be helped than harmed by further tests or treatment to reduce the risk of a disease or its complications [1].

It is different from a diagnostic test in that it identifies those at increased risk rather than those having a disorder. Screening is termed 'mass' screening when it is applied to the whole population or 'targeted' screening when it is aimed at specific parts of the population. 'Opportunistic' screening (or case finding) is applied to those who seek medical attention for another, perhaps unrelated, condition.

Should we establish a new screening programme?

Screening incurs harms as well as benefits. Screening tests may wrongly identify healthy people as having a disease (false positives), detect disease which would never have had any harmful clinical implications or lead to interventions which themselves carry risk of harm. Screening will result in some unnecessary diagnostic tests, which may have harmful physical effects as well as cause worry and concern for individuals. Those who are detected as having a disease early may feel labelled by that condition. This can also lead to psychological harm but the overall psychological impact of screening is not easy to determine as, for example, a false positive may be reassuring for some and extremely worrying for others. In addition, there are opportunity costs to be paid during the screening, on diagnosis and treatment. These come primarily in the form of time and money for an attendance, which may prove to have been unnecessary for the individual. Policy is shifting towards informed choice so that patients have the potential risks and benefits of the screen explained clearly to them through good-quality information to ensure the resulting choice reflects the decision maker's values. The effects of informed choice may be to reduce emotional distress and increase motivation to change behaviours. However, it may also decrease uptake but not consistently across the population as not everyone will have the skills to access or interpret information. This could increase inequity [2].

This potential for harm leads to ethical debates when a population who believe themselves healthy are offered an intervention which may determine that they are, in fact, at higher risk of disease. As relatively high coverage is needed to produce health gains this leads to target-setting for coverage rates and incentives to encourage screening. Those offered screening may find it difficult to make an informed decision about participation as it is not easy to weigh the harms and benefits that accrue over a long period and it is difficult for individuals to understand health outcomes which have a low probability of occurrence. Explaining the pros and cons of screening is not always easy for health professionals and, increasingly, decision support aids are being developed to help individuals make these complex decisions [3].

Thus, it is important to weigh up the benefits and harms of a potential screening programme before implementing it and to evaluate the effects carefully. There are established criteria for doing this. Initially outlined by Wilson and Jungner in 1968 [4], they have been updated variously since to take account of more rigorous standards of evidence required and an increased awareness of the potential for harm. The criteria used for evaluating the viability, effectiveness and appropriateness of a screening programme can be split into four categories relating to the condition, the test, the treatment and the programme itself. We use examples of UK screening programmes to illustrate these criteria.

The condition

The condition screened for should be an important problem. A population-wide intervention such as screening will only be effective if it can prevent significant disease. For rare conditions without major health effects screening would not be worthwhile.

Breast cancer is a heterogeneous group of diseases and is the most common cancer in women (around 22% of all cancer cases). There are over a million cases worldwide per year and incidence is around four times higher in more-developed countries than less-developed ones. There are around half a million cases of cervical cancer worldwide per year (around 3000 in the UK) and mortality is nearly three times higher in less-developed regions compared to more developed regions. Thus, both breast and cervical cancer give rise to a high burden of disease (see Figure 9.1) although the incidence of cervical cancer may become too low to meet this criterion in the UK.

From the charts in Figure 9.1, which three cancers would you suggest should be considered for screening programmes in women in the UK, based solely on the burden of disease?
The three cancers with the highest incidence and highest death rates for women are breast, lung and colorectal. In men, prostate cancer has the highest incidence followed by lung and colorectal. Lung cancer, followed by prostate and colorectal, has the highest death rate.

The natural history of the condition sought should be adequately understood and there should be a recognisable latent or early symptomatic stage. To make gains in morbidity or mortality it must be possible to identify an early stage of disease so that early intervention can prevent progression. For example, in cervical cancer the presence of abnormal cells provides a pre-cancerous stage which is detectable and the likelihood of these abnormalities progressing to cancer is known.

All practicable, cost-effective primary prevention measures should have been implemented. It is better to prevent the onset of disease rather than have to detect it early and then treat. Thus, screening programmes are more often established for conditions where preventive measures have not led to significant reductions in disease prevalence or incidence, such as cancers.

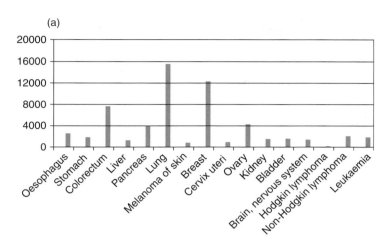

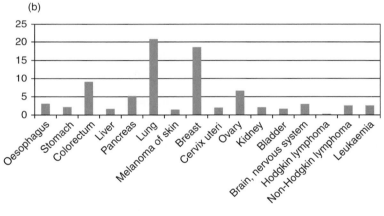

Figure 9.1   Estimated number of female cases and death rates from selected cancers in 2008, UK (from GLOBOCAN 2008; see globocan.iarc.fr/). (a) Cases. (b) Age-standardised death rate per 100,000 population.

The main risks for the development of sight-threatening diabetic retinopathy are high blood glucose, hypertension, smoking and elevated blood lipid levels. In the UK, all of these have received significant attention in recent years regarding their place in prevention of a range of diseases. Other risk factors such as duration of diabetes and age are not modifiable by individuals [5]. Owing to this situation and the severe impact of retinopathy on sight, screening via digital imaging of the retina was introduced by the NHS in 2005.

The test

There should be a suitable test available which is simple, safe, precise and validated. As screening only identifies those at increased risk it is necessary to have a clearly valid test for the condition so that those who do not need further investigation can be reassured and those that do can be rapidly referred for diagnosis and treatment. The population distribution of screening test values should be known and an agreed 'cut-off' value identified so that those people warranting further investigation can be identified.

The test or examination should be acceptable to both the public and to professionals. Screening programmes depend, for their effectiveness, on high proportions of the target population complying with screening offers. If the screening or diagnostic test is not acceptable this will reduce the effectiveness of the programme as many will not attend.

There should be an agreed policy on further diagnostic investigation. Those who receive a positive screen result must be informed of the choices available to them and access to diagnostic services should be available equitably for the whole screened population.

Cervical cancer develops from altered cells in the cervix and microscopy can be used to detect abnormal cells (dysplasia) at early stages. A screen for cervical abnormalities involves a smear or brush of the cervix and examination of the removed cells under a microscope. The standard test used to be a smear (Papanikolaou) test but a test based on liquid-based cytology (LBC) was recently introduced. The sensitivity of screening for cervical cancer has improved with a move to LBC where samples are taken using a brush and suspended in a liquid medium. Women with abnormalities are then investigated further using colposcopy and any areas of abnormal cervix can be biopsied or removed.

When screening for Down's syndrome, combinations of ultrasound scanning and serum biochemistry tests are used to determine women at increased risk of delivering a baby with an anomaly. If an increased risk of Down's syndrome is detected an invasive diagnostic test can be performed enabling genetic-marker identification on fetal cells collected via either amniocentesis or chorionic villus sampling (CVS). However, these carry an excess risk of miscarriage (1/100 procedures for amniocentesis and approximately 2/100 procedures for CVS). These screening and diagnostic tests are considered unpleasant by some but have been shown over time to be acceptable. However, there are concerns about whether this is consistent across all parts of the population. Some women may not be comfortable with intimate examinations for cultural reasons. For example, this may explain why a number of studies have found lower screening uptake in Asian populations [6].

The treatment

There should be an accepted and effective treatment for patients with recognised disease, facilities for treatment should be available and such treatment optimised by all healthcare providers. Implementing a screening programme which raises hopes and uncovers demand for treatment services that do not exist or that do not have a firm evidence base would be unethical and an uneconomical use of resources.

There should be an agreed policy on whom to treat as patients, including management of borderline disease. Treatment policies for cancers are, in the main, in place well before screening is established. Treatments may, however, be invasive and unpleasant and this must be explained clearly before screening is undertaken. In some screening programmes, the 'treatment' becomes more of an issue. For example, abdominal ultrasound of men aged 65 to detect and treat large abdominal aortic aneurysms has been shown to decrease aneurysm-related mortality by 42% [7]. However, the surgical aneurysm repair carries a 6% risk of dying within 30 days of surgery. The diagnosis or treatment may not be acceptable to those being screened and the attitudes of health-care staff to treatment options has an impact on an individual's decision whether or not to accept screening.

The programme

There should be robust evidence that the screening programme is effective in reducing mortality or morbidity. Evidence from randomised controlled trials of screening programmes should be considered before initiating a screening programme. Much screening activity, for example in childhood, is no longer undertaken for lack of evidence that it is effective [8].

There should be evidence that the programme is acceptable to the public and professionals and that the benefits outweigh the harms. All elements of the screening programme from invitations through to treatment should be acceptable and the outcomes of the programme in terms of morbidity and mortality should outweigh the physical and psychological harms caused by the test, diagnostic procedures and treatment.

The cost of early diagnosis and treatment should be economically balanced in relation to the total expenditure on health-care. Within a limited health-care budget all health and health-care spend must be justified in terms of cost-effectiveness. Implementation of a screening programme must be demonstrated to be an efficient use of health-care funds in comparison to other interventions possible for specific conditions.

The programme must be adequately resourced. As well as all the staffing and other resource implications of the testing, diagnosis and treatment, screening programmes require significant money for management and monitoring, quality assurance and long-term evaluation. All these resource implications must be determined before the programme is established.

Following successful trials in Sweden, breast cancer screening was introduced in the UK in 1990. Women aged between 50 and 70 years are invited for a mammogram and two X-ray views are taken to maximise the chance of detecting abnormalities. Women are recalled every 3 years. Mammographic screening has been shown to reduce mortality in women aged 50–69 years by an estimated 35% [9]. Among women screened regularly over a 10-year period between the ages of 50 and 70, it is estimated that one life is saved for every 400 women screened and 1400 lives are saved each year in England [10]. In younger women (aged 40–49 years) screening is of less benefit and screening more frequently than every 3 years is not predicted to improve mortality [11]. In the UK, the Government proposes to increase the age range for breast screening to 47–73 years and, due to the limited evidence of benefit, this is being rolled out as a randomised controlled trial to investigate the net effects (see: www.controlled-trials.com/ISRCTN33292440).

In the UK, the National Screening Committee oversees the introduction of new screening programmes and robust evidence for all of the criteria is needed for a new programme to be established. Thinking back to our question earlier about screening for the major cancers in the UK, we can see why some of these diseases are not screened for.

Many of the criteria for assessing the need for a population programme have not been met for prostate cancer, for example. In particular, there is a lack of knowledge about the epidemiology and natural history of the disease, a poor level of accuracy in the screening tests, and a lack of good-quality evidence concerning the effectiveness and cost-effectiveness of treatments for localised prostate cancer. In addition, the evidence suggests that a screening programme would not reduce deaths [12]. There is currently little evidence on the effectiveness of screening for either ovarian or lung cancer in those at risk and a number of studies are investigating potential screening tests.

Examples of effective screening programmes

Screening can be targeted at various stages of the life course. Some examples of screening programmes established in the UK at each life stage are given in Table 9.1.

Other forms of 'screening'

There are a number of other situations in which healthy individuals are tested that lie outside our definition of population screening. The underlying difference here is that this kind of testing relates to the need of the individual, rather than to reducing mortality or morbidity in populations, see Box 9.1.

Another interesting, if controversial, example is immigration screening. In the UK, immigrants and those wishing to stay in the UK for longer than 6 months are screened for tuberculosis; immigrants to the USA are screened for a range of infectious diseases including HIV, tuberculosis, gonorrhoea, syphilis and leprosy. While this detects disease in the individuals, it is termed screening as the intention is to protect the resident population from the effects of communicable diseases. Evidence for the effectiveness of this form of screening is contested [13].

 Can you think of reasons why HIV screening of immigrants from high risk areas may not protect the host population?

Table 9.1 Screening programmes in the UK, 2011*

Life stage	Population offered screening	Diseases screened for
Antenatal	All pregnant women	Anaemia
		Bacteriuria
		Blood group
		Rhesus D status
		Red cell antibodies
		Hepatitis B
		Human Immunodeficiency Virus (HIV)
		Rubella
		Syphilis
		Down's syndrome
		A range of foetal anomalies detectable by ultrasound scan e.g. Spina bifida, Sickle cell disease
		Thalassaemia
Newborn	All newborn babies	Congenital hypothyroidism
		Phenylketonuria (PKU)
		Cystic fibrosis
		Sickle cell disease
		Medium Chain Acyl Dehydrogenase Deficiency (MCADD)
		General physical examination with particular emphasis on the eyes, heart and hips
		Automated hearing screen
Children	All children	Growth abnormalities (height and weight at school entry)
		Visual impairment (between 4th and 5th birthdays)
		Hearing loss in school-age children
Adults	Women of certain ages	Breast cancer (aged 50–70)
		Cervical cancer (aged 25–64)
	All older people aged 60–69	Colorectal cancer
	Diabetics	Sight-threatening retinopathy
	Men aged 65	Abdominal aortic aneurysm

*Source: National Screening Committee, http://www.nsc.nhs.uk/

Box 9.1 Not screening....

- Pre-employment checks (e.g. sight tests for drivers)
- Infection control (e.g. food handlers being cleared of an *E. coli* infection)
- To determine suitability for clinical interventions (e.g. pre-operative assessments)
- Research studies
- Fitness test prior to starting an exercise regime

Evaluating screening programmes

Screening test performance

No screening test can be 100% perfect. It only picks up those people thought to be at increased risk of disease and some of these may not in fact develop the condition.

It is important in population terms to be able to predict the numbers of false results (either false negatives or false positives) and to judge the best screening test for a particular condition. It is also important on an individual basis to be able to predict how likely a test result is to reflect the true status of the patient.

Two measures used are *sensitivity* and *specificity*. Sensitivity is the proportion of truly diseased persons, as measured by the gold standard, who are identified as diseased by the test under study; specificity is the proportion of truly non-diseased persons, as measured by the gold standard, who are identified as non-diseased by the test under study. A sensitive test will identify all (or almost all) the true positives, but in doing so will wrongly identify some truly negative cases as positive ('false positives'). A specific test will only identify positives if it is certain (or almost certain) that they are truly positive, but in doing so will wrongly identify some truly positive cases as negative ('false negatives'). A sensitive test keeps the false-negative rate low, and a specific test keeps the false-positive rate low. In the design of tests, it is usual that as tests are made more specific they become less sensitive, and vice-versa. A balance is needed and the calculated sensitivities and specificities are used to determine the best screening test for each condition.

Calculating sensitivity and specificity

In calculating these measures one needs to know the numbers screened and the numbers deemed later to have the disease by a 'gold standard' diagnostic test. These are the people termed 'test' and 'true' positives and negatives.

The 2×2 in Table 9.2 illustrates this: a is the number of people who truly have the disease who have a positive test result (true positives); b is the number of people who

Table 9.2 Generic 2 × 2 table showing the possible outcomes of a screening test and used to calculate its validity

		'TRUE'		
		Positive	Negative	
'TEST'	Positive	a	b	a + b
	Negative	c	d	c + d
		a + c	b + d	a + b + c + d

Box 9.2 Sensitivities and specificities

Sensitivity = a/ (a + c)
False positive rate = b/ (b + d) (or 1 − specificity)
Specificity = d/ (b + d)
False negative rate = c/ (a + c) (or 1 − sensitivity)

Table 9.3 A 2 × 2 table showing results of a urine analysis glucose tolerance test for diabetes

		'TRUE' Gold standard diagnostic		
'TEST' Result of urine test for glucose		Positive	Negative	
	Positive	6	7	13
	Negative	21	966	987
		27	973	1000

truly do not have the disease who have a positive test result (false positives); c is the number of people who truly have the disease who have a negative test result (false negatives); and d is the number of people who truly do not have the disease who have a negative test result (true negatives).

For example, urine analysis can be used to screen for the likelihood of diabetes. The validity of this test has been considered [14].

Using terms from the 2 × 2 table sensitivity, specificity and false test rates can be calculated using formulae from Box 9.2.

Use the formulae in Box 9.2 to calculate the sensitivity and specificity for the results of a glucose tolerance test shown in Table 9.3.
Sensitivity = 6/27 = 22%, specificity = 966/973 = 99%.

This test is very specific but not very sensitive. This means that, at a population level, it is not very effective at picking up positive cases of diabetes but is quite good at identifying people who do not have diabetes. It is unlikely that a test with such a low sensitivity would be used as a widespread screening tool without further information being available for the clinician to inform decision making following the test. More information is needed and can be provided by calculating the predictive values and a likelihood ratio for the test.

Let us consider cervical and aortic aneurysm screening and their reported validity as examples. Sensitivities for conventional smear testing and liquid-based cytology

> ### Box 9.3 Predictive values
>
> Positive predictive value $= a/(a + b)$
> $$= 6/13 = 46.2\%$$
>
> Negative predictive value $= d/(c + d)$
> $$= 966/987 = 97.8\%$$

have been calculated as 72% and 80%, respectively. Thus, liquid-based cytology is associated with a 12% improvement in sensitivity [15]. The validity of aneurysm screening is more complicated because the ultrasound scan used to screen for risk of aneurysm rupture is actually the gold standard test itself. In this case, validity is reported as the variation in an ultrasound operator's ability to measure the size of an aneurysm (less than 0.3 cm inter-operator variability) and as a false-negative rate (risk of rupture following a normal scan) of 0.56 per 1000 person years [16].

Predictive values and likelihood ratios

The sensitivity and specificity of a test do not depend on the prevalence of the disease in question. In other words, they are the same, no matter which population you screen. However, screening tests can vary considerably in their ability to predict the true disease state of an individual. This is termed the predictive value and depends on how prevalent the disease is. Take the diabetes test again as an example.

The prevalence of the condition in the example in Table 9.3 is 2.7% (27 true positives in a population of 1000). In this case the predictive values can be calculated – see Box 9.3.

This can be interpreted to mean that a patient with a positive urine test result has a 46.2% chance of really having diabetes but a patient with a negative result has a 97.8% chance of NOT having diabetes. In this case the test is good at ruling out diabetes but not so good at ruling it in!

What difference does it make to this prediction if the prevalence of the condition is higher? Table 9.4 shows the same sensitivity and specificity but in a population where the prevalence of diabetes is 15% (150 cases out of 1000).

 Use Table 9.4 to calculate the positive and negative predictive values of the test in this population.

Positive predictive value = 33/41 = 80%, negative predictive value = 842/959 = 88%.

This demonstrates that when there is already a greater likelihood of the disease being present (a prevalence of 15% compared to 2.7%) the test is a better predictor, both of true negatives and true positives. This begs a question. What if we already

Table 9.4 A 2 × 2 table for a urine glucose test as a screen for diabetes in high (15%) prevalence population

		'TRUE' Gold standard diagnostic		
'TEST' Result of urine test for glucose		Positive	Negative	
	Positive	33	8	41
	Negative	117	842	959
		150	850	1000

suspected the patient might have diabetes from other information? We might be testing an elderly patient who has come to clinic complaining of increased urination, tiredness and excess thirst. An individual clinician might then have a higher index of suspicion and trust a positive result more. Because this is the way people really think in real situations, sensitivities and specificities (and even predictive values) are not always useful tools on a patient-by-patient basis.

Here, *likelihood ratios* can be useful. We start before the test with a probability that the patient has the condition we are interested in. This is called the pre-test probability. A positive likelihood ratio tells us how much more likely it is that a condition is present when the test result is positive. A negative likelihood ratio tells us how much more likely the patient is not to have the condition after a negative test result and we can use these to amend our pre-test estimate of the odds into a post-test odds and thus work out the probability that an individual patient has or does not have the condition being tested for. Boxes 9.4 and 9.5 show a worked example. Say we thought our elderly, potentially diabetic, patient already had a 50% chance of having diabetes from his symptoms (a probability of 0.5 or 50:50 odds, i.e. odds of 1:1 – this is called the pre-test odds). The negative likelihood ratio is calculated in Box 9.4 using the sensitivity and specificity for the test in Table 9.3. We use this to alter our first estimate of the odds (which was 1) so that the probability of the patient having diabetes can be calculated (Box 9.5).

In this case, even though the test was negative, there is still a 44% chance that the patient has diabetes. This value is lower than our initial pre-test probability of 50%, but a negative test result here is unlikely to deter further diagnostic tests.

The positive likelihood ratio of 22 is so high that with a positive result we would be pretty certain our patient had diabetes and would be likely to initiate treatment. Box 9.6 summarises when these concepts are useful in practice. See the Internet Companion for useful on-line calculators.

Estimates of positive predictive value in the UK Breast Screening Programme range from 6% to 8% for prevalent screening, meaning that 6% to 8% of women recalled for further tests after their first screening have cancer. The positive predictive value is higher for incident screens (women who are having their second or subsequent mammogram) and has been estimated at between 12% and 14% [17].

Box 9.4 Likelihood ratios

Using sensitivity = 22%, specificity = 99%

Negative test

$$\begin{aligned}
\text{Negative likelihood ratio} &= (1 - \text{Sensitivity})/\text{Specificity} \\
&= (1 - 0.22)/0.99 \\
&= 0.78/0.99 \\
&= 0.79
\end{aligned}$$

Positive test

$$\begin{aligned}
\text{Positive likelihood ratio} &= \text{Sensitivity}/(1 - \text{Specificity}) \\
&= 0.22/(1 - 0.99) \\
&= 22
\end{aligned}$$

Box 9.5 Using post-test odds and likelihood ratios

Assuming a negative test for our elderly patient....

$$\begin{aligned}
\text{Post-test odds} &= \text{Pre-test odds likelihood ratio} \\
&= 1 \times 0.79 \\
&= 0.79
\end{aligned}$$

$$\begin{aligned}
\text{Post-test probability} &= \text{Post-test odds}/(\text{Post-test odds} + 1) \\
&= 0.79/(0.79 + 1) \\
&= 0.44 (44\%)
\end{aligned}$$

Box 9.6 When to use.....

- *Sensitivities and specificities*
  When we want to know how good the test is and to determine which the best test for any condition is.
- *Predictive values*
  When we want to know how the test utility varies across populations.
- *Likelihood ratios*
  When we want to interpret test results for individual patients where we have additional information on the likelihood of a disease being present before we do the test.

> **Box 9.7 Monitoring screening programmes**
>
> Information which can be used to judge the effectiveness of a screening programme includes:
> - clinical or laboratory expertise of those responsible for screening tests
> - coverage achieved
> - number of referrals
> - number referred who attend for specialist diagnosis
> - number of test positives who are confirmed as true positives
> - number of false positives
> - number of true cases missed
> - number of cases effectively treated
> - the impact of the screening programme on other related services
> - the delays between different steps of the programme and resulting anxiety
> - the quality, accuracy and readability of the information provided to patients about the programme
> - the extent of the benefit accruing to those effectively treated
> - the cost of the programme, the cost per case detected and the value of the benefits obtained
> - coverage by different population groups to determine inequalities in access
> - the training required to initiate the programme and maintain high standards.

Monitoring screening programmes

Criteria based on those of Wilson and Jungner are generally used to determine whether to put a screening programme in place but they do not guarantee that a screening programme will work in practice. The programme must be evaluated to ensure that it is safe and acceptable in the short term and meets its aims of morbidity or mortality reduction in the long term. In the UK, all new screening programmes are established with quality assurance programmes that consider a range of short-term outcomes (see Box 9.7). As well as determining a test's validity, it is necessary to consider potential sources of bias and health-related long-term outcomes.

Sources of bias in screening

Selection bias
We hope that screening programmes attract the population we intended to screen but those who respond to our invitations may be systematically different from the target population in some way. We have already mentioned that Asian populations tend to have lower uptake rates for screening and early analysis of the UK bowel cancer

Figure 9.2   Lead time bias.

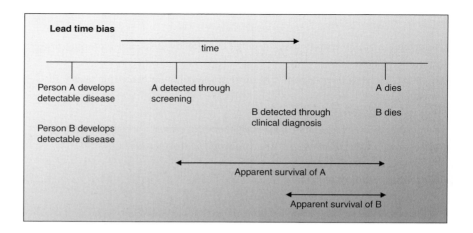

screening programme shows that uptake is lower in more deprived populations, and in younger men [18]. Such studies and statistics demonstrate to those running the screening programme that efforts are needed to minimise selection biases among the individuals who are screened.

Lead time bias

Lead time bias occurs when detection by screening seems to increase disease-free survival but only because disease has been detected earlier and not because screening is actually delaying death or disease. Figure 9.2 shows how this works: person A and B develop disease, then die at the same time; however, it appears that A lives longer than B because she found out about her disease earlier through screening. This is one reason why it is important to evaluate a programme using mortality as an outcome and compare screened and unscreened populations. Where there is a lead time bias reduced improvements in mortality will be demonstrated.

Length time bias

Length time bias occurs if the screening programme is better at picking up milder forms of the disease. Figure 9.3 shows this. Length time bias means that people who develop disease that progresses more quickly or is more likely to be fatal (person A) are less likely to be picked up by screening and their outcomes may not be included in evaluations of the programme. Thus the programme looks to be more effective than it is. The programme evaluation must compare the type of disease which is picked up through screening with that picked up by routine diagnosis. Where length time bias occurs the screening programme will systematically identify disease which has a better prognosis.

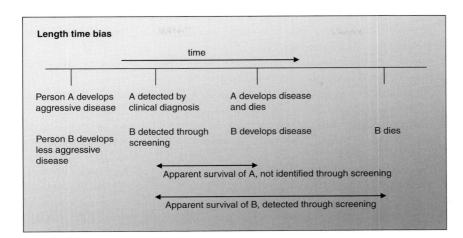

Figure 9.3   Length time bias.

Conclusion

We have seen that screening is an important public health intervention which has been demonstrated to have had a major impact on mortality for certain conditions. However, screening carries risks to individuals and is a good example of an area of public health where the needs of individuals and the needs of populations may conflict. Professionals working in screening, whether counselling individuals on screening choices or supporting screening at a population level, need to be aware that their beliefs colour the way we communicate with people.

REFERENCES

1. UK National Screening Committee, What is screening? See: www.screening.nhs.uk/screening.
2. T. M. Marteau and A. L. Kinmonth, Screening for cardiovascular risk: public health imperative or matter for individual informed choice? *British Medical Journal* **325**, 2002, 78–80.
3. C. von Wagner, A decision aid to support informed choice about bowel cancer screening in people with low educational level improves knowledge but reduces screening uptake. *Evidence Based Nursing*, doi:10.1136/ebn1142.
4. J. M. G. Wilson and G. Jungner, *Principles and Practice of Screening for Disease*, Geneva, WHO, 1968.
5. P. Scanlon, Risk factors for the development of diabetic retinopathy and sight threatening diabetic retinopathy, Annual Evidence Update on Diabetic Retinopathy, September 2010.
6. A. Szczepura, C. Price and A. Gumber, Breast and bowel cancer screening uptake patterns over 15 years for UK south Asian ethnic minority populations, corrected for differences in socio-demographic characteristics. *BMC Public Health*, **2**, 2008, doi: 10.1186/1471-2458-8-346.

7. H. A. Ashton, M. J. Buxton, N. E. Day *et al.*, The multicentre aneurysm screening study (MASS) into the effect of abdominal aortic aneurysm screening. *The Lancet* **360**, 2002, 9345; ProQuest Medical Library, p. 1531.

8. D. M. B. Hall, *Report of the Joint Working Party on Child Health Surveillance: Health For All Children*, 3rd edn, Oxford, Oxford University Press, 2003.

9. H. Vainio and F. Bianchini (eds.), *IARC Handbooks of Cancer Prevention, Volume 7: Breast Cancer Screening*. Lyon, IARC Press, 2002.

10. Advisory Committee on Breast Cancer Screening, Screening for breast cancer in England: past and future. NHSBSP Publication No. 61, Sheffield, NHS Cancer Screening Programmes, 2006.

11. The Breast Screening Frequency Trial Group, The frequency of breast cancer screening: results from the UKCCCR Randomised Trial. *European Journal of Cancer* **38**, 2002, 1458–64.

12. S. Selley, D. Gillatt, J. Coast, A. Faulkner and J. Donovan, Diagnosis, management and screening of early localised prostate cancer. *Health Technology Assessment* **1**, 1997, no. 2.

13. R. Coker, Compulsory screening of immigrants for tuberculosis and HIV. *British Medical Journal* **328**, 298–300.

14. D. K. G. Andersson, E. Lundblad and K. Svardsudd, A model for early diagnosis of type 2 diabetes mellitus in primary health care. *Diabetic Medicine* **10**, 1993, 167–73.

15. J. Karnon and J. Peters, Liquid-based cytology in cervical screening: an updated rapid and systematic review. Technology assessment report commissioned by the HTA Programme on behalf of The National Institute for Clinical Excellence. The School of Health and Related Research (ScHARR), The University of Sheffield, January 2003.

16. NHS Abdominal Aortic Aneurysm Screening Programme, NHS AAA Screening Programme (NAAASP) Standard Operating Procedures (SOPs) and Workbook Version 2.2, May 2010.

17. R. G. Blanks, S. M. Moss and J. Patnick, Results from the UK NHS breast screening programme 1994–1999. *Journal of Medical Screening* **7**(4), 2000, 195–8.

18. C. von Wagner, G. Baio, R. Raine *et al.*, Inequalities in participation in an organized national colorectal cancer screening programme: results from the first 2.6 million invitations in England. *International Journal of Epidemiology* **40**(3), 2011, 712–18.

10

Health protection and communicable disease control

Jan Yates and Padmanabhan Badrinath

Key points

- The term 'health protection' covers threats to health such as infectious diseases, environmental hazards such as chemical releases and radiological incidents, natural disasters and terrorism.
- Health-protection actions depend upon the nature of the infecting organism (pathogen) or hazard, the transmission route and the response of the host to the hazard. Individuals can help to protect themselves by being aware of the nature of different risks and the methods by which individuals are exposed.
- Vaccines are an effective way to protect whole populations against some infectious diseases.
- Surveillance of infectious diseases is important to identify outbreaks, monitor levels of disease, plan control measures, monitor outcomes of control programmes and enable efficient targeting of resources.
- The public health effects of communicable disease are controlled through actions that affect hosts for the disease, transmission, susceptibility of the population, disease identification and disease treatment.
- Environmental health involves the reduction, investigation and control of potential health hazards, which arise from an environmental or man-made origin.
- Emergency planning and response is increasingly important as a mechanism to plan for and control the health effects of large-scale disasters and emergencies, including natural disasters and terrorist attacks.

Introduction

Health protection refers to threats to health such as infectious diseases, environmental threats, natural disasters and the threats from terrorist acts. Health protection

Essential Public Health, Second Edition, ed. Stephen Gillam, Jan Yates and Padmanabhan Badrinath.
Published by Cambridge University Press. © Cambridge University Press 2012.

may also overlap with action tackling the determinants of health, especially legislative aspects such as workplace smoking bans or speed restrictions and even lifestyle choices and the health issues of ageing populations such as increasing levels of chronic disease (which we now know may also be due to infections).

Thus, a generic framework for dealing with a health protection issue might be:

- identify the threat to health;
- quantify the risk to health;
- implement immediate and long-term, effective, control measures to mitigate the risk.

This chapter will outline the public health aspects of communicable disease control and touch on some of the other areas now included within health protection in the UK. Important health protection terms are included in the glossary.

Patterns of communicable disease

Based on the demographic transition, it was widely believed until recently that infectious diseases, especially childhood diseases, were an historic problem in developed countries. As a country develops the burden of disease shifts from a primarily infectious one (such as diarrhoea and pneumonia) to non-communicable such as long-term conditions and cancer. The eradication of smallpox, the development of public health and medical interventions such as safe water supplies and vaccines appeared to signal their continuing decline. However, the WHO Global Burden of Disease project (2004) portrays a different picture. Globally, 51% of the years of life lost are due to communicable diseases but in low-income countries the figure is 68% (and 80% in the African region) compared to 8% in high-income countries. In Africa, southeast Asia and the eastern Mediterranean this years-of-life-lost burden is greater than that for non-communicable diseases and injuries combined, fourfold higher in Africa. Whilst interventions to moderate the burden of infectious diseases have been shown to be cost-effective (for example, a measles vaccination costs less than $1 per vaccination and less than $25 per quality-adjusted life year gained [1]), the resurgence of diseases once thought to be coming under control, such as tuberculosis (TB), illustrate an on-going failure to tackle basic causes as well as the natural ingenuity of causative micro-organisms. The lack of political and pharmaco-industrial will to develop low-cost remedies for 'unprofitable' diseases like leishmaniasis and TB also remains an obstacle. In the UK, deterioration has been seen in the field of sexually transmitted infection including human immunodeficiency virus (HIV), chlamydia, syphilis and gonorrhoea.

New challenges continue to arise. Global pandemics such as HIV/AIDS and influenza have graphically underlined the continued importance of health inequalities and poverty as determinants of ill health. Health-care associated infections (HCAI) are of increasing importance to health. *Clostridium difficile* is a major cause of nosocomial diarrhoea, having been recognised in the 1970s and identified as the causal organism in 1978 [2]. Different patterns of drug resistance continue to emerge and are linked in part to increasing use of anti-microbial or parasitic agents in medicine and animal husbandry; examples here are malaria, extensively drug-resistant *Mycobacterium tuberculosis*, methicillin- or vancomycin-resistant *Staphylococcus aureus* (MRSA) and *Salmonella* species. Finally, more exotic threats to human health such as variant Creutzfeld-Jakob's disease, avian and swine influenza and severe acute respiratory syndrome (SARS) have further fuelled media interest in communicable disease.

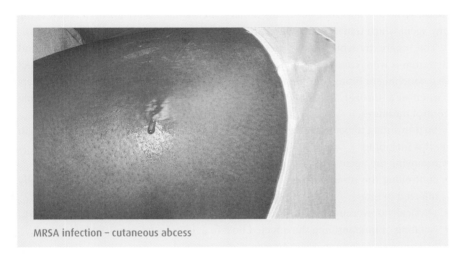

MRSA infection – cutaneous abcess

Controlling communicable diseases

In many ways the public health challenges associated with infectious diseases are similar to those associated with other diseases: identify the burden of disease (identify the threat and quantify the risk), consider how to prevent or treat it, and take appropriate action (implement control measures). However, there are some elements of dealing with infectious agents which set this field apart. Interactions between the cause (agent), host and environment are also important. For example, *Mycobacterium tuberculosis* is the direct cause of tuberculosis but crowded housing and poor nutrition also increase the risk of infection. However, causes of communicable disease have the ability to replicate. These agents are transmissible, can alter and evolve, as can the host's response to them. This host response is something we can use as a target for control when we utilise vaccines. Also, in contrast to much of public health, timescales in communicable disease control can be relatively short and there may be little time to initiate effective control measures. Thus, we often need to balance enforcement of control measures and education. The sporadic nature of outbreaks raises the importance of surveillance systems to spot problems early.

Controlling transmission of infectious agents

Infection can be defined as the entry and multiplication of an infectious agent in the body of man or animals. Control of infection relies on determining opportunities to interrupt transmission from reservoir to host. The organism causing the infection is termed an agent or pathogen and may be a protozoan, e.g. *Cryptosporidiosis*; a virus, e.g. polio, influenza; a bacterium, e.g. *Escherichia coli*; or a larger organism, e.g. worms, mites, some of which may be vectors rather than the disease organism (a vector being any agent which transmits an infectious agent, e.g. mosquitoes transmitting malaria).

The means by which agents are transmitted from reservoir to host varies and determines what control methods are appropriate. In general, transmission is direct (e.g. touching or biting), indirect (e.g. via food or water) or airborne (e.g. via droplets carried in a sneeze). Table 10.1 shows some modes of transmission with possible control measures.

So preventing transmission is easy in theory and there are a number of clear ways to do this including:

- removing the agent (e.g. kill headlice, treat infections);
- controlling the reservoir (e.g. animal control of rabies, disinfection of potentially infected fomites);
- physically preventing transmission from the reservoir (e.g. barrier contraception);
- isolating or quarantining the infected host (e.g. in hospital-acquired infections);
- preventing infection in a new host (e.g. vaccination).

Box 10.1 shows how individual control might work.

> ### Box 10.1 Individual control of infections
>
> Chlamydial infection
>
> *Chlamydia trachomatis* causes one of the most common sexually transmitted infections in Europe with rates in sexually active young people of between 5 and 10%. Symptoms may be those of genital tract inflammation but the majority of cases are asymptomatic. Untreated, chlamydial infection can lead to pelvic inflammatory disease, sub-fertility and poor reproductive outcomes. Individual control simply involves safe-sex practice and testing to enable cure before long-term effects are felt. However, as a public health programme, *Chlamydia* screening is hard to implement across a young population who may not perceive a risk.

However, difficulties arise when preventing transmission. One of these is where reservoirs of infection exist in animals (for example, rabies, *Salmonella*) or the environment (for example, *Cryptosporidium* and *Legionella*). Smallpox provided the

Table 10.1 Modes of transmission of communicable diseases and possible control measures

Mode of transmission	Examples of agents transmitted in this way	Possible control measures
Direct person-to-person transmission – physical contact with human reservoir	Sexually transmitted infections such as Chlamydia Head lice MRSA Chicken pox Measles	Isolation of cases Hygiene Barrier contraception Treat cases, e.g. with pediculocides, antibiotics
Airborne person-to-person transmission – respiratory	Influenza Measles TB	Isolation/quarantine of cases Treat cases Chemoprophylaxis Vaccination Hand washing
Direct person-to-person transmission – blood to blood	HIV Hepatitis B	Needle exchanges Safe sharps and clean-up practices Screening of blood products Sterilisation Safe operating practices including decontamination
Direct person-to-person transmission – transplacental	HIV Hepatitis B Rubella CMV Listeria	Vaccination Chemoprophylaxis
Indirect faecal–oral transmission from human or animal reservoirs	Salmonella, E. coli or Campylobacter Polio Typhoid Hepatitis A	Good hygiene Isolation of cases Vaccination
Indirect transmission through contamination of food or water (often also faecal–oral)	Salmonella, Cryptosporidium, Legionella (also respiratory transmission of aerosolised bacteria)	Good hygiene practices for food safety (hand washing is of central importance) Separation of raw and cooked food, clean water and sewage Destruction of contaminated goods Production controls assurance Legislation Good management of water supply systems/effective cleaning and maintenance
Direct transmission through physical contact with animal reservoirs	Rabies	Avoidance Vaccination of animals Vaccination of humans

Table 10.1 (*cont.*)

Mode of transmission	Examples of agents transmitted in this way	Possible control measures
Indirect transmission through physical contact with the environment	Tetanus	Hygiene Disinfection and wound management Vaccination
Indirect transmission through fomites (objects harbouring a disease agent)	Influenza Norovirus	Disinfection or destruction of fomites such as clothing or utensils
Indirect transmission through insect vectors	Malaria Yellow fever Lyme disease West Nile virus	Eradication/control of vector Chemoprophylaxis Vaccination Barriers, e.g. mosquito nets

World Health Organisation's (WHO's) greatest triumph partly because man is the only reservoir and an effective vaccine was available.

Control is problematic where it depends upon changing behaviours (e.g. controlling sexually transmitted infection relies on individual and cultural attitudes to behaviours such as condom use).

Organisms which have become resistant to some antimicrobial drugs are now being found in patients in both hospital and community settings. Organisms include MRSA, *Mycobacterium tuberculosis*, *Clostridium difficile* and certain strains of *E. coli*. While some organisms are naturally more resistant to antimicrobials (such as *M. tuberculosis*, which has thick cell walls) resistance can also occur through changes in an organism's genes or be introduced by transmission of resistance genes from other organisms. It is still possible to treat most drug-resistant infections but the treatment options become limited and it is better to prevent the development of resistance. Resistance is particularly problematic in the care of hospital inpatients who are especially susceptible to infections. In general, solutions to the reduction of HCAI, including those due to drug-resistant organisms, are multifactorial and include: surveillance, clear infection control standards, maintaining clean hospital environments, strict antibiotic prescribing practices and isolation of infected patients.

Systems have to be in place to ensure that the control measures which prevent individuals transmitting or contracting infections are applied across large numbers of people. This type of control aims to reduce morbidity and mortality from these diseases in populations. Whilst it would be ideal from a human point of view to *eradicate* infectious diseases (as we have with smallpox), pragmatism dictates that our control objectives cannot always be so ambitious. In some cases we aim to *eliminate* infection from large geographical regions by preventing transmission but accept that the organism still persists in our environment. We have achieved this to a large extent with *Salmonella enteritidis* in eggs through the vaccination of chicken flocks to eliminate the organism (British eggs from *Salmonella*-free flocks carry a 'Lion' mark and the US Food and Drug Administration have an Egg Safety Rule requiring producers to comply with control measures), and pasteurisation to eliminate milk as a vehicle for transmitting *M. tuberculosis* and *E. coli* O157. Lastly, we may accept that a disease cannot be eliminated or eradicated but aim to *contain* it so that it does not present a significant public health problem. Winter outbreaks of influenza are an example of where a disease is contained to minimise its impact on the population.

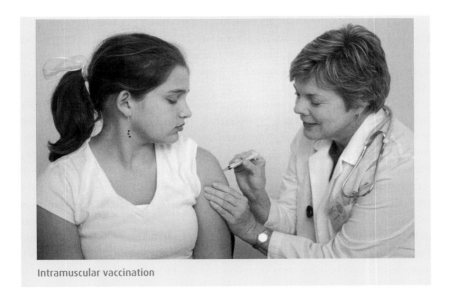

Intramuscular vaccination

Protecting populations through vaccination

The term vaccination derives from the historical origins of the process for inoculation with vaccinia virus against smallpox (first described by Edward Jenner in 1798). Whilst immunisation is, strictly speaking, the protection (making immune) of an individual by the administration of a vaccine, the terms 'immunisation' and 'vaccination' tend now to be used synonymously by many people.

Vaccination is used to make large proportions of populations actively immune to bacterial or viral diseases such that the host is able to generate an active antibody immune response to combat an infectious agent. The agent administered (usually by injection) can be living but modified (e.g. yellow fever), a suspension of killed organisms (e.g. whooping cough (pertussis)), or an inactivated toxin (such as tetanus). The aim is to generate an immune response in those vaccinated, which will protect them from serious disease should they later be challenged with that organism. Killed organisms provide a limited immunity and may have to be given as a starter dose with boosters to provide optimal protection. Vaccines can also be given in pulses (repeated doses over time) to maximise immunity. Live, attenuated vaccines such as the oral polio vaccine provide better cover. These tend to be for viral infections. Sometimes a temporary, passive immunity can be generated with antibodies, for example immunoglobulins against varicella are given to pregnant women who may have come into contact with chicken pox. In this case the body does not produce its own antibodies but depends upon pre-produced antibodies.

Immunisation may be general or targeted. General vaccination aims to eradicate, eliminate or contain infection similarly to other control methods. For example, mass measles vaccination resulted in a 78% drop in measles deaths between 2000 and 2008 worldwide. However, targeted vaccine programmes can sometimes be more effective than mass vaccination. Box 10.2 shows smallpox as an example. Influenza is another example of vaccination that is targeted at those most at risk and aims to contain infection.

No vaccine is 100% effective as individuals mount different immune responses, which last varying amounts of time. However, it is not necessary for every person to be immune. *Herd immunity* is the degree to which a population is resistant to an infection as high general levels of immunity protect the non-immune. Herd immunity is an important concept in health protection and can be thought of as the immunity of a community. The basic reproductive rate (R_0) is the mean number of new cases generated by each case of a disease and can be imagined as the potential for growth of a disease epidemic. If $R_0 > 1$, a disease will continue to spread unless control measures are initiated. The R_0 of measles is 12–18, for example. However, if there is adequate herd immunity (i.e. enough people have been vaccinated and had a good response), the reproductive rate becomes less than one and the incidence of cases falls. This is why the coverage rate for vaccinations is considered important. If fewer people are vaccinated the herd immunity drops and outbreaks of a disease occur. The proportion of a population which needs to be vaccinated to prevent sustained spread is given by $1 - 1/R_0$.

Box 10.2 Targeted vaccination – smallpox

When the incidence of smallpox was high the dangers of vaccination (the vaccine causes death in approximately one in a million people) were vastly outweighed by the protection and reduction in mortality provided by the vaccine. As the occurrence of the disease declined, mass vaccination was not warranted but when an outbreak occurred all susceptible individuals in the defined area around the outbreak were vaccinated to contain the spread of disease (termed ring vaccination) [3].

What proportion of the population needs to be vaccinated to provide herd immunity for measles?

Proportion = $1-1/R_0$

$= 1-1/18$

$= 96\%$

This is occurring in the UK with measles. Although the WHO recommended coverage above 95% [4] in the UK coverage falls below 90%. Low uptake and incomplete coverage of vaccination in earlier years (partly due to low vaccine stocks and partly due to public apprehension around the MMR vaccine fueled by negative media coverage) have resulted in an upswing in the number of measles outbreaks occurring in the UK.

The population need for a vaccine is determined by consideration of the characteristics of the disease and then vaccines are developed through clinical trials in much the same way as new drugs are. For example, a vaccine for meningococcal group C was introduced to the UK in 1999 because meningococcal disease, whilst quite rare (815 cases reported in England and Wales in 1998), is so devastating that a vaccine programme was considered cost-effective. The incidence has now fallen significantly (10 cases in 2009).

The aims of vaccination programmes vary depending on the disease and whether the control intended is eradication, elimination or containment. In general, vaccine coverage in the more-developed regions is higher. This means that more booster vaccinations may be given in less-developed countries in attempts to improve coverage. Not all infectious diseases have effective vaccines (for example, Dengue fever) and not all countries need programmes for all the vaccines available. For example, hepatitis B vaccination is currently given in many countries where the infection is endemic and primarily transmitted in childhood but not in the UK as the incidence is insufficiently high to justify widespread vaccination. Thus, knowing the burden of diseases in various populations determines the vaccine policy developed. Hence, vaccination schedules differ by country depending on the local epidemiology of vaccine-preventable diseases.

Can you list four characteristics that should determine the ideal immunization schedule for a country or region?

Four features of a good immunization schedule are: epidemiological relevance, immunological effectiveness, operational feasibility and social acceptability. Ensuring adequate vaccine for targeted diseases is a major industry and public health can provide useful advice to those developing and manufacturing vaccines through support for clinical vaccine trials as well as supporting the delivery of vaccines to target audiences, for example by managing the maintenance of a cold chain where necessary. This can be particularly problematic in developing countries. Public and professional attitudes to vaccination as well as the complexity of decision making when individual risk and community benefit are involved mean that public health workers also have a role in educating the public and professionals about vaccination. At a national level, the management of programmes also includes vaccine funding and surveillance to monitor vaccination uptake and targets.

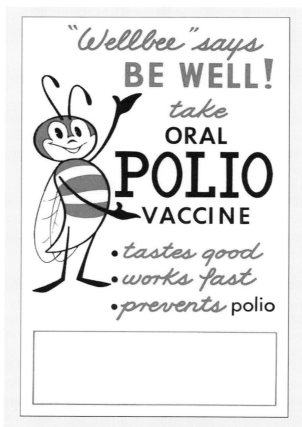

1963 Poster encouraging polio vaccination in the United States. Due to a comprehensive vaccination programme, the last cases of naturally acquired paralytic polio in the USA were in 1979

The 2011 vaccination schedule for the UK is given in Table 10.2. Use the Internet to find current vaccination schedules for the USA and India. Think about what action would be needed if a new vaccine was to be added to the schedule. More information about immunisation can be found on the World Health Organization website.

Identifying threats, planning and monitoring control measures – surveillance

The practice of surveillance, monitoring diseases through measuring morbidity and mortality, arose in the fourteenth and fifteenth centuries with the Black Death. In this

Table 10.2 2011 UK vaccination schedule

Age	Vaccine
Neonates	BCG (high-risk groups only)
	Hepatitis B (high-risk groups only)
2, 3 + 4 months	Three-dose primary course of: diphtheria/tetanus/pertussis/inactivated polio vaccine/*Haemophilus influenza* type b (DTaP/IPV/Hib)
	Meningococcal *C* (MenC)
	Pneumococcal conjugate vaccine (PCV) given at 2 and 4 months
12–13 months	One-dose primary course of: measles/mumps/rubella (MMR)
	PCV
	Hib/MenC
3 years 4 months–5 years	One-dose booster of: lower-dose (d) or full-dose (D) diphtheria/tetanus/pertussis/inactivated polio vaccine (dTaP/IPV or DTaP/IPV)
	MMR
13–18 years	One-does of booster of: dTa/IPV
Girls aged 12 to 13 years	Three-does course of human papillomavirus (HPV) types 16 and 18 (as protection against cervical cancer)
65 years	Influenza
	Pneumococcal polysaccharide vaccine (PPV)
Any age	Boosters for tetanus and polio if appropriate
	Influenza, pneumococcal vaccine, Hib, MenC, Hepatitis B (medical or lifestyle risk groups)
	Travel vaccines

case, authorities wanted to be aware of ships with infected people aboard in order to prevent them coming ashore and infecting others. Surveillance can be defined as the on-going, systematic collection, collation and analysis of data and the prompt dissemination of the resulting information to those who need to know so that action can be taken.

Surveillance is used to identify individual cases of disease so that action can be taken to prevent spread (for example, excluding food handlers from work if they contract food poisoning). This can also be used over time to detect changes in trend or distribution in order to initiate investigative or control measures. A microbiology laboratory, for example, might notice several cases of legionella infection and trigger an investigation into the possible source in order to prevent further cases. Trends in infection which are continuously monitored through surveillance systems can indicate changes in risk factors or that certain elements of a population are at increased risk (for example, a rise in sexually transmitted infections in young women). This allows interventions to be targeted appropriately. Knowing the epidemiology of infectious diseases in close to real time through surveillance can help to evaluate current control measures such as vaccination programmes. A fall in incidence may

Box 10.3 What makes a good surveillance system?

Clear objectives. The system can then be evaluated to ensure that it is relevant to the needs of the population covered.

Clear case definitions. Clear definitions are needed for the conditions under surveillance so that the same thing is counted accurately all the time. Data need to flow from clear sources to a clear collection point.

Easy reporting mechanisms. These will maximise the number of cases reported and useful, timely feedback to reporters encourages participation and enables action.

allow control measures to be relaxed. For example, it is no longer necessary to vaccinate against smallpox. Lastly, and very importantly, surveillance allows new infections to be detected and hypotheses produced regarding their causes. Many countries have communicable disease surveillance programmes, which carry out these functions.

Surveillance is, however, resource-intensive and it is important to make it as simple as possible to get the maximum amount of data reported (see Box 10.3). Reports generally come from individuals dealing with the diseases in question – clinicians and public health professionals or from information on laboratory diagnoses. The type and importance of the disease determines the type of surveillance. In some cases, reporting is mandatory; 'notifiable diseases' in the UK and the USA must be reported by doctors. It may, however, be preferable for surveillance to be voluntary and anonymous. Such is the case for HIV in the UK, which is monitored in annual surveys and where it is not possible to identify an individual patient from the data collected. In some infections, as with the HIV surveillance, it is not practical to collect details of every case. Representative samples can be taken and the true rates of disease extrapolated from them.

Containing infection – outbreak investigation

When preventative measures fail (or when control was only ever going to contain the disease, not eradicate or eliminate infection), then control measures must be used retrospectively to contain the infection to as few people as possible. The management of an outbreak of a food-borne illness is a good example of how outbreaks are investigated and control measures implemented although the methods used can be applied to any infectious disease. How such an investigation might progress is described here and it highlights the stages and important points of such an investigation. In reality, the stages will not always occur in order. See Figure 10.1 and the report in Figure 10.2.

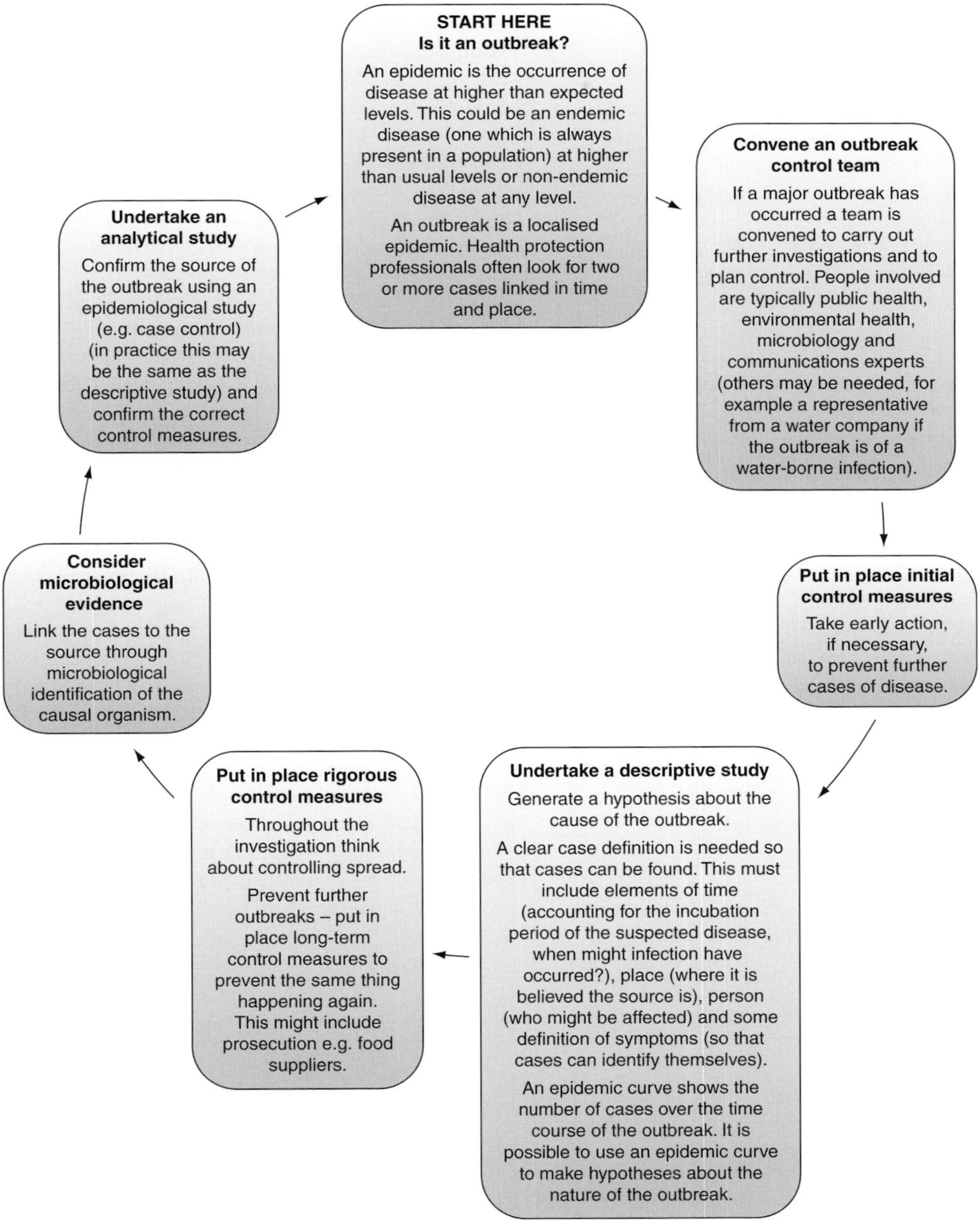

START HERE
Is it an outbreak?

An epidemic is the occurrence of disease at higher than expected levels. This could be an endemic disease (one which is always present in a population) at higher than usual levels or non-endemic disease at any level.

An outbreak is a localised epidemic. Health protection professionals often look for two or more cases linked in time and place.

Convene an outbreak control team

If a major outbreak has occurred a team is convened to carry out further investigations and to plan control. People involved are typically public health, environmental health, microbiology and communications experts (others may be needed, for example a representative from a water company if the outbreak is of a water-borne infection).

Undertake an analytical study

Confirm the source of the outbreak using an epidemiological study (e.g. case control) (in practice this may be the same as the descriptive study) and confirm the correct control measures.

Consider microbiological evidence

Link the cases to the source through microbiological identification of the causal organism.

Put in place initial control measures

Take early action, if necessary, to prevent further cases of disease.

Put in place rigorous control measures

Throughout the investigation think about controlling spread.

Prevent further outbreaks – put in place long-term control measures to prevent the same thing happening again. This might include prosecution e.g. food suppliers.

Undertake a descriptive study

Generate a hypothesis about the cause of the outbreak.

A clear case definition is needed so that cases can be found. This must include elements of time (accounting for the incubation period of the suspected disease, when might infection have occurred?), place (where it is believed the source is), person (who might be affected) and some definition of symptoms (so that cases can identify themselves).

An epidemic curve shows the number of cases over the time course of the outbreak. It is possible to use an epidemic curve to make hypotheses about the nature of the outbreak.

Figure 10.1   Outbreak investigation stages.

Local pub in outbreak close down shocker!

Last week, on Sunday 6th August, 17 unlucky people all had a lovely lunch at the Golden Lion but over the next few days came down with serious vomiting and diarrhoea!

The local health protection team rushed to take action and, after deciding an outbreak of food poisoning was the likely cause formed an outbreak control team to sort it out.

On Sunday, Dr Christopher Jones, the public health specialist in charge told us "We are working with the environmental health officer and microbiologist to find the cause and prevent more people becoming ill. In the meantime the pub will not be serving food."

The landlord, Bob, waited with baited breath for the results of the initial investigation. Bob told us "The food hygiene people have been round, took the leftovers from Sunday lunch and checked all our kitchens were cleaned thoroughly and our staff trained in food safety. I don't know yet what's happened but we'll be open again soon!"

Dr Jones' team asked all the local GPs to find any other cases for them – anyone who had eaten at Bob's place between the 4th and the 6th – and produced this descriptive graph of who got sick when.

This shows there was one source of the bug, i.e. people who attended the Sunday lunch became ill. The experts say if people were then infecting each other, the chart would show more little peaks after the first big one.

We interviewed Dr Stephen Smith, the microbiologist, on Tuesday. He had the unenviable job of trying to identify the bug responsible from all the samples of stools the sufferers were kind enough to give him.... lovely! Dr Smith says "This is important because we need to try to link the organisms causing the sickness with any found in the foodstuffs. Also, control measures vary dependent upon the causal organism. E coli 0157, for example, is an important cause of food poisoning, and due to its serious nature is followed up carefully. All those who come into contact with a known case are investigated. In particular, food handlers, those caring for vulnerable people and those with poor personal hygiene are excluded from work or school until it is clear they are no longer carrying the organism. In this case, we have found the same bug in the stool samples and the beef from Sunday lunch so we've found the problem."

Dr Jones contacted the paper again on Friday to tell us the outcome of his full investigation. "We have carried out a full analytical study and determined that the undercooked roast beef was the cause. The landlord of the Golden Lion has cooperated fully, the kitchens have been thoroughly cleaned and some of his staff have had food hygiene training. The environmental health department are not planning to prosecute and the pub is now open for business again."

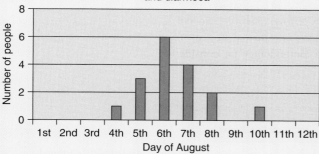

Epidemic curve for Golden Lion outbreak of vomiting and diarrhoea

Figure 10.2 An outbreak of food poisoning, as reported in a 'daily local newspaper'.

Table 10.3 Examples of sources, pathways and receptors for some environmental hazards

SOURCE	PATHWAY	RECEPTOR
Chemical spillage from tanker crash	Air	Grazing cattle
	Ground	Man
	Rivers	Allotment vegetables
Oil dump into the ocean	Ocean water	Wild fowl
		Fish
Factory fire, ash and smoke	Air	Man
		Wild life
		Crops

Environmental public health

Environmental hazards to health include chemicals released into the air, contaminated water sources or industrial accidents. The medical model of control applied to communicable disease control serves less well in these circumstances. Here, the environmental model (also called the pollutant linkage model and source–pathway–receptor model) is used. Methods to control the hazard are determined by identifying the source, the pathway and the receptor (Table 10.3).

The receptor need not be human – it may be animal or vegetable. Pathways can be air, water or ground. An example might be the release of a toxic chemical into the environment due to a road accident and a tanker spillage. The crashed tanker is the source. Pathways for this hazardous chemical to become a problem may be through the air if it is a fine powder or volatile liquid, through the ground if it leaks onto a porous surface such as fields, or through water if it enters a water course. From here it may reach a variety of receptors – plant life through soil or water, and then animal life directly or via eating the plants. Animal life may also be affected directly from exposure to airborne matter. This model provides a methodology for considering where the path from source to receptor can be interrupted or contamination prevented.

So we can think about containing an environmental hazard in a similar way to containing the hazards from communicable diseases – consider how the hazard transmits its effects to us and find ways to interrupt this.

In addition to this, there are more complex areas of environmental health that a public health practitioner might be called upon to contribute to. See the following exercise for examples of these.

Table 10.4 Environmental hazards

	Source	Pathway	Potential health effects
1	Nuclear waste spillage	Water, ground or air	Radiation poisoning
2	Gastro-intestinal disease organisms in flood water	Water, food	Intestinal infection/food poisoning
3	Radiation from radio masts	Air	Increase in leukaemia incidence
4	Earthquake	Ground	Physical injury from falling buildings
5	Volcanic ash	Air	Respiratory effects
6	Loud neighbours or new airport runway	Air	Psychological distress
7	Poor workstation posture	N/A	Repetitive strain injury
8	Terrorist chemical attack	Air or water	Toxic effects dependent upon chemical used
9	Poor building design	N/A	Low physical-activity levels and adverse health effects
10	Second-hand smoke in public places	Air	Increased lung cancer, coronary heart disease
11	Exposure to radon in the home	Air	Lung cancer

Table 10.4 shows some environmental hazards which a public health practitioner may be called upon to control. In each case the receptor of interest is humans. For each hazard, what approaches to control might be relevant?

1. The best control measure for prevention of radiation poisoning is avoidance so removing people from the risk area for a period of time is important. Specialist decontamination may also be possible depending on the radiation source.
2. Specialist decontamination, aid, provision of bottled water, drainage.
3. An epidemiological analysis of the likelihood of an increase in disease being due to chance alone often proves no link.
4. Adequate emergency health facilities, search and rescue.
5. Relocation.
6. Mediation or environmental/health impact assessment is a set of tools to ascertain the extent of likely health effects and mitigate these via new policy.
7. Workplace assessment, provision of supports such as foot rests.
8. See emergency planning section below for how emergencies are planned for and dealt with.
9. Impact assessment during planning stages to provide healthy building design.
10. Legislation.
11. Installation of radon-protection measures such as membranes under floors.

It is important to note that some environmental hazards result from occupational sources and the effects of these and their modification are often dealt with by specialist occupational health practitioners. Some important areas of occupational health in a range of countries including the UK, Australia and the USA include the protection of the workforce from infectious diseases (e.g. hepatitis C in health-care workers), occupational cancers and mental disorders (e.g. work-related stress), physical injuries (e.g. related to poor workstation posture, physical trips and falls and lifting injuries) and chemical injuries (such as asbestosis and chemical burns).

In each case the tools needed are those already highlighted in previous chapters, the effective use of epidemiological methods and risk assessment. A good public health toolkit will contain all the necessary spanners and wrenches needed to get to grips with the investigation of an environmental health issue.

Preparing for emergencies

Another specialist area within the field of health protection is disaster or emergency planning and response. There are a variety of interpretations of the words 'disaster' and 'emergency'. The UK Civil Contingencies Act of 2004 states that an emergency is an event or situation which threatens serious damage to human welfare; an event or situation which threatens serious damage to the environment; or war, or terrorism, which threatens serious damage to security. The United Nations International Strategy for Disaster Reduction states that a disaster is a serious disruption of the functioning of a community or a society causing widespread human, material, economic or environmental losses, which exceed the ability of the affected community or society to cope using its own resources.

Figure 10.3 shows the cycle of action which surrounds the planning for and response to disasters.

Imagine how the disaster cycle could be used to deal with a range of disaster scenarios. You could think, for example, about floods, volcanoes, terrorist attacks, the emergence of a new disease, a breakdown in fuel supply, a hurricane.

Box 10.4 Quantifying risk

- Risk (probability of harmful consequences)
- Hazard (phenomenon which has the potential to cause harm)
- Vulnerability (capacity of a community to cope)

  Risk = Hazard × Vulnerability [5]

Figure 10.3   Disaster cycle.

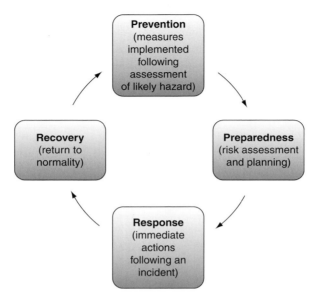

Beginning with preparedness, quantifying the scale of the risk to populations (Box 10.4) is important in prioritising planning and is dependent upon the nature of the hazard and the vulnerability of communities.

Sometimes the scale of the hazard is expressed as hazard × exposure and the vulnerability of a community may be assessed as the balance between its various vulnerabilities and its capacities. An additional factor may be added, deficiencies in preparedness, which becomes a multiplier in the equation. An example of using this framework is included in the Internet Companion.

Three main types of emergency are planned for: those which creep up on us like a rising tide, those that hit with a 'big bang' and those which emerge completely out of the blue. In many countries this planning process is highly organised. In the UK, the Civil Contingencies Secretariat of the Cabinet Office co-ordinates the planning process and in the USA the Federal Emergency Management Agency is part of the Department of Homeland Security and leads the process. Other governments have similar bodies such as the Indian Ministry of Home Affairs National Disaster Management Division. In the process of planning for disasters the role of the health sector is to identify threats, deal with mass casualties and deaths as well as, potentially, mass vaccination. With partners in local government, the emergency services and those in the armed forces, health-care organisations form the front line in responding to a wide range of incidents and have the primary responsibility for protecting health and maintaining health-care services during the emergency and restoring health afterwards. All agencies must also plan to maintain business continuity during times of disaster when the workforce may be significantly depleted due to illness, death or

---

Box 10.5 Disaster planning for a flu pandemic

We can use the disaster cycle to illustrate elements of how public health workers plan for and respond to an emergency such as a flu pandemic.

Prevention
Minimisation of opportunities for a highly pathogenic strain of animal influenza to acquire the ability to transmit to humans (e.g. slaughter or vaccination of bird flocks to prevent H5N1 transmission to humans).

Preparedness
Business continuity planning to deal with illness and absenteeism in the health-care sector:
- stockpiling of anti-viral drugs and plans for distributing them;
- media awareness campaigns;
- worldwide surveillance of circulating virus strains.

Response
Rapid, co-ordinated development of case definitions and diagnostic tools:
- rapid development of treatment guidelines, vaccines, etc.;
- identification of at-risk staff and implementation of increased safety measures;
- isolation and treatment of cases;
- development of supply chains for antiviral drugs and vaccines;
- staff sharing to enable learning and cover of necessary functions;
- development of alternative access for maintaining urgent and intensive care when some centres may be closed due to mass infection;
- management en masse of infected casualties.

Recovery
Additional services to manage increased waiting lists due to cancelled procedures:
- cover arrangements for any staff who have worked overtime;
- provision of counselling for staff.

---

absenteeism. Box 10.5 illustrates how the health sector plans for a flu pandemic, a disaster for planning purposes as it could kill large numbers of people. In the 2009 H1N1 pandemic, fewer infections and deaths were experienced than were planned for but many of the measures planned for were instigated during the pandemic wave to reduce the anticipated impact.

Conclusion

The field of health protection encompasses the disciplines and services which respond to threats to human health. In the UK, health protection is seen as one third of public health alongside health improvement and health-care quality but in reality the three domains are inseparable and always overlapping. The tools we have covered in other chapters in this section must be applied to the domain of health protection and the skills specific to health protection are applicable in other domains of public health.

REFERENCES

1. D. S. Shepard., J. A. Walsh, E. Kleinau, S. Stansfield and S. Bhalotra, Setting priorities for the Children's Vaccine Initiative: A cost-effectiveness approach. *Vaccine*, **13** (8), 1995, 707–14.
2. J. G. Bartlett, N. Moon, T. W. Chang, N. Taylor and A. B. Onderdonk, Role of *Clostridium difficile* in antibiotic-associated pseudomembranous colitis. *Gastroenterology* **75**, 1978, 778–82.
3. D. T. Karzon, Smallpox vaccination: The end of an era. *Acta Medica Scandinavica* **197**, 1975, 29–38. doi: 10.1111/j.0954–6820.1975.tb14805.x.
4. Eliminating measles and rubella and preventing congenital rubella infection: European Region strategic plan 2005–2010. *WHO European Region*, 2005.
5. The World Health Organization, *Risk Reduction and Emergency Preparedness: WHO Six Year Strategy for the Health-Sector and Community Capacity Development*, Geneva, WHO, 2007, p. 8. See: http://www.who.int/hac/techguidance/preparedness/emergency_preparedness_eng.pdf.

11

Improving quality of care
Nicholas Steel and Stephen Gillam

Key points

- Good-quality health-care makes a large contribution to public health, both by increasing life expectancy and improving quality of life.
- Quality can be defined; it is multidimensional. The different dimensions of quality can be measured, but some (e.g. clinical effectiveness) are easier to measure than others (e.g. professionals' empathy for patients).
- Problems with quality of care are widespread, with many people either not receiving effective health-care, or receiving care that is ineffective or harmful.
- Evaluation of an intervention attempts to determine objectively whether the activity in question is meeting its objectives.
- Assessing the impact of public health interventions in the short term can present particular challenges.
- Clinical governance refers to the systems through which NHS organisations and staff are accountable for the quality of patient care.

Introduction

As we saw in the introductory chapter, effective health-care makes a large and increasing contribution to preventing disease and prolonging life, by reducing the population burden of disease. However, only the right kind of health-care can improve health. Health-care interventions that are powerful enough to improve population health are also powerful enough to cause harm if incorrectly used. The last part of the planning cycle to which you were introduced in Chapter 6 concerns evaluation. How can public health specialists know whether their interventions are having the desired effect? Clinicians can monitor the impact of their treatments on an individual patient

Essential Public Health, Second Edition, ed. Stephen Gillam, Jan Yates and Padmanabhan Badrinath.
Published by Cambridge University Press. © Cambridge University Press 2012.

basis but how do we examine the impact of a new service? In this chapter, we will look at what we mean by quality of care and consider one well-known framework for its evaluation. We will consider ways in which quality of care is promoted across the NHS.

What is quality and can it be measured?

The science of quality measurement in health-care is still young, but it is already generally accepted that quality of health-care can be defined, and that elements of quality can be measured. Some dimensions of quality, such as clinical effectiveness, are more straightforward to define and measure quantitatively than 'softer' dimensions such as patient-centred health-care. As quality measurement becomes commonplace in health-care, there remain concerns that attempts to measure something as complex as quality will inevitably undermine professionalism and the doctor–patient relationship. Paradoxically, measurement may thus reduce overall quality of care. A more widely held view is that measurement is an essential component of quality improvement. If we do not measure quality, we cannot know whether health services are achieving the level of population health benefit of which they are potentially capable.

Quality has been defined as: 'the degree to which health services for individuals and populations increase the likelihood of desired health outcomes and are consistent with current professional knowledge' [1]. 'Desired health outcomes' is a key phrase as it deliberately does not specify who is doing the desiring. It implicitly accepts that different people will want different outcomes.

A 72-year-old woman with osteoarthritis of her left hip is booked for a total hip replacement operation. She also suffers from diabetes and mild high blood pressure.
- **List as many aspects of good-quality of care in this situation as you can**.
- **Who should be involved in assessing quality of care?**
- **Describe the likely concerns of the different individuals and groups involved in this situation**.

Desired health outcomes may be different for managers, patients and clinicians [2]. Managers may be rightly concerned with efficiency, and seek to maximise the population health gain through best use of an inevitably limited budget. Clinicians are usually more focused on effectiveness, and want the treatment that works best for each of their patients. Patients clearly want treatment that works, and also place a high priority on how the treatment is delivered. Coulter has described the following health-care aspirations of patients [3]:
- fast access to reliable health advice;
- effective treatment delivered by trusted professionals;
- participation in decisions and respect for preferences;
- clear, comprehensible information and support for self care;

- attention to physical and environmental needs;
- emotional support, empathy and respect;
- involvement of, and support for, family and carers;
- continuity of care and smooth transitions.

Dimensions of quality and their evaluation

Quality in health-care means doing the right thing, at the right time, in the right way, to the right person – and having the best possible results. A more formal framework is provided by Maxwell who described six dimensions to quality [4]:
- effectiveness (achieves intended benefit);
- acceptability (satisfies reasonable expectations);
- efficiency (making the best use of available resources);
- accessibility (those who need services will receive them);
- equity (resources are fairly shared);
- relevance (treatments are appropriate to their particular target groups).

These six dimensions of quality are often simplified to three: clinical effectiveness, patient safety and patient experience. These three are used by the Department of Health in England [5], and by NICE in the development of quality standards (http://www.nice.org.uk/guidance/qualitystandards/moreinfoaboutnicequalitystandards.jsp).

Of course, it is not only health professionals who are interested in the quality of care they provide – as media interest in medical mishaps reminds us. Managers in hospitals and health authorities are charged to monitor quality as part of clinical governance (see page 194 below). Whether as users or voters, the general population have a great interest in the quality of health-care, and patients' priorities may differ from the priorities of health-care providers. Patients may place clear information, caring communication and outcomes that improve activities of daily living higher up their list than technical aspects of care, which may be difficult to assess.

Evaluation has been defined as 'a process that attempts to determine as systematically and objectively as possible the relevance, effectiveness and impact of activities in the light of their objectives' [6]. A successful evaluation will tell us whether the intervention makes a difference, and whether the difference is worth the cost.

Where do we start when thinking about evaluation of a delivery system in the NHS? Avedis Donabedian, a guru in quality-improvement circles, distinguished four elements [7]:
- structure (buildings, staff, equipment);
- process (all that is done to patients);
- outputs (immediate results of medical intervention);
- outcomes (gains in health status).

Thus, for example, an evaluation of the national screening programme for colorectal cancer may consider:

- the volume and costs of new equipment (colonoscopic, radiographic, histopatho-logical), staff and buildings (structure);
- the numbers of patients screened, coverage rates within a defined age range, numbers of true and false positives (process);
- number of cancers identified, operations performed (outputs);
- complication rates, colorectal cancer incidence, prevalence and mortality rates (outcomes).

This distinction between process and outcome measures is helpful for at least two reasons. First, because for many interventions it may be difficult to obtain robust data on health outcomes unless large numbers are scrutinised over long periods. For example, evaluating the quality of hypertension management within a general practice, you may be reliant on process measures (e.g. the proportion of the appropriate population screened, treated and adequately controlled) as a proxy for good outcomes. The assumption here is that evidence from larger-scale studies showing that control of hypertension reduces subsequent death rates from heart disease will be reflected in your own practice population's health experience. Second, one of the biggest problems in evaluating large-scale public health inter-ventions is the effect of the many different factors influencing outcomes: back-ground 'noise'. For example, assessing the impact of mass media campaigns on smoking prevalence might be complicated by the impact of new laws to prevent smoking in public places, changes to the national curriculum, increased taxation on cigarettes or background decline in the population prevalence of smoking. Similarly, it is difficult to measure the contribution of fruit and vegetable provision to, for example, reduction in bowel cancer rates, due to the multifactorial nature of the determinants of bowel cancer.

Thinking about the care provided for people with a particular disease, evaluation – like resource allocation – can also be considered in terms of different elements of their care: prevention, diagnosis, treatment and rehabilitation.

Use a structure, process, output, outcome model to consider what measures might be relevant to the evaluation of the following services:
1. **Smoking cessation service.**
2. **Immunisation programmes.**
3. **Breast screening programme.**
4. **Cardiac rehabilitation services.**
5. **Hip replacement for osteoarthritis.**
6. **Chronic-disease management (e.g. diabetes in general practice).**
7. **National programmes to Roll Back Malaria.**

Examples of measures that might be relevant for evaluation
1. Smoking cessation service:
   - number of smokers seen and counselled;
   - prescriptions for nicotine replacement therapy dispensed;

- quit rates, costs (of material/staff etc.);
- trends in smoking prevalence;
- death rates from smoking-related diseases.

2. Immunisation programmes:
   - numbers of vaccines administered;
   - proportion of target population covered;
   - costs (of vaccines distributed, maintaining cold chain, other disposables, staff deployed etc.);
   - disease incidence rates over time.

3. Breast screening programme:
   - numbers of mammograms carried out;
   - abnormality detection rates;
   - false positives at lumpectomy;
   - proportion of target population covered, breast cancer incidence (falling or rising?);
   - long-term mortality trends;
   - costs.

4. Cardiac rehabilitation services:
   - numbers passing through programme;
   - numbers as a proportion of all patients admitted with diagnosis of myocardial infarction (MI), and as a proportion of all of those meeting appropriate referral criteria;
   - percentages of patients in programme receiving recommended interventions post MI (aspirin, beta blockers, statins if not contraindicated);
   - impact on patients' quality of life;
   - costs;
   - long-term re-infarction rates.

5. Hip replacement for osteoarthritis:
   - numbers of operations performed;
   - lengths of stay;
   - infection or other complication rates;
   - readmission rates;
   - proportion of patients requiring surgical revision;
   - costs (prostheses, hospital stay and rehabilitation);
   - numbers on waiting lists;
   - length of waiting;
   - prevalence of unmet need within local community;
   - patient satisfaction surveys;
   - impact on quality of life/activities of daily living.

6. Chronic disease management (e.g. diabetes in general practice):
   - numbers on disease register;
   - proportion receiving annual check (e.g. retinal screening);

- proportion meeting appropriate standards for criteria of good care (e.g. blood pressure below 140/90 mm Hg, glycosylated haemoglobin (HbA1c) less than 53 mmol/mol (7%), etc.);
- proportion of patients with management plan;
- costs;
- rates of disease-related complications.

7. National programmes to Roll Back Malaria:
   - numbers of people treated with artemesinin-based medications;
   - measures of distribution of insecticide-treated bednets;
   - numbers/level of staff trained;
   - spending on malaria-related activities in health and education sectors;
   - outcomes – morbidity and mortality rates (especially in high-risk groups such as mothers and children).

Remember that readily available measures of quality are not necessarily the most important and the most important elements of quality may not be easily measurable. For example, with their interest in equity of provision, public health specialists need to consider the accessibility of services particularly to disadvantaged groups.

Can you think of other factors that might complicate the evaluation of public health interventions?

The evaluation might be complicated by the complexity of the determinants of disease and of interventions designed to prevent them, as well as by the long time lag between some interventions and their expected effect (e.g. efforts to improve food labelling will not swiftly affect obesity levels).

Is there a problem with quality?

We have seen that health-care is a powerful tool for improving public health. Like all powerful tools, it can have adverse as well as positive effects. Problems with health-care fall into one of three broad categories: underuse, overuse and misuse, all of which are amenable to public health action [8]. Effective health-care can be underused, so that people miss out on opportunities to benefit from it. It can be overused, wasting resources by delivering care to those who do not need it, or where the potential for harm exceeds the benefit. Misuse is where patients suffer avoidable complications of surgery or medication. An example of misuse is a patient who suffers a rash after receiving penicillin as treatment for an infection, despite having a known allergy to penicillin.

We know that some effective health-care is underused. Many effective interventions are only received by half the people who should receive them [9]. There is also great variability in the quality of care experienced by different populations, by illness, age, sex, race, wealth, geographic location and insurance coverage. This problem of inequalities or disparities has been the focus of considerable policy attention, helped by Julian Tudor Hart's devising of his famous Inverse Care Law 'as a weapon' over thirty years ago [10] (see also Chapter 15):

The availability of good medical care tends to vary inversely with the need for it in the population served. This ... operates more completely where medical care is most exposed to market forces, and less so where such exposure is reduced. The market distribution of medical care is a primitive and historically outdated social form, and any return to it would further exaggerate the maldistribution of medical resources.

We also know that care is overused. Wennberg first documented the wide variations in care received by similar populations. He showed that health-care is often driven by the availability of specialist services, rather than by the health needs of the population, with no detectable difference in health outcomes [11]. This variation in quantity of health-care with no apparent relationship with quality implies that some health-care is over-used. People are receiving more care than they have the capacity to benefit from.

Harm resulting from misuse of health-care is a major problem. Adverse drug events have been shown to cause considerable morbidity, mortality and cost in the UK and USA [12]. About 850,000 'adverse events' occur in the NHS each year involving 10% of admissions and costing an estimated 2 billion pounds per year. Four hundred people die or are seriously injured in events involving medical devices. Nearly 10,000 people are reported to experience serious adverse reactions to drugs. Two infective agents alone, methicillin-resistant *Staphylococcus aureus* and *Clostridium difficile*, contribute to the deaths of around 9000 people annually in England [13].

Four reasons have been identified for the widespread problems with quality [1]:

1. The growing complexity of science and technology. Our ability to deliver safe effective health-care cannot keep up with the rapid advances in science and medical treatments.
2. The increase in chronic conditions. People are now living longer, and chronic conditions are the major cause of disability and death, and consume the majority of health-care resources in developed countries.
3. Poorly organised delivery systems. Most health-care systems are still designed to deal primarily with acute health problems, and lack an effective chronic care model.
4. Constraints on exploiting the revolution in information technology.

None of these reasons for widespread quality problems lays the blame on individual clinicians making mistakes. They emphasise that quality is a property of health systems, and not simply of the health professionals in the system. Human beings will always make occasional mistakes, and experience from other industries has shown that dramatic quality improvement can occur when systems are designed that do not rely on humans avoiding mistakes. A graphic recent example was provided during the inquiry into multiple failures at the Mid Staffordshire Foundation NHS Trust ([14]; see Internet Companion). Some of the main approaches used to improve quality in health-care are described in the next section.

Table 11.1 Approaches to quality improvement in health-care

Type of approach	Example
Regulation and standards	American Board of Medical Specialties in USA General Medical Council in UK
Education, audit, development and dissemination of best practice	Health-care organisations, Royal Colleges, professional organisations
Market and financial	Payment of British general practitioners according to achievement of performance indicators

How can quality of care for populations be improved?

Many different approaches to quality improvement in health-care have been tried in the past, with varying levels of success. They can be broadly classified into three groups, as summarised in Table 11.1.

Regulation and standards

A robust regulatory framework is important for assuring a basic standard of health-care, and regulation of medical professionals is a central component of quality improvement in nearly all countries. Historically, regulation has been primarily associated with the medical profession, but is increasingly used for non-medical health professionals. Sutherland and Leatherman have described the three main purposes of professional regulation: to set minimally acceptable standards of care, to provide accountability of professionals to patients and payers, and to improve quality of care by providing guidance about best practice [15].

In the UK, the General Medical Council regulates doctors, with a specialist register for public health and a separate regulatory system in place for non-medical public health specialists. These are currently adapting to a new environment where greater levels of public accountability are required. The Care Quality Commission (http://www.cqc.org.uk/) assesses the performance of health-care organisations in England. In the USA, the American Board of Medical Specialties oversees certification of doctors. The requirements are a mixture of accredited training, cognitive examination, competency-based evaluation, audit and clinical performance, and certification needs to be renewed every 6 to 10 years. Certification status has been shown to be associated with higher quality of care [15]. Accreditation of US hospitals for Medicare reimbursement takes place through the Joint Commission on Accreditation of Health-care Organisations.

Standards of care can be set out in guidelines such as those published by the National Institute for Health and Clinical Excellence (NICE) and the Scottish

Intercollegiate Guidelines Network (SIGN) in the UK, and the US Preventive Services Task Force (USPSTF) in the USA.

A good example of the method by which standards of care are developed is the RAND/UCLA appropriateness method [16]. This was developed in response to the lack of randomised controlled clinical trial data on many interventions, and the problems with interpreting sometimes contradictory trial results for use in routine care. It combines research data with clinical expertise, and involves the following stages:

1. Identifying clinical area(s) of care for quality assessment.
2. Conducting a systematic review of care in the relevant clinical area(s).
3. Drafting quality indicators.
4. Presenting draft quality indicators and their evidence base to a clinical panel for a modified Delphi process. The Delphi process typically involves asking panel members to anonymously rate the draft indicators for validity, over two rounds with face-to-face discussion between rounds.
5. Approving a final set of indicators.

The quality standards produced by methods such as this can be used to assess the quality of care in a single clinic or a whole health system. An example of quality assessment on a very large scale is the payment of incentives to general practitioners in the UK on the basis of their performance against quality indicators. Table 11.2 gives examples of indicators from the 2009–10 revision of the British general practitioners' contract [17].

Table 11.2 Examples of clinical domains and indicators for UK general practitioners 2009–10 [17]

Clinical domain	No. of indicators	Example of indicator in each clinical domain
Hypertension	3	The percentage of patients with hypertension in whom there is a record of the blood pressure in the previous 9 months
Asthma	4	The percentage of patients aged 8 and over diagnosed as having asthma from 1 April with measures of variability or reversibility
Depression	3	In those patients with a new diagnosis of depression, recorded between the preceding 1 April to 31 March, the percentage of patients who have had an assessment of severity at the outset of treatment using an assessment tool validated for use in primary care
Chronic kidney disease (CKD)	5	The percentage of patients on the CKD register with hypertension who are treated with an angiotensin converting enzyme inhibitor (ACE-I) or angiotensin receptor blocker (ARB) (unless a contraindication or side effects are recorded)
Smoking indicators	2	The percentage of patients with any or any combination of the following conditions: coronary heart disease, stroke or transient ischaemic attack (TIA), hypertension, diabetes, chronic obstructive airways disease (COPD), CKD, asthma, schizophrenia, bipolar affective disorder or other psychoses who smoke whose notes contain a record that smoking cessation advice or referral to a specialist service, where available, has been offered within the previous 15 months

Education, audit, development and dissemination of best practice

The dominant approach for health professionals has been education and audit. Education and audit are common requirements for regulation, but go beyond the requirements of regulation in that they seek to go beyond a minimum standard, and strive for excellence. Education has traditionally been professionally led, and is seen by many as an obligation of professional status. Professional organisations, such as the Royal Colleges in the UK, have been influential in setting high standards and encouraging audit.

The clinical audit cycle refers to the monitoring of performance against pre-defined standards (Figure 11.1). Measurement of one's performance against defined criteria can be demanding but the real challenge is to make necessary adjustments and re-evaluate your performance – in other words to complete the cycle.

Professionals have, of course, not had a monopoly on education, and the evidence-based medicine movement and the Cochrane Collaboration have been very important in improving the quantity and quality of information on the effectiveness of health-care interventions. The Plan–Do–Study–Act (PDSA) cycle (Figure 11.2) takes audit one stage further, and is widely used in health-care. The PDSA cycle has four stages, designed to help with the development, testing and implementation of quality improvement plans. The stages are first, to develop a plan and define the objective (plan). Second, to carry out the plan and collect data (do), then analyse the data and summarise what was learned (study). The final stage is to plan the next cycle with necessary modifications (act). For further information see the Institute for Health-care Improvement's website (http://www.ihi.org/ihi).

Figure 11.1   The audit cycle.

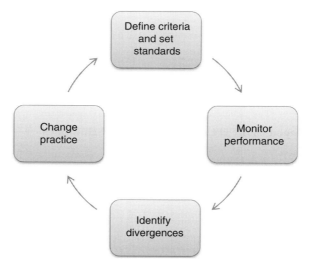

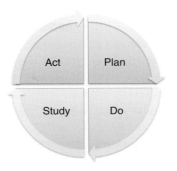

Figure 11.2 The plan–do–study–act cycle.

An example of this approach is in patient safety. The UK National Patient Safety Agency (NPSA) aims to improve the safety and quality of care for NHS patients (http://npsa.nhs.uk/). As well as making sure that incidents are reported in the first place, the NPSA promotes an open culture across the health service, encouraging doctors and other staff to report incidents and 'near misses', when things almost go wrong. A key aim is to encourage staff to report incidents without fear of personal reprimand and know that by sharing their experiences others would be able to learn lessons and improve patient safety. The NPSA also supports local organisations in addressing their concerns about the performance of individual doctors and dentists, through its responsibility for the National Clinical Assessment Service (NCAS).

The first rule of quality assurance based on experience in private production systems and public services across the world is: when things go wrong and mistakes are made the problem arises more often from faulty systems than from faulty individuals ('bad apples'). In *An Organisation with a Memory*, the Department of Health laid down its approach to risk management in the NHS borrowing on experience in the airline industry [18]. It declared the need for:

1. Unified mechanisms for reporting and analysis when things go wrong.
2. Mechanisms for ensuring that, where lessons are identified, the necessary changes are put into practice.
3. Much wider appreciation of the value of the systems approach in preventing, analysing and learning from errors.
4. A more open culture in which errors or service failures can be reported and discussed.

In your experience, how 'open' is the culture of health-care? How does increasing litigation affect the way in which doctors practice medicine and their willingness to share adverse events?

Market and financial

Market-based approaches have been most used in the USA, and rely on an informed consumer exercising choice. An example is the Consumer Assessment of Health-care Providers and Systems programme. Public release of performance data alone has met with limited success in improving quality, perhaps due to lack of data to inform real choice, or perhaps because the data are not used by the public. However, data publication can be effective as part of a larger initiative. An example is the publishing of risk-adjusted mortality rates from coronary artery bypass grafting for hospitals and surgeons in New York State [19]. Importantly, the data were used to inform quality improvement efforts which were associated with state-wide reduction in mortality. Similar effects were not seen where data publication was not accompanied by improvement efforts. (Following the Bristol inquiry, cardiothoracic surgeons have pioneered similar systems in the UK.)

Payment for performance is perhaps the dominant model internationally. Examples are the payment of a substantial portion of salary to British general practitioners according to their performance against quality criteria (see Table 11.2), and financial incentives to providers from the US Centers for Medicare and Medicaid Services. CQUIN (Commissioning for Quality and Innovation) is an initiative that incentivises hospitals financially in England to improve the quality of care they deliver.

We have seen that approaches to quality improvement can be grouped into three broad categories: regulation, education and market-based. Whichever combination of these is used, the level in the health-care system at which quality improvement approaches are applied is important. Previously, most quality improvement took place in single clinics, in patients with single diseases. Multilevel approaches to change have greater chances of success, by impacting on individuals, groups or teams, the organisation as a whole, and the larger environment and system level [20]. For example, the reduction in mortality seen in New York discussed above was effective because it was implemented at a health-system level. Changes at the system level made it easier for individual hospitals and teams to drive through beneficial changes. The importance of change at a system level has already been mentioned.

System-level approaches to quality improvement

A common criticism of much of what health professionals do to try and improve the quality of their care is that it is piecemeal and poorly coordinated. Variable quality of care, particularly in the poorest, least healthy and least well-resourced parts of the country, have long been a fact of NHS life. In this section, we consider some widely used approaches at system level to improve quality: clinical governance, lean and six sigma, and significant-event audit.

Clinical governance

The term 'clinical governance' (borrowing on notions of corporate governance from the private sector) refers to the framework through which NHS organisations and their staff are accountable for the quality of patient care. Clinical governance has been defined as: 'a system through which NHS organisations are accountable for continuously improving the quality of their services and safeguarding high standards of care by creating an environment in which excellence in clinical care will flourish' [21].

An element of clinical governance which has the potential to have a rapid impact on patient care is clinical audit, which has been described above. Good governance is central to public health practice, and in the UK the Faculty of Public Health has set out a framework for 'good public health practice', to 'assist the public, public health professionals, colleagues and employers to better understand what 'good practice' should look like' (http://www.fph.org.uk/good_practice).

Lean and six sigma

The business world has given us powerful examples of quality-improvement initiatives that consider the whole system, and two that have been successfully adopted into health-care are 'six sigma', invented by Motorola, and Toyota's 'lean' technique. The lean technique entails assessing every process for its value to the patient, to cut waste and inefficiencies and improve patient care [22]. The idea behind six sigma is simple: we should not accept the current common error rates of 50% in health-care, nor 10% or even 1%, but strive for near-perfect error rates of less than 1 in 3.4 million [23]. Proponents of six sigma argue that these error rates are achievable in health-care, just as in manufacturing, and cite anaesthesia as an example of an area that has seen dramatic improvements in safety. Table 11.3 gives examples of the defect rates (which relate to a particular sigma level) in different industries.

Table 11.3 Sigma levels and defect rates in different industries [8, 23]

Defects per million	Sigma level	Health-care examples	Other industry examples
3.4	6		Publishing: one misspelled word in all books in a small library
5.4		Deaths caused by anaesthesia during surgery	
230	5		Airline fatalities
6210	4		Airline baggage handling Restaurant bills
10,000		1% of all hospitalised patients injured through negligence	
66,800	3		Publishing: 7.6 misspelled words per page in a book
350,000	2	36% of patients with depression not diagnosed/treated adequately; 35% of heart attack survivors not given beta-blockers	

Significant-event audit and root-cause analysis

Significant-event audit (SEA) has been described as the processes by which 'individual cases, in which there has been a significant occurrence (not necessarily involving an undesirable outcome for the patient), are analysed in a systematic and detailed way to ascertain what can be learnt about the overall quality of care and to indicate changes that might lead to future improvements' [24]. It is often linked to root-cause analysis (RCA) (see e.g. http://www.nrls.npsa.nhs.uk/resources/?entryid45=75602), and the aim is to:

- Gather and map information to determine what happened.
- Identify problems with health-care delivery.
- Identify contributory factors and root causes.
- Agree what needs to change and implement solutions.

Conclusion

The risks of quality improvement should be considered. What are the opportunity costs of quality improvement? Do the benefits outweigh the costs? Disparities in access to health-care are a problem in all countries, and any quality-improvement programme may worsen disparities unless the improvement has proportionally greater benefit for the relatively disadvantaged population. The most important part of any quality-improvement initiative is a group of committed people who consistently seek to make health-care better. The particular technique chosen is probably much less important than the dedication of the people involved.

REFERENCES

1. Institute of Medicine (IOM) Committee on Health Care in America. *Crossing the Quality Chasm: A New Health System for the 21st Century*, Washington, DC, National Academy Press, 2001.
2. N. Steel, Thresholds for taking antihypertensive drugs in different professional and lay groups: questionnaire survey. *British Medical Journal* **320**, 2000, 1446–7.
3. A. Coulter, What do patients and the public want from primary care? *British Medical Journal* **331**, 2005, 1199–201.
4. R. Maxwell, Quality assessment in health. *British Medical Journal* **288**, 1984, 1470–2.
5. Secretary of State for Health. *High Quality Care For All: NHS Next Stage Review Final Report*, Department of Health, 2008.
6. J. M. Last, *A Dictionary of Epidemiology*, 4th edn., Oxford, Oxford University Press, 2001.
7. A. Donabedian, Explorations in quality assessment and monitoring. In *The Definition of Quality and Approaches to its Assessment*, Ann Arbor, MI, Health Administration Press, 1980, vol. 1.

8. M. Chassin and R. W. Galvin, The National Roundtable on Health Care Quality. The urgent need to improve health care quality. *Journal of the American Medical Association* **280**, 1998, 1000–5.

9. N. Steel, M. Bachmann, S. Maisey *et al.*, Self reported receipt of care consistent with 32 quality indicators: national population survey of adults aged 50 or more in England. *British Medical Journal* **337**, 2008, a957.

10. J. Tudor Hart, Commentary: three decades of the inverse care law [comment]. *British Medical Journal* **320**, 2000,18–19.

11. E. S. Fisher, D. E. Wennberg, T. A. Stukel *et al.*, The implications of regional variations in Medicare spending. Part 1: The content, quality, and accessibility of care. *Annals of Internal Medicine* **138**(4), 2003, 273–87.

12. Committee on Quality of Health Care in America IoM, *To Err is Human: Building a Safer Health System*, Washington, DC, National Academy Press, 2000.

13. National Audit Office, *Reducing Healthcare Associated Infections in Hospitals in England*, London, The Stationery Office, 2009.

14. The Mid Staffordshire NHS Foundation Trust Independent Inquiry. See: http://www.midstaffsinquiry.com/.

15. K. Sutherland and S. Leatherman, Does certification improve medical standards? *British Medical Journal* **333**, 2006, 439–41.

16. R. H. Brook, M. R. Chassin, A. Fink *et al.*, A method for the detailed assessment of the appropriateness of medical technologies. *International Journal of Technology Assessment in Health Care* **2**, 1986, 53–63.

17. NHS Employers and the General Practitioners Committee, *Quality and Outcomes Framework Guidance for GMS Contract 2009/10. Delivering Investment in General Practice*, London, NHS Employers, 2009.

18. Department of Health, *An Organisation with a Memory*. London, The Stationery Office, 2000.

19. M. R. Chassin, Achieving and sustaining improved quality: lessons from New York State and cardiac surgery. *Health Affairs (Millwood)* **21**(4), 2002, 40–51.

20. F. B. Ferlie and S. M. Shortell, Improving the quality of health care in the United Kingdom and the United States: A framework for change. *The Milbank Quarterly* **79**(2), 2001, 281–315.

21. G. Scally and L. J. Donaldson, Clinical governance and the drive for quality improvement in the new NHS in England. *British Medical Journal* **317**, 1998, 61–5.

22. D. Jones and A. Mitchell, *Lean Thinking for the NHS*, London, NHS Confederation, 2006.

23. M. R. Chassin, Is health care ready for six sigma quality? *The Milbank Quarterly* **76**(4), 1998, 565–91.

24. M. Pringle, C. P. Bradley, C. M. Carmichael, H. Wallis and A. Moore, Significant event auditing. A study of the feasibility and potential of case-based auditing in primary medical care. *Occasional Papers of the Royal College of General Practitioners* **70**, 1995, i–71.

Contexts for public health practice

Introduction to Part 2 – what do we mean by contexts in public health?

Jan Yates

As we discussed in regard to leadership (Chapter 1), the context in which the public health tools are used has a bearing on the choice of tool and how it is implemented. In the second part of *Essential Public Health: Theory and Practice* we will consider a range of contemporary contexts in which public health is practiced and illustrate how the tools we have described are applied.

First, the individual context. Throughout Part 1 of this book we have provided examples of where the public health tools we describe have been used. However, you the reader may be left wondering, "How would I use that skill?" "How is that relevant to my job?"

All the editors are employed (in part) as Consultants in Public Health within the NHS. Our jobs require us to use all the public health tools at our disposal in the fulfilment of our duties. We use epidemiological tools and demographic information to understand and describe the populations for which we are responsible. We lead teams and multi-agency networks to prioritise and drive changes in health and health improvement policy and practice. We develop strategies to encourage behaviour change in patients, the public and professionals. We focus on and evaluate the quality of screening programmes, their evidence base, equity of provision and safety. We are part of a health-protection on-call system, which responds to incidents and emergencies out of hours that have a potential population health impact. All the tools in Part 1 are part of our daily routines and essential to the outcomes we must achieve.

Many of those who practice public health and need to access these tools are not so explicitly aware of their own public health role, or of the tools they are using. We hope you will be, and the following examples demonstrate how the public health tools are employed in a range of health care-related roles.

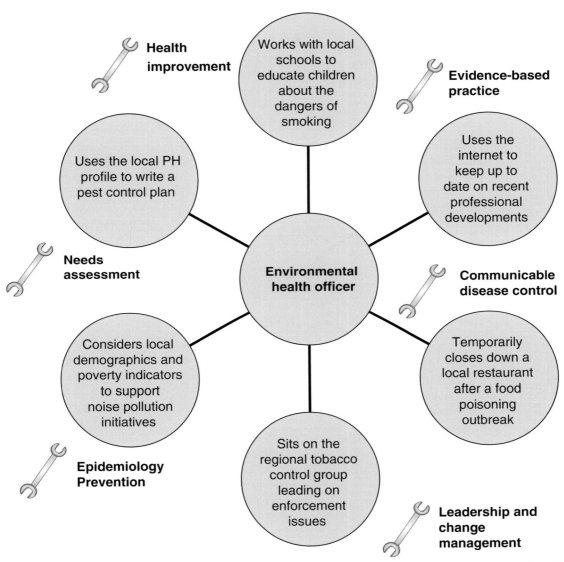

Figure 1 Examples of how different professionals apply public health tools

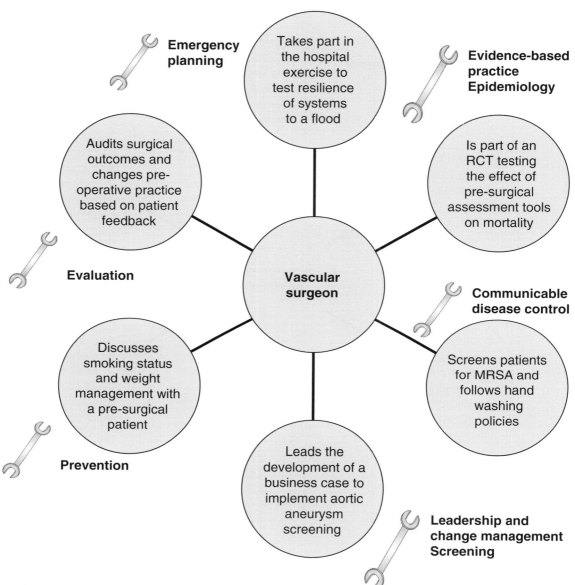

Figure 1   (cont.)

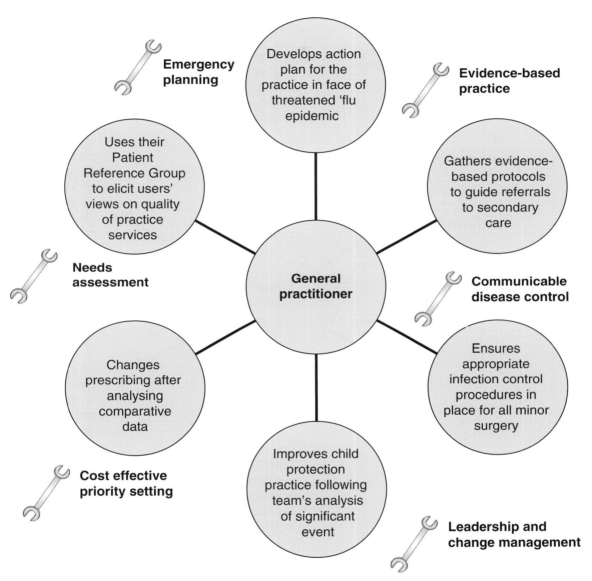

Figure 1   (cont.)

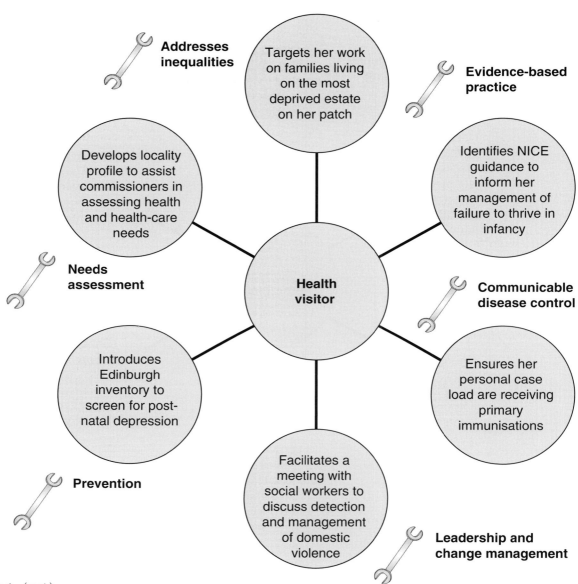

Figure 1   (cont.)

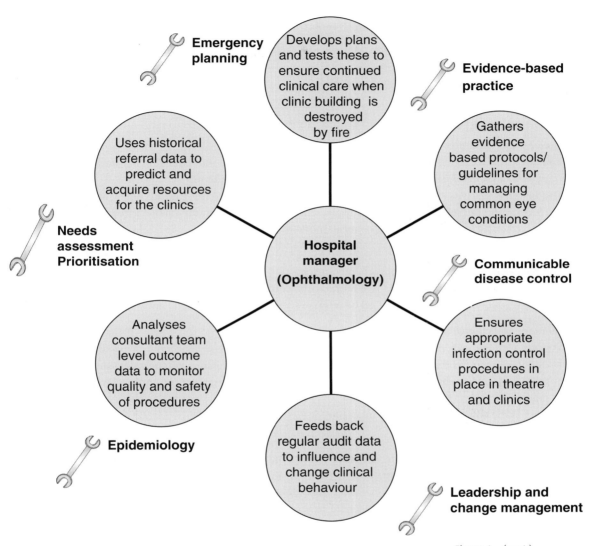

Figure 1   (cont.)

Can you think of examples of how a medical student could apply some of the public health tools?

You might have thought of various examples. See Box 1 for a couple in each category.

Box 1 Examples of the application of public health tools

- **Evidence-based practice**:

    You have seen a case of heart failure in a 65-year-old man and you wanted to find out how to manage the patient based on the current best available evidence for this condition.

    You help the vascular surgeon you are working with prepare a business case for a new abdominal aortic (AAA) screening service within your hospital and write a section on the evidence of the effectiveness of this screening in reducing aortic aneurysm mortality.

- **Communicable disease control**:

    You have seen a case of meningococcal meningitis in a 6-year-old school boy and appreciate the need to notify the local public health team to enable contact tracing and appropriate prophylaxis.

    You wash your hands or use alcohol gel between every patient contact and on entry and exit to every ward.

- **Leadership and change management**:

    You are working as a part of team to complete a project as part of your work in paediatrics. There is disagreement on the content of the work and the way it is progressing. You take the lead, put forward a reasonable argument and help your team to complete the assignment on time, which secures good grades.

    You act as the editor for a university magazine.

- **Health improvement**:

    During your community placement you come across a young smoker. You take the time to talk to him about the hazards of smoking and sign post him to the local stop-smoking services.

    An obese patient you see in a pre-operative assessment clinic is deemed unsuitable for anaesthesia until they have lost weight. You take the time to question the presiding nurse on the access to weight-management services locally for this patient.

- **Decision making**:

    You are constantly presented with various choices and you develop the ability to analyse the costs and consequences of your actions and arrive at an appropriate decision.

    The hospital you are working in sets up a new service to provide a general physician in the emergency department to manage patients who are not severe enough to need hospital emergency care. You recognise that one of the drivers for this new service is the need to reduce the costs of health-care overall in a resource-limited system and a decision has been taken that the benefits of this model are likely to outweigh the costs of employing additional staff.

As well as there being variety in the nature of those who practice public health, the population for which public health tools are employed varies considerably. There are nuances of implementation when public health is used to describe, improve and protect health across the life course and we consider these in the first three chapters of Part 2 – on children, adults and older people.

It is also imperative to remember that public health is not practiced in a vacuum. It is inseparable from the political, economic, social and environmental factors which influence it, and which it seeks to influence. The last four chapters in Part 2 describe these factors in more detail as we consider the policy context in which public health must exist, the global nature of the practice and two key challenges – inequalities and sustainability.

The tools which we have described in Part 1 are all applied in the contexts we describe in Part 2 but the practitioner must be flexible, tenacious and innovative to achieve the optimal public health outcomes in such a complex environment – as you shall see. The spanner icon is used in the following chapters to identify some of the places where the tools in Part 1 apply.

12

The health of children and young people

Kirsteen L. Macleod, Rachel Crowther and Sarah Stewart-Brown

Key points

- Child public health is important in its own right, but also because children represent the future.
- Although child health has improved greatly over the last century, great disparities still exist between the health of children in different social groups and relative poverty remains a key determinant of child health both in the UK and worldwide.
- Family relationships are an important determinant of many risk factors for poor health across the life course and play a key role in the transmission of social inequalities.
- Other challenges facing child public health in the twenty-first century include the rise in emotional and behavioural disorders, childhood obesity, chronic disease and disability, the continuing globalisation and commercialisation of children's lives, and climate change.
- The promotion of child health requires action at the level of the individual, family, school and society and demands cross-disciplinary and intersectoral collaboration.

Children and their health

Why is child public health important?

Childhood is important in its own right, but children also represent the future: they are the adults (and the parents) of tomorrow. Because of their vulnerability, children deserve particular care and protection from society, and their right to this protection,

Essential Public Health, Second Edition, ed. Stephen Gillam, Jan Yates and Padmanabhan Badrinath.
Published by Cambridge University Press. © Cambridge University Press 2012.

Figure 12.1   Returns to a unit pound invested. Reproduced with permission from Heckman, James J. (2008). Schools, skills and synapses, *Economic Inquiry*, **46**(3), 289–324.

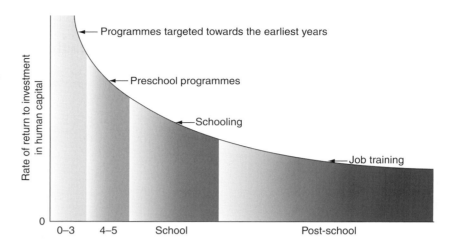

enabling them to flourish, enjoy life, health, identity, education and other fundamental goods, is enshrined in the United Nations Convention on the Rights of the Child. Although most countries are signatories to this convention, many children worldwide – and some in the UK – are still denied basic rights through accident of birth, or through the ignorance or inadequacy of adults.

Another compelling reason to promote health in childhood is provided by the growing body of research showing the extent to which physical and emotional development in infancy and childhood influence adult health and social functioning [1]. This research has played a part in expanding the status of child public health both in the UK and other parts of the developed world. Today, in contrast to previous decades, 'a good start in life' is regarded as central to many public health and social policy initiatives [2–4]. The economic arguments in favour of investment in childhood are now very strong and the earlier in life the investment is made, the greater the financial return to society [5] (see Figure 12.1).

Child public health shares many of the tools, approaches and skills of other areas of public health practice but it is also a distinct subspecialty, reflecting the changing developmental stages of children and their dependence on adults for much of this period. Because adults are often keen to offer children conditions that they felt they deserved but were denied in their own childhood, and because children are rightly seen as vulnerable, child public health can also blaze new trails for the wider cause of public health. Social inequity is more obviously unfair to children, who play no part in creating the circumstances under which they live, and social inequity was a feature of child public health practice long before it was recognised as an important issue in adult public health. Sustainable development and climate change are important for the whole of society, but their relevance is nowhere more obvious than to child public health. Positive health outcomes like emotional and social well-being first appeared in policy for children [6]; now these goals are firmly embedded in adult health policy [2,4].

Adapting Acheson's well-known definition, Kohler has defined child public health as 'the organised efforts of society to develop healthy public health policies to promote child and young people's health, to prevent disease in children and young people and to foster equity for children and young people, within a framework of sustainable development' [7]. It involves:

- *A concern and advocacy for the health and well-being of all children and young people in the population*: whether local, national or international, with a particular emphasis on health inequalities and enabling children's voices to be heard.
- *Promoting health in the broadest sense*: including physical, mental and social well-being.
- *Assessing health needs*: including understanding patterns of health and illness in children; identifying factors which affect children's health and exploring ways of modifying these.
- *Implementing and managing a wide range of public health interventions*: including screening and immunisation programmes; advice on the commissioning of health-care for children; and community-based health promotion initiatives, including support for parents and parenting, Surestart and Healthy Schools.
- *Identifying childhood antecedents of future disease or disability and developing preventive interventions.*
- *Seeing children in context*: as members of families, communities and wider social networks [8].
- *Co-operation between a wide variety of individuals and organisations*: including specialist public health practitioners and many different professionals who work in health, education, social services and a range of other fields.

The child population

Using tools such as those outlined in Chapters 2 and 8 we can consider the demography and health status of the child population.

Demography

According to mid-2010 estimates, there were approximately 11.6 million children under the age of 16 in the UK. In common with most developed countries, the UK is currently witnessing a decline in its child population (see Chapter 2) and the 2001 census showed that for the first time we now have more people aged over 60 than under 16. As a proportion, the under-16 population fell from 25% in 1971 to 20% in 2001, and is projected to fall to 17% by 2031 (see www.statistics.gov.uk).

According to the most recent UK Census of 2001:

- one in three households in the UK contains dependent children and one in nine households contains children under 5;
- 10% of children are from an ethnic minority group;

- 19% of boys and 17% of girls have a minor disability (of which emotional and behavioural problems are the most common) or long-standing illness (of which asthma is the most common);
- 11 per 10,000 boys and 5 per 10,000 girls have a more severe disability (of which autism is the most common specific condition).

Main causes of mortality and morbidity in children

Health
status

Over the last century, children in the UK have become healthier and their life expectancy has increased. Due to social and environmental – and to some extent medical – advances, many of the scourges of the nineteenth and early-twentieth centuries have more or less vanished. But in their place are new problems and disorders, which reflect changes in society over this period. Instead of life-threatening infectious diseases and high infant mortality rates, we now have high levels of emotional and behavioural problems and childhood obesity, which threaten longevity, and high rates of survival for premature babies, many of whom will need care and support throughout their lives.

Historically, public health experts have followed a medical model, measuring health negatively in terms of levels of disease, disability and mortality. While the value of refocusing on the positive is clear and there are moves afoot to develop valid measures [9], examination of health trends will continue to rely on disease-based measures for some time to come.

Some of the leading concerns in terms of morbidity and mortality in the UK today – and much of the rest of the developed world – are set out in Table 12.1.

Comparison of mortality rates and causes of death reveals the extent of the differences between the most and the least privileged children across the globe. Most of the world's child population lives in the poorest countries, where child and infant mortality rates are highest (Chapter 17). According to UNICEF, in the least-developed countries in the world (which together have a child population of 340 million), 10% of children can expect to die before their first birthday and almost 16% before their fifth birthday – compared to 0.6% and 0.7% respectively for children in the UK [16].

Communicable
disease
control

The main causes of death worldwide and in the UK are very different (see Table 12.2). Many deaths in the developing world are potentially preventable by means of simple interventions – ensuring clean water supplies, and providing immunisation and basic health-care (especially during pregnancy and childbirth).

Causes of death for children in the UK vary by age and sex. Boys have a higher mortality rate than girls at all ages, but especially in adolescence, when they account for two thirds of deaths. Much of the steep rise in mortality rates in this age group is due to deaths from injury and poisoning. Leading causes of mortality among older age groups are shown in Table 12.3.

Table 12.1 Key child public health challenges in the UK for the twenty-first century

Social and health inequalities. The UK has a poorer record on *child poverty* than most other European countries. Although Government action to tackle child poverty in the UK has met with some success, a child in the UK still has nearly twice the chance of living in a relatively low income family than was the case a generation ago.

Childhood obesity. This is one of the most significant public health challenges of the twenty-first century. Prevalence has increased sharply in recent years and this trend threatens to curtail the life expectancy of current and future generations of children, as well as creating a significant financial burden for the NHS. (See case study later in chapter.)

Emotional and behavioural/mental health problems. Prevalence is rising in children and young people [10]. Impacts may include educational failure, unemployment, unhealthy lifestyles and problems in interpersonal relationships in adulthood. These problems have implications (e.g. stress, violence) for parents and siblings, future partners and children, teachers and wider society (through their impact on social capital, delinquency and youth crime). *Suicide* rates are higher for older teenagers (15–19 year olds) than younger children (10–14 year olds) and higher in boys than girls. Suicide rates for 10–19 year olds were falling between 1997 and 2003 [11].

Substance misuse. This includes alcohol, tobacco, drugs and glue-sniffing. Binge drinking, and the continuing rise in smoking rates among teenage girls, are worrying trends [12]. Regular smoking amongst 11–15 year olds declined from 13% in 1996 to 6% in 2007, and remained at this level in 2009. However, 66% of adult smokers start before they are 18, making teenage smoking a significant child public health issue [13].

Teenage pregnancy. Public health and education policy has been successful in helping to reduce the teenage pregnancy rate in the past decade. The under-18 conception rate in England fell to 40.4 per 1000 in 2008 – a reduction of 13.3% since 1998 [14]. However, the UK still has one of the highest rates in Europe, and the impact on health and well-being is substantial, both for teenage mothers and their children.

Sexually transmitted infections are a related problem [12]. There has been an increasing trend in these preventable infections amongst 15–24 year olds [15] and health protection efforts focus mainly on reducing the risk of transmission through safe-sex practices, contraception and encouraging early testing.

Accidents and injuries. Despite considerable progress in recent years, injuries remain a significant cause of morbidity and mortality especially among adolescents, and the UK has the highest rates for injuries to child pedestrians in Europe. Non-accidental injury, and other types of *child abuse and neglect* are also important – the NSPCC estimates that there are 100 fatal cases per year, and recent high-profile cases have made clear that identifying fatal abuse is fraught with difficulties.

Poor vaccine uptake. For example, poor uptake of MMR, due to media scares about links to autism and mistrust of government advice, has resulted in significant risk of outbreaks of measles and greater exposure of pregnant women to rubella.

Disabilities. These are increasing in prevalence, partly due to improved care and survival of premature and small-for-date babies, and of care for children with *chronic illnesses* such as asthma and diabetes.

Determinants of health in children

Children's health is affected by a wide range of factors, from the intra-uterine environment and genetic inheritance to international business interests and cross-governmental agreements operating across the globe. Epidemiological studies (see Chapter 3) have provided evidence for some of the main factors and these are explored in more detail below.

Epidemiology

Table 12.2 Main causes of death among children under 5 (in 2008)

UK	Worldwide
Population	Population
13.5 million children under 18 (0.6% of world child population), 3.5 million under 5	2.1 billion children under 18, 613 million under 5
Deaths	Deaths
Approx. 4300 deaths per year (under-5 mortality rate 5 per 1000 live births)	8.8 million deaths per year (under-5 mortality rate 60 per 1000 live births)
Causes of death	Causes of death
55% occur in newborns:	68% of deaths are caused by infectious diseases:
• prematurity, low birthweight etc. (perinatal conditions) (36%)	• pneumonia (18%)
• congenital anomalies (26%)	• diarrhoea (15%)
• sudden infant death (14% – but 25% of deaths under a year)	• malaria (8%)
• birth asphyxia (7%)	• neonatal infection (6%)
Other main causes include:	Other main causes include:
• injury and poisoning (4%)	• complications of pre-term delivery (12%)
• respiratory disease (2%)	• birth asphyxia (9%)

Sources: Black *et al.*, 2010 [17] WHO, 2011 [18].

Table 12.3 Main causes of death among older children in the UK

Rates per million	Cause of death	Boys	Girls
5–9 years:	Cancer	46	30
	Injury and poisoning	30	22
	Diseases of nervous system	20	20
	Congenital anomalies	12	8
	Respiratory disease	9	11
	All deaths	141	111
10–14 years:	Injury and poisoning	67	28
	Cancer	39	17
	Diseases of nervous system	21	23
	Congenital anomalies	11	11
	All deaths	176	117
15–19 years:	Injury and poisoning	329	114
	Cancer	53	34
	Diseases of nervous system	38	23
	Congenital anomalies	23	10
	Circulatory disease	16	13
	All deaths	555	267

Source: Department of Health, 2004 [19].

Individual and congenital factors

Genetic factors play a direct role in conditions such as cystic fibrosis, Down's syndrome and sickle cell disease. They have also been shown to be predictive of other conditions such as diabetes or juvenile chronic arthritis, but their contribution is minor compared to environmental factors (e.g. conduct disorder and depression). Gene–environment interaction effects are increasingly being demonstrated, for example between genes predisposing to depression and parenting [20,21], making what once seemed a simple picture both more complicated and more amenable to public health intervention. Intra-uterine life also affects both child health (e.g. via birth weight or insults such as rubella virus or teratogenic drugs) and health in later life. Even parental mental health problems during pregnancy have been shown to predict key health outcomes in the child [22]. See Chapter 15 for more detail on this 'life course' explanation of adult health in the context of health inequalities.

Ethnicity

Children's ethnic background plays a part in determining their health. Here, socio-economic factors contribute (see below), but genetic and cultural determinants also have a role to play, together with the impact of racism, intolerance and stigma. For example, infant mortality rates in the UK are higher for babies of mothers born in Pakistan, the Caribbean, and most parts of Africa; but babies born into black and minority ethnic families are more likely to be breast-fed, and those whose mothers were born in Africa or Asia are less likely to die of sudden infant death syndrome. Children seeking asylum in the UK live in particularly difficult circumstances and have often experienced war, torture, separation from friends and relatives, and fear and danger in transit.

Parenting

The family constitutes a child's immediate environment and has a profound influence on health and well-being. Maternal age and income, family structure, siblings and birth order all play a part, but parenting and family relationships are particularly important. Good relationships can buffer the detrimental health effects of stress and adverse life events throughout the life course and poor parenting contributes to the development of conduct disorder, delinquency, educational failure, criminal activity, poor mental health, cardiovascular disease risk and premature mortality [20,23].

The critical importance of parenting for resilience and the resulting impact on the incidence of common mental-health problems has only recently been appreciated and started to influence policy [24]. Other long-term studies illustrating the interconnectedness of mental and physical health show links to lifestyles related to poor health, cardiovascular disease risk and premature mortality [25].

Mechanisms underpinning these effects have been elucidated from studies in both man and animals which show how early stressful experiences play a role in shaping the emotional and social brain, affecting future resilience and setting the scene for the quality of future relationships [20]. Parenting is to some extent socially patterned, but differences within social groups are greater than the differences between them. However, because of its role in supporting educational and social development, parenting plays a key role in perpetuating social inequalities and cycles of disadvantage. A recent cross-party government report on childhood poverty [26] has concluded that little progress will be made in combating its effects until parenting is changed.

Aspects of parenting which seem to play a role include parental behaviour (boundary setting, praise, encouragement and positive discipline, as opposed to derogation, criticism, hitting and shouting) and relationship skills (sensitivity and attunement, especially in infancy, appropriate expectations, affection, as opposed to insensitivity, neglect, aggression and hostility) as well as the more obvious components of offering children a range of experience and supporting their intellectual development [23]. There is now a wide range of evidence-based ways to improve parenting from low-cost interventions suitable on a universal basis to highly intensive programmes necessary for very high-risk families [27]. Abuse and neglect are extreme examples of poor parenting and have the greatest long-term impact. They are very often associated with other key and relatively intractable determinants of problem parenting – parental mental illness, drug or alcohol misuse [28]. Lesser degrees of suboptimal parenting are associated with less risk, but because such parenting is common, the population-attributable risk for adult health may be substantial.

Family structure

Family break-up and conflict can seriously affect children's well-being. The 2001 Census indicated that globally the UK has the second largest proportion of children living in single-parent families and step families (the USA has the largest). Single-parent or reconstituted families (which now house 23% and 10% of children, respectively) have many disadvantages for some children, among which are poverty and lack of male role models. The outcome of family break-up may be an improvement for children if conflict is resolved and they continue to receive loving care, but in many families break-up creates rather than solves conflict and it is this which is damaging [29].

Child care

Child care and working patterns have changed over time: more young children spend more time in day care. While there are benefits from contact with other children, and from age three for emotional and social development, day care is stressful for children [30]. Current evidence suggests that the quality of day care has a significant impact on children's development [31] and only a small proportion of the day care on offer in this country meets appropriate quality standards. It is very difficult, in day-care settings, to provide the limited number of close, secure relationships infants need to develop secure attachments, and it is doubtful if day care in the first year of life can ever be as good as care in all but the most disadvantaged homes.

Peer relationships

Later, when children go to school (and in some cases spend long hours in after-school care), peer relationships become increasingly important. The health effects of bullying frequently receive adverse publicity in the wake of teenage suicides, but long-term studies show an impact on adult mental health too [32]. Good relationships within the family provide a template for children to build good relationships with peers and protect them to some extent from the impact of bullying [33]. School ethos also has a role to play, and health-promoting school programmes with a focus on positive mental health can be important in supporting and enabling change [34].

Poverty and deprivation

Poverty has a profound influence on child health, in the UK and worldwide, and income inequality [35] accounts for much of the variation in morbidity and mortality in children across the country (Chapter 15). Both *absolute* and *relative* poverty are important:

- **Absolute poverty** is defined in terms of a family's ability to purchase essential goods (such as housing, heating, food, clothing and transport). There are various so-called 'consensus measures' of absolute poverty, which define a generally accepted minimum income for a family of a particular size.
- **Relative poverty** is defined in relation to the average income in a particular population: the European Union definition of relative poverty includes all families whose income is at or below 50% of the national average (sometimes called the 'poverty line').

Tackling absolute poverty by increasing the income of the very poor to minimally acceptable levels is potentially more straightforward than tackling relative poverty, which means achieving a more thorough redistribution of wealth. The effects of relative poverty, however, are generally accepted to be more powerful and more pervasive: their impact can be seen at every geographical level.

As average wealth has increased in the UK, the distribution of wealth has become more unequal – and the numbers living in relative poverty have increased. In 2008, it was estimated that 20.9% of children in England were 'living in poverty', defined as the percentage of children in households with a reported income of less than 60 per cent of the median income [36]. Within the UK there are also significant socio-economic inequalities between north and south, deprived inner cities (where, in the worst locations, up to three quarters of children live in poverty), the more affluent suburbs and rural areas (where there are also pockets of poverty, and isolation can be a real problem).

LIVERPOOL JOHN MOORES UNIVERSITY
LEARNING SERVICES

The last UK government pledged to halve child poverty between 1998–99 and 2010, and eradicate it by 2020. While some progress has been made, the risk of a child living in relative poverty today is still twice the level it was a generation ago [37]. Importantly, the new UK coalition government has continued to support initiatives to prevent the deleterious impact of childhood poverty. As well as parenting and social-policy interventions to support families, measures to redistribute wealth are likely to be needed if real inroads are to be made.

Communities, social capital and stigma

Most of the research on social capital relates to adult health (see Chapter 15) and shows that local community networks, social cohesion and social trust make a difference to health. These factors are likely to have an effect on children's health and well-being too, if only through effects on their parents' health. Social capital describes the 'glue' which holds communities together and offers some protection against the adverse health effects of poverty and deprivation. However, strong social capital in one group may mean social exclusion and stigma for others and may thus adversely affect children from marginalised and minority groups. These include the very poor, travelling families, asylum seekers, ethnic and religious minorities, as well as children with disabilities or chronic illnesses, all of whom may be less able to access services and participate in community life.

Physical environment

Children's physical environment is important too. Damp housing increases the risk of asthma; overcrowding predisposes to infectious diseases, domestic violence and accidents [38]. Traffic danger and air quality are other important factors, and the condition of the local environment – buildings, streets, parks, facilities and infrastructure – has a profound influence on the lives children lead. Access to green spaces and the opportunity for free play outdoors has come to be recognised as important for children's mental health and development [39].

Behaviour and lifestyle choices

Changes in the quality and quantity of food consumed and the amount of exercise taken by children have generated the current epidemic of childhood obesity. Parents influence children's lifestyles both by making choices for them in early life and by shaping habits which children may follow later when choosing for themselves. Socio-economic and environmental factors also play a role: for example, local availability of food; the information on food labels; and local provision of safe outdoor play areas. Many foods which are cheap and readily available are high in fat, calories, sugar and salt. Physical education provision can be poor in schools, especially where playing fields are absent, and parents are often reluctant to allow children to play outside because of fear of traffic or assault. The amount of sleep children get and the hours they spend viewing television have been shown to be key predictors of childhood obesity [40].

Exposure to substances such as tobacco, alcohol and illegal drugs are also important factors. Smoking in pregnancy increases the risk of low birth weight, stillbirth and infant death, and smoking in the same household as a young child increases the risk of sudden infant death and respiratory problems. Many forms of risk behaviour are increasing among adolescents, including binge drinking, drug use, sexual behaviour, accidents and deliberate self-harm.

Media and the commercial world

The wider world has more and more impact on children as the broadcast and printed media, and particularly the internet, encourage the development of globalisation and consumerism. Examples include the marketing of unhealthy food and expensive consumer goods to children and the promotion of infant formula to mothers in the poorest countries. Trends towards increasing exposure to television, even in the background, and other screen-based activities, are now being discouraged both by those with an interest in child development and those with an interest in obesity [41].

Public services

Access to public services is important for children's health. As well as *health services* (including preventive, acute and community services), *education* has a significant impact on self-esteem and well-being in children and on later health; *social services* may provide vital support for families with difficulties, or protection for children at risk; *leisure services* such as sporting facilities and youth clubs can benefit physical, mental and emotional health; and *transport services* such as cycle lanes, traffic calming and safe routes to school also play a role in promoting health.

Health promotion and health policy for children

Child health promotion

Chapter 8 discussed the tools used in health improvement in detail and these are highly relevant to promoting and improving children's health across the population – a fundamental goal of child public health. In common with health promotion for adults, child health promotion involves action at national level (policy development, legislation, etc.) as well as local level (parenting support, community development, realignment of services). Some examples are given below for each of the five 'pillars' of the 1986 Ottawa Charter for Health Promotion:

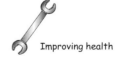

Improving health

- *Building healthy public policy*. For example: health impact assessment for proposed new roads, which takes into account child health concerns such as air pollution and asthma and the risk of road traffic accidents; banning advertising of foods containing high fat and high sugar to children on television; banning physical punishment of children; ban on smoking in public places.
- *Creating supportive environments*. For example: preserving and developing green spaces, encouraging walking and cycling to school; promoting food co-operatives and farmers' markets, which make healthy food more easily available to local families; clear food labelling.
- *Strengthening communities*. For example: enabling parents and children to contribute to decision making about issues they feel are important to their health, such as community safety, leisure provision and the quality of the local environment (e.g. street lighting); supporting voluntary sector provision and community development initiatives.
- *Re-orienting health services*. For example: reducing inequalities in access to child health services; ensuring services meet local needs and are child-centred; developing ambulatory care; increasing provision of support for parenting so that all families can access it; increasing provision of mental health promotion initiatives in schools.
- *Developing personal knowledge and skills*. For example: offering programmes to support children's emotional and social development in schools; ensuring children are introduced to key health knowledge in sound programmes at an appropriate age.

Child health promotion can therefore operate in many different ways and at many different levels. Many child health promoting policies are essentially intersectoral and involve a wide range of people working in partnership towards the common goal of improving children's health and well-being, including all those involved in healthcare as well as other fields of public and private life. Some activities led by different organisations or groups are set out in Table 12.4.

Case study: childhood obesity

The threat of the childhood obesity 'epidemic' to public health has been widely recognised in recent years and was famously dubbed by one Chief Medical Officer as 'a ticking time bomb'. The UK has one of the highest rates of childhood obesity in Europe and is not far behind the USA, which has the highest rate worldwide.

The National Child Measurement Programme (NCMP), operated jointly by the departments of Health and Education, measures the height and weight of all children entering Reception and Year 6. This helps to inform local planning and delivery of services (see the National Obesity Observatory website for more information).

In 2008/2009, the programme data showed that almost a third of 10–11 year olds and over a fifth of 4–5 year olds were overweight or obese. In the UK, the prevalence of

Table 12.4 Examples of health-promotion activity in different sectors

Health professionals – including doctors, nurses, midwives, health visitors, dentists, pharmacists, orthoptists.

Roles include:

- Child health surveillance
- Immunisation and screening
- Advice and support to parents and carers on health and parenting

Other statutory agencies – including social services, education, transport, planning and leisure departments, youth services, careers and training advice, the police and probation services.

Roles include:

- Supporting families and parenting and protecting children
- Helping all children to reach their potential
- Ensuring that children live in safe and healthy environments
- Supporting and advising young people as they approach adulthood

Voluntary, third-sector or not-for-profit organisations – including NSPCC, Save the Children, National Children's Bureau, charities working with specific groups (e.g. children with disabilities, bereaved children, asylum seekers, travellers or young carers) and informal local groups (such as mother-and-toddler groups or youth drop-in centres); organisations offering parenting support.

Roles include:

- Supporting families and parenting and protecting individual children
- Advocacy and lobbying for policy change and service improvement
- Identifying unmet needs (locally, nationally or internationally) and working with statutory agencies, communities and individuals to meet them
- Providing information and services (e.g. respite care, after-school clubs, parenting programmes)

The commercial world – including employers, local retailers and multinational businesses, manufacturers, providers of leisure facilities.

Roles include:

- Offering family-friendly employment practices
- Helping to make healthy choices easier (e.g. enforcing age restrictions on the sale of tobacco and alcohol, reducing salt and fat content in processed food)
- Improving children's safety in public places
- Promoting physical activity
- Philanthropic support for community initiatives

Local communities – including faith groups, residents' associations, parent–teacher associations (PTAs), parent support groups.

Roles include:

- Identifying local priorities (e.g. traffic-calming measures, parks and green spaces)
- Developing local networks and projects to support children and families
- Promoting community safety

National and international organisations – including governments, non-governmental organisations, UNICEF, WHO.

Roles include:

- Promoting healthy public policy
- Protecting and promoting children's rights across the globe

obesity rose between 1995 and 2007 by approximately 6% in boys to 17.1% and by 4.2% in girls to 16.4%.

If the increase continues, parents' life expectancy may exceed their children's, with obesity becoming the main cause of premature death in the UK. Some children are more at risk than others. Girls have higher rates than boys: up to 30% of girls aged 2–15 are overweight or obese in some areas of England. According to the NCMP, there is a higher prevalence of obesity in children from most minority ethnic groups than White British children, although this varies for age and sex. Prevalence is highest at reception age in Black African boys and girls and, for Year 6 children, it is highest in Bangladeshi boys and girls from African and Other Black groups.

Changes in energy intake (diet) and output (physical activity) both play a part in creating this problem. Children in England eat on average double the required amounts of saturated fat, salt and sugar per day, and 40% of boys and 60% of girls get less than the recommended hour of physical activity a day.

Overweight and obesity affects children's physical, mental and social well-being. The consequences may include:

- the development of risk factors for heart disease such as hyperinsulinaemia, high blood pressure and type 2 diabetes, previously only seen in adults, which is now seen (albeit rarely) in obese children;
- low self-esteem, social isolation and bullying;
- reduced participation in sport and physical activity, creating a vicious cycle;
- poorer educational achievement;
- up to 25% risk of becoming an obese adult, which carries serious long-term health risks. The risk is highest if both parents are overweight.

Childhood obesity is a complex problem, which requires collaborative, multi-sectoral action to tackle both the input and output sides of the energy equation. The 2010 White Paper 'Healthy Lives, Healthy People: Our Strategy for Public Health in England' set out details of the UK government's plans to prevent and treat obesity in children.

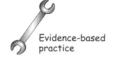
Evidence-based practice

The evidence on interventions to reverse or prevent obesity in individual children is not encouraging [40]. Interventions which do show some impact include a component focusing on parenting and family relationships [42–44]. In 2006, the National Institute for Health and Clinical Excellence (NICE) published a clinical guideline (CG43) on the identification, assessment and management of overweight and obesity in adults and children. This offered evidence-based guidance for interventions within the NHS, and for local authorities, schools and the public.

Tables 12.5 and 12.6 illustrate how action might be planned at different levels, and by different agencies, to tackle childhood obesity.

Further case studies on parenting and healthy schools are available in the Internet Companion.

Table 12.5 Tackling childhood obesity: examples of action at individual, community and policy levels

Level	Input (food and nutrition)	Output (physical activity)
Individual	Classroom activities which focus on healthy eating and food preparation	Exercise prescriptions, cycle-proficiency training, wider provision of physical activities in school to appeal to 'non-sporty' children
	Programmes for parents providing knowledge and skills relating to food and its preparation, physical activity and behaviour management	
Community	Community gardens, farmer's markets and local food co-operatives; healthy school food	Improved access to leisure facilities (e.g. free swimming for children) and green spaces
Policy	Improved food labelling, reducing fat and sugar content of ready meals	Transport policy measures to promote walking and cycling (e.g. cycle lanes, traffic calming)
	Ban advertising of high-sugar, high-fat foods to children	

Table 12.6 Tackling childhood obesity: examples of action by different agencies

Agency	Input (food and nutrition)	Output (physical activity)
Schools	Changing to healthy school meals and vending machines (selling fruit and other healthy snacks, not crisps and chocolate and fizzy drinks)	Developing safe routes to school and 'walking buses'
Local authorities	Allotment schemes to encourage local people to grow their own fruit and vegetables	Improving street safety and outdoor play spaces
Media	Campaign highlighting healthy eating – e.g. local restaurants with 'lite' menu; recipe ideas; 'Change 4 Life'	Disseminating information about local sports teams' outreach programmes to young people
Commercial world	*Food manufacturers*: reducing sugar, salt and fat content of food	*Leisure providers*: helping to widen access to sports facilities
	Supermarkets: promoting 'Five a day' message and offering ranges of fruit and vegetables to appeal to children	Sponsorship of local sports teams
National government	Food-pricing policies to promote healthy rather than 'junk' foods; setting nutritional standards for school catering	Investing in school sport, cycle lanes, leisure facilities and sports clubs

Health policy for children

A number of key documents have shaped health policy for children in the UK. Many of these – such as the Children Act and 'Every Child Matters' [45] – apply not just to the health sector but to all agencies working with children. Others – such as the 2010 Public Health White Paper 'Healthy Lives, Healthy People' [2] – include children but also cover the rest of the population. This policy document recognises the significance of child public health and the central importance of ensuring children get 'the best start in life'. The National Service Framework (NSF) for children, young people and maternity services [6], published in 2004, sets out the previous government's vision for health- and social-care services for children and young people and includes eleven standards which should shape children's services in future.

Conclusion

We have demonstrated in this chapter that tackling the public health challenges faced by children provides a good exemplar of the use of public health skills in a particular population context. However, we have also described ways in which, due to the vulnerability of children, the nature of the determinants of ill health and their impact on health in later life, the public health challenges for this population are distinct and need to be given special attention.

REFERENCES

1. S. Stewart-Brown, Child Health and Adult Health. In M. Blair, S. Stewart-Brown, A. Waterston, R. Crowther (eds.), *Child Public Health*, Oxford, Oxford University Press, 2010.
2. Department of Health, Healthy Lives Healthy People: Our Strategy for Public Health in England (White Paper), London, HM Government, 2010. Available at: http://www.dh.gov.uk/en/Publicationsandstatistics/Publications/PublicationsPolicyAndGuidance/DH_121941.
3. M. Marmot, Strategic Review of Health Inequalities in England Post-2010 (The Marmot Review), London, University College, 2010. Available at: http://www.ucl.ac.uk/gheg/marmotreview.
4. Department of Health, No health without mental health: A cross-government mental health outcomes strategy for people of all ages, London, HM Government, 2011. Available at: http://www.dh.gov.uk/prod_consum_dh/groups/dh_digitalassets/documents/digitalasset/dh_124058.pdf.
5. J. Heckman, Schools, skills and synapses. *Economic Inquiry* **46**(3), 2008, 289–324.
6. Department of Health, National Service Framework for children, young people and maternity services (guidance document), London, HM Government, 2004.
7. L. Kohler, Child public health: a new basis for child health workers. *European Journal of Public Health* **8**, 1998, 235–5.

8. U. Bronfenbrenner, *The Ecology of Human Development: Experiments by Nature and Design*, Cambridge, MA, Harvard University Press, 1979.

9. J. Macheson, Measuring What Matters: National Statistician's Reflections on the National Debate on Measuring National Well-being, Office for National Statistics, 2011. Available at: http://www.ons.gov.uk/ons/guide-method/user-guidance/well-being/index.html.

10. B. Maughan, A. C. Iervolino and S. Collishaw. Time trends in child and adolescent mental disorders. *Current Opinion in Psychiatry* **18**, 2005, 381–5.

11. K. L. Windfuhr, D. T. While, I. M. Hunt *et al*, Suicide in juveniles and adolescents in the United Kingdom. *Journal of Child Psychiatry and Psychology* **49**, 2008, 1165–75.

12. C. Currie, K. Levin and J. Todd, Health Behaviour in School-aged Children: World Health Organization Collaborative Cross-National Study (HBSC): Findings from the 2006 HBSC Survey in Scotland, Child and Adolescent Health Research Unit, The University of Edinburgh, 2008. Available at: http://www.st-andrews.ac.uk/cahru/publications/reports.php.html.

13. E. Fuller, Smoking, Drinking and Drug Use Among Young People in England, National Centre for Social Research, 2009. Available at: http://www.ic.nhs.uk/pubs/sdd08fullreport.

14. Department of Children, Schools and Families, Teenage Pregnancy Strategy: beyond 2010, London, HM Government, 2010. Available at: https://www.education.gov.uk/publications/standard/publicationdetail/page1/DCSF-00224-2010.

15. Health Protection Agency, Sexually Transmitted Infections and Young People in the United Kingdom: 2008 Report. Available at: http://www.hpa.org.uk/web/HPAwebFile/HPAweb_C/1216022461534.

16. UNICEF, *State of the World's Children 2011*, New York, NY, UNICEF, 2011. Available at: http://www.unicef.org/sowc2011/pdfs/Table-1-Basic-Indicators_02092011.pdf.

17. R. E. Black, S. Cousens, H. L. Johnson *et al.*, Global, regional, and national causes of child mortality in 2008: a systematic analysis. *Lancet* **375**, 2010, 1969–87.

18. World Health Organization, *World Health Statistics 2011*. Geneva, The WHO, 2011.

19. Department of Health, *Choosing Health; Making Healthier Choices Easier*, London, HM Stationery Office, 2004.

20. Centre on the Developing Child at Harvard University, A science-based framework for early childhood policy: using evidence to improve outcomes in learning behaviour and health for vulnerable children. 2007. Available at: http://www.developingchild.harvard.edu.

21. A. Caspi, K. Sugden, T. E. Moffitt *et al.*, Influence of life stress on depression; moderation by a polymorphism in the 5-HTT gene. *Science* **301**, 2003, 386–9.

22. B. R. Van Den Bergh, E. J. Mulder, M. Mennes and V. Glover, Antenatal maternal anxiety and stress and the neurobehavioural development of the fetus and child: links and possible mechanisms. *Neuroscience and Biobehavioural Reviews* **29**, 2005, 237–58.

23. S. Gerhardt, *Why Love Matters; How Affection Shapes a Baby's Brain*, London, Routledge, 2004.

24. S. Weich, J. Patterson, R. Shaw and S. Stewart-Brown, Family relationships in childhood and common psychiatric disorders in later life: systematic review of prospective studies. *British Journal of Psychiatry* **194**, 2009, 392–8.

25. R. Repetti, S. Taylor and T. Seeman, Risky families: early social environments and the mental and physical health of offspring. *Psychological Bulletin* **128**, 2002, 330–6.

26. F. Field, The Foundation Years: preventing poor children becoming poor adults. The report of the independent review of poverty and life chances, London, HM Government, 2010.

27. S. Stewart-Brown and A. Scharder-McMillan, Parenting for mental health: what does the evidence say we need to do? Report of Workpackage 2 of the DataPrev project. *Health Promotion International* **26**, 2011, i10–i28.

28. S. Stewart-Brown and A. Schrader MacMillan, Promoting the mental health of children and parents: evidence and outcomes for home and community based parenting support interventions. Report of Workpackage 2 of the DATAPREV Project European Community 6th Framework Research Programme, 2010. Available at: http://wrap.warwick.ac.uk/3239/.

29. P. R. Amato, L. S. Loomis and A. Booth, Parental divorce, marital conflict and offspring wellbeing during early adulthood. *Social Forces* **73**(3), 1995, 895–915.

30. A. C. Dettling, S. W. Parker, S. Lane, A. Sebanc and M. R. Gunnar, Quality of care and temperament determine changes in cortisol concentrations over the day for young children in childcare. *Psychoneuroendocrinology* **25** (8), 2000, 819–36.

31. M. R. Burchinal, J. E. Roberts, R. Riggins, Jr. *et al*. Relating quality of center-based child care to early cognitive and language development longitudinally. *Child Development* **71**, 2000, 338–57.

32. L. Arseneault, E. Walsh, K. Trsesniewski *et al.*, Bullying victimisation uniquely contributes to adjustment problems in young children: a nationally representative cohort study. *Pediatrics* **118**, 2006, 130–8.

33. A. Sroufe, E. Egland and E. Carlson, One social world: integrated development of parent child and peer relationships. In B. Laursen and W. A. Collins (eds.), *Relationships as Developmental Contexts. Minnesota Symposium on Child Psychology*, London, Lawrence Erlbaum Associates, 1999.

34. K. Weare, *Promoting Mental, Emotional and Social Health: a Whole School Approach*, London, Routledge, 2000.

35. D. Acheson and N. Spencer, *Poverty and Child Health*, Abingdon Radcliffe Medical Press, 2000.

36. HM Revenue and Customs. Personal tax credits: Related statistics – child poverty. NI116: The proportion of children in poverty, 2008. Available at: www.hmrc.gov.uk/stats/personal-tax-credits/child_poverty.htm.

37. D. Hirsch, Estimating the costs of child poverty, York, Joseph Rowntree Foundation, 2008. Available at: http://www.jrf.org.uk/sites/files/jrf/2313.pdf.

38. D. Wilkinson, Poor housing and ill health – a summary of research evidence, The Scottish Office, Central Research Unit, Housing Research Branch, 1999.

39. Faculty of Public Health, *Thinking Ahead: Why We Need to Improve Children's Mental Health and Wellbeing*, London, FPH, 2011.

40. J. J. Reilly, J. Armstrong, A. R. Dorosty *et al.*, Early life risk factors for obesity in childhood: cohort study. *British Medical Journal* **330**, 2005, 1357–9.

41. C. D. Summerbell, V. Ashton, K. J. Campbell *et al.*, Interventions for treating obesity in children (Cochrane Review). *Cochrane Library*, Issue 4, 2003.

42. University of York NHS Centre for Reviews and Dissemination, The prevention and treatment of childhood obesity. *Effective Health Care* **7** (6), 2002.

43. W. Robertson, M. Thorogood, N. Inglis, C. Grainger and S. Stewart-Brown. Two year follow-up of the 'Families for Health' programme for the treatment of childhood obesity. *Child Care Health and Development*, April 2011. doi: 10.1111/j.1365–2214.2011.01237.x.

44. P. M. Sacher, M. Kolotourou, P. M. Chadwick, *et al.*, Randomized controlled trial of the MEND Program: A family-based community intervention for childhood obesity, *Obesity* **18**, 2010, S62–S68.

45. Government Green Paper, Every Child Matters, Norwich, The Stationery Office, 2003.

13

Adult public health

Veena Rodrigues

Key points

- Adults aged 15 to 64 years account for a sizeable proportion of the population (over 60%) both worldwide and within the UK.
- Non-communicable diseases are the leading causes of death in developed countries whereas in developing countries, communicable diseases, maternal, perinatal and nutritional conditions and injuries are the leading causes of death.
- Within the UK, cancers, cardiovascular diseases, diabetes mellitus, mental illness and obesity are significant public health problems in this age group.
- Although national policies are already in place to tackle these conditions, concerted health-improvement efforts with engagement of local populations are required to make a significant impact on the burden of ill health.

Introduction

Approximately 66% of the world's population in 2010 was estimated to be aged between 15 and 64 years, with a male:female ratio of 1.02. In less-developed regions of the world, this age group comprises 65% of the total population whereas in the more developed regions it comprises about 68% [1].

In 2009, 65% of the UK population were aged between 15 and 64 years. Although the total UK population increased by 10% between 1984 and 2009, the proportion of the population aged 15–64 years increased only by 1% [2]. The old-age dependency ratio (number of people aged 65 or more for every 100 people aged 15–64) in the UK was 24 in 2009; this is close to the EU average but is projected to rise to 39 by 2035 as the population ages (see Chapter 14).

Demography

Essential Public Health, Second Edition, ed. Stephen Gillam, Jan Yates and Padmanabhan Badrinath. Published by Cambridge University Press. © Cambridge University Press 2012.

Figure 13.1 Determinants of health. Source: G. Dahlgren and N. Whitehead, Policies and strategies to promote social equity in health. Stockholm, Institute of Futures Studies, 1991; reproduced with permission.

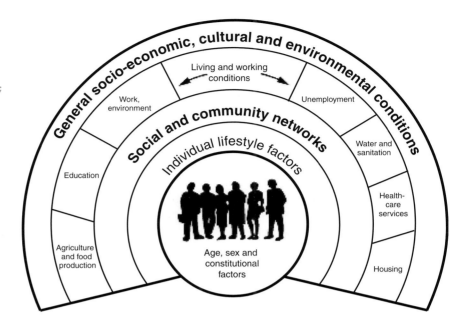

Determinants of health

There are several factors that determine the health of the adult population (Figure 13.1). According to this model, determinants of health work at various levels. These are:

- *Individual lifestyle factors*, which can be grouped into fixed factors such as age, sex and genetics, and modifiable factors such as diet, physical activity, cigarette smoking and alcohol consumption.
- *Social and community networks* (interactions between friends, family and other members of the community) play an important role in maintaining people's health and are particularly important in maintaining good mental health.
- *Living and working conditions* such as education, agriculture and food production, work environment, housing, water and sanitation, and unemployment also have a role.
- *General socio-economic, cultural and environmental conditions* such as standard of living, mean income levels, the place of women in society, employment rates, levels of deprivation and inequalities prevalent in society as a whole have an impact on adult health.

Causes of mortality and morbidity

Health status

Adult mortality rates have been declining in most countries, but the relative importance of a range of causes differs across developed and developing countries, with non-communicable diseases predominating in developed countries and communicable diseases, maternal, perinatal and nutritional conditions, and injuries being leading causes of mortality in developing countries [3]. However, population ageing and changes in risk-factor distributions in many developing countries have resulted in an acceleration of the epidemic of non-communicable diseases.

In the UK, life expectancy at birth was 77.7 years for males and 81.9 years for females in 2009. Although it has increased steadily over the previous 20 years, the increase has been higher in males than females (5.3 years versus 3.8 years).

In 15 to 64 year olds, neoplasms account for 39% of the deaths, followed by diseases of the circulatory system (22%) [4]. In terms of the burden of ill health in this age group, apart from cancers and cardiovascular diseases, conditions such as obesity, diabetes and mental illness are significant public health problems. In this section, for each major condition, the burden of disease, risk factors and potential public health action is described. More information on these conditions can be found on the Internet Companion.

Cancer

Burden of disease

Each year, 7.6 million people worldwide die from cancer and 11.3 million people are diagnosed with cancer [5]. In 2009, there were more than 156,000 deaths due to cancer in the UK (Figure 13.2). Cancer mortality is highest among people aged 65 and over but still significant in those under 65. In 2008, cancers accounted for 36% of all deaths in the under 65s compared with 25% in the over 65s [6].

Risk factors

Many of the known risk factors for cancers are avoidable and cancer risk could be decreased further by making changes to individual lifestyles. Risk factors include smoking, ultraviolet radiation, physical inactivity, obesity, diet, alcohol and infections.

Prevention

Secondary prevention includes raising awareness of signs and symptoms, effective treatment and, importantly, screening. Screening was discussed in detail in Chapter 9 and has been estimated to save around 1400 [7] lives per year in England due to breast cancer screening and 1300 due to screening for cervical cancer [8]. Studies have shown that screening can reduce bowel cancer mortality by 15% in those screened. A national bowel cancer screening programme was rolled out in 2006 following a successful pilot and achieved nation-wide coverage in 2010 [9].

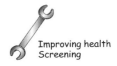
Improving health
Screening

Implications for policy

In England, the NHS Cancer Reform Strategy [10] describes a comprehensive action to tackle cancer through better prevention and treatment. It continues national policy

Figure 13.2   European age-
standardised mortality rates by
sex for lung, breast, prostate and
bowel cancer, UK 1971–2008.
Source CancerStats, info.
cancerresearchuk.org.

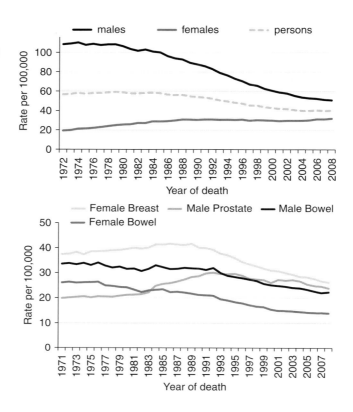

aims for reduction of smoking rates, early diagnosis, e.g. promoting screening, and provision of high-quality treatment and care throughout the country, e.g. establishing national standards for cancer services and specialist palliative care.

Cardiovascular diseases

Burden of disease

Cardiovascular diseases (CVD) are one of the leading causes of death within adults in the UK and accounted for over 191,000 deaths in 2008. Of these, around 88,000 were from coronary heart disease and another 43,000 from stroke [11]. Cardiovascular diseases caused more than 50,000 premature deaths in the UK in 2008 and among the under 75s it is responsible for more than one in four deaths among men and one in five deaths among women. It is estimated that there are around 2.7 million people living in the UK who have or have had either angina or a heart attack, and the Health Survey for England [12] and the General Household Survey [13] suggest that morbidity appears to be rising, particularly in older age groups. Rates of treatment for CVD vary widely across the UK. For example, in England in 2010, there was a greater than 10-fold variation in the percentage of people suffering a stroke who were treated within 24 hours [14].

Health
status

Table 13.1 Risk factors for CVDs

Non-modifiable risk factors for CVD	Modifiable risk factors for CVD
Older age	High serum cholesterol
Male gender	Hypertension
Ethnicity	Smoking (mortality is 60% higher in smokers and 80% higher in heavy smokers as compared to non-smokers [15])
Family history	Second-hand smoke
Genetic predisposition	Diet high in fat, salt and low in fruit and vegetables
	Obesity (particularly central obesity)
	Diabetes
	Physical inactivity (< 2.5 hours moderate-intensity activity per week) [16]
	Hypertension
	High blood-cholesterol levels

These inequalities have implications for the provision of both medical and preventative interventions [11], which include a high financial burden to health-care services, both for acute and chronic care. Overall, CVDs are estimated to cost the UK economy just under £26 billion a year (around 57% is due to direct health-care costs, 24% to productivity losses and 19% to the informal care of people with CVD).

Risk factors

Although treatments for these diseases continue to be developed and improved, the proportion of people dying from heart attacks remains high and most heart disease is potentially preventable. Epidemiological studies have identified a number of risk factors for cardiovascular diseases (Table 13.1).

Prevention

The modifiable risk factors are of potential public health importance and hence national public health targets aim to reduce the prevalence of these risk factors in the population.

A key intervention to reduce the impact of CVD is preventing and stopping smoking. Ways to achieve this include smoking cessation interventions, which support smokers to quit (see Chapter 8 for more details), tobacco taxation and legislation to ban smoking in public places. In 1994, the Committee on Medical Aspects of Food and Nutrition Policy [16] recommended targets for reducing *saturated fat, total fat* and increasing *fruit and vegetable consumption*. Progress towards the targets has been disappointing. *Salt* consumption also remains well above the levels (6 g per day) recommended. A reduction in the salt content of processed foods and drinks is required if the target is to be met. Apart from being an independent risk factor for heart disease, *obesity* is also a major risk factor for hypertension, raised serum cholesterol and diabetes. See below for more details on preventing obesity. The Chief Medical Officer's report [17] recommended that adults in England should participate in a minimum of 30 minutes of moderate-intensity activity (such as brisk walking, cycling or climbing the stairs) on five or more days of the week. Risk of heart disease is directly related to *blood cholesterol levels*; these can be reduced by drugs, physical activity and by reducing consumption of saturated fat. The 2011/12 English Quality and Outcomes Framework for general practice sets a secondary prevention target for cholesterol of < 5.0 mmol/l [18].

Implications for policy

Policy develops over time as improvements in outcome are monitored. In the UK, a report on the impact of the National Service Framework (NSF) for coronary heart disease [19] highlighted the need for further improvements in prevention of heart disease, and reduction in inequalities of access, particularly among those with chronic vascular conditions as compared to acute conditions. Improvements had been seen in faster treatment of heart-attack patients, higher numbers of revascularisation operations performed with shorter waiting times and the setting up of rapid-access chest-pain clinics across the country to improve the speed with which people with suspected angina can be assessed.

Diabetes mellitus

Burden of disease

Between 1996 and 2009, the number of people with diagnosed diabetes increased from 1.4 million to 2.6 million in the UK [20]; of these, the majority (85%) have Type 2 diabetes. It is estimated that up to half a million more people could have undiagnosed diabetes. The rising number of people diagnosed with diabetes is thought to be due to the ageing population and the increasing prevalence of obesity in the UK.

Diabetes is a significant cause of morbidity and mortality. People with diabetes have a lower life expectancy and they are more likely to develop coronary heart disease and stroke. Diabetes is the leading cause of blindness among those of a working age in the UK and people with diabetes spend over a million days in hospital each year. If undiagnosed, untreated or not managed effectively, diabetes has a high risk of complications. Often, complications begin before diagnosis (50% of individuals have evidence of complications on diagnosis of Type 2 diabetes) [20]. However, if managed effectively, complications of diabetes can be reduced considerably and life expectancy can be increased.

Risk factors

Risk factors for Type 2 diabetes are shown in Table 13.2. Type 1 diabetes almost always occurs in individuals under the age of 40 years, whereas Type 2 diabetes

Table 13.2 Risk factors for diabetes [20]

Ethnicity (African-Caribbean or South Asian)
Older age
Genetic predisposition
Overweight and obesity
Physical inactivity

generally tends to occur in those over the age of 40. Changing lifestyle factors are resulting in Type 2 diabetes being detected in younger individuals. In the UK, the prevalence of diabetes is at least six times higher among individuals from Asian communities and about three times higher in individuals from African and African-Caribbean communities. Diabetes often appears before the age of 40 among these individuals. A genetic predisposition is known to exist in both types of diabetes, although the disease is determined by complex gene–environment interactions. Around 80–90% of individuals with Type 2 diabetes are overweight. The risk of developing diabetes is 10 times higher among obese individuals.

Prevention

The pattern of risk factors means that effective primary prevention should focus on increasing physical activity levels, improving diet and nutrition and reducing overweight and obesity. Secondary prevention includes increased awareness of symptoms, follow-up and regular testing of individuals known to be at increased risk of developing diabetes, and opportunistic screening of people with multiple risk factors for diabetes. The risk of complications due to diabetes is high, which makes tertiary prevention important. Early detection and treatment of microvascular complications (retinopathy, nephropathy, neuropathy) can prevent impairment. Control of hypertension, reduction of cholesterol levels and smoking cessation in people with diabetes reduces their risk of developing both microvascular complications and cardiovascular disease, and regular recall and review of people with diabetes improves the subsequent outcomes.

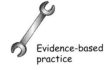

Evidence-based
practice

Implications for policy

In the UK, an NHS report on the national diabetes strategy, published in 2010 [21], found that although, nationally, considerable improvements to service provision have been made and results are being delivered, treatment and care for people with diabetes still requires focus and consistency.

Table 13.3 Classification of BMI

Classification	BMI (kg/m^2)
Underweight	<18.5
Healthy weight	18.5–24.9
Overweight	25.0–29.9
Obese	30.0 or more

Obesity

Burden of disease

Obesity is caused by a sustained imbalance between energy intake (higher) and energy expenditure (lower). The main measures for assessment of obesity are:

1. **Body mass index (BMI).** This is measured as weight (kg) divided by height squared (m^2), and classified into four categories as shown in Table 13.3.

   The risk of morbidity and mortality rises with increases in BMI over 25, the risk of co-morbidities being very severe in individuals with morbid obesity, i.e. BMI of 40 or more.

2. **Waist circumference.** Central obesity is also correlated with disease risk, with cut-off points indicating risk of co-morbidities. For the general adult population this is >40 inches for men and >35 inches for women. But in south Asian populations the cut-off points are lower at >35 and >32 inches respectively.

3. **Waist–hip ratio.** This is calculated as the waist circumference (m) divided by the hip circumference (m). Values of 0.95 or more among men and 0.85 or more among women are correlated with a higher risk of disease.

Obesity is a significant public health problem in the UK and shows an increasing trend. Figures from the Health Survey for England [22] indicate that almost two thirds of adults are either overweight or obese with nearly a quarter of adults being obese. The levels of obesity have risen from 19.8% in 1993 to 23% in 2009. The relative increase is much higher among women as compared to men. However, many individuals are unaware that they may have a weight problem.

Obesity is associated with increased mortality and morbidity and a decreased quality of life. Health problems associated with obesity are shown in Table 13.4.

Risk factors

Risk factors for obesity are shown in Table 13.5. The rise in global obesity has been linked to environmental and behavioural changes (e.g. sedentary lifestyle, easy access to high-calorie, low-cost foods) brought about by economic development, modernisation and urbanisation.

Table 13.4 Effect of obesity on health

Greatly increased risk of	Moderately increased risk of	Slightly increased risk of
Type 2 diabetes	Coronary heart disease	Breast cancer in post-menopausal women, colon cancer
Insulin resistance	Hypertension	Polycystic ovaries
Gall bladder diseases	Stroke	Risk of anaesthetic complications
Dyslipidaemia	Osteoarthritis (knees and hips)	Impaired fertility
Breathlessness	Hyperuricaemia and gout	Low back pain
Sleep apnoea	Psychological factors	Reproductive hormone abnormalities

Table 13.5 Risk factors for obesity [23]

Older age
Female gender
Lower socio-economic status
Black Caribbean and Black African ethnicity (obesity is low in Chinese populations)
Physical inactivity

The metabolic syndrome, a condition characterised by obesity and insulin resistance, confers an increased risk of diabetes, heart disease and stroke. Almost a quarter of the adult population in the UK are estimated to have this condition.

Prevention

The *population* approach to primary prevention seeks to lower the risk of becoming overweight or obese in the whole community. It consists largely of two elements: promoting a balanced diet and increasing physical activity levels in the community. The UK government recommendations on diet are based on the recommendations of the Committee on Medical Aspects of Food Policy. These include advice to eat at least five portions of fruit and vegetables per day, decrease consumption of saturated fats to less than 11% of total energy consumption, decrease salt to less than 6 grams per day, and increase dietary fibre to 18 grams per day.

United Kingdom government recommendations on physical activity for adults are a total of at least 30 minutes of physical activity (moderate intensity) per day at least five times a week. This could be achieved through everyday activities such as walking, gardening and swimming or through sport or structured exercise and, increasingly, an approach to support people to make small changes is being used (www.nhs.uk/Change4Life).

The *high-risk* approach to primary prevention concentrates on individuals who have an increased chance of becoming overweight or obese, such as individuals from lower socio-economic classes, individuals from south-Asian communities (increased risk of diseases caused by obesity), Black Caribbean and Black African individuals (higher prevalence of obesity), people with physical disabilities affecting mobility and people with learning difficulties.

For secondary prevention in those already overweight or obese, for *weight management* to be effective and sustainable, a combination of advice on diet and physical activity, and motivation and support to make and maintain these changes, are essential. For some individuals, drug treatment and surgery may be additional options to be considered.

Implications for policy

Obesity is becoming increasingly important in UK health policy. Guidance on the management of overweight and obesity in primary care in the UK was published in early 2006 by the Department of Health [24]. Clinical guidelines on the prevention and management of obesity (including drugs and energy) have been published by the National Institute for Health and Clinical Excellence (NICE) [25]. A new national Public Health Responsibility Deal [26] has been produced following the publication of the White Paper 'Healthy Lives, Healthy People' [27] to encourage organisations and businesses to play their part in improving the health of the public and tackling the health inequalities related to food, physical activity, alcohol and workplace health with the intention of complementing government action on the same.

Local action should focus on developing or reviewing strategies to tackle obesity using a multifactorial approach involving a range of stakeholders which provide opportunities for healthy lifestyles to be the norm and support treatment through traditional and novel forms of care.

Mental health

Burden of disease

Definitions of mental health include concepts such as psychological well-being, autonomy, competence, inter-generational dependence, and actualisation of one's intellectual and emotional potential. Although it is difficult to define mental health comprehensively, it is generally agreed that mental health is broader than a lack of mental disorders.

The World Health Organization defines mental health as 'a state of well-being in which the individual realises his or her own abilities, can cope with the normal stresses of life, can work productively and fruitfully, and is able to make a contribution to his or her community'.

Table 13.6 Risk factors for mental health problems [30]

Age
Female gender for depression
Exposure to violence, conflict and disasters
Stressful life events
Ethnic minority status
Low socio-economic status
Genetic predisposition

The terms mental illness or mental disorder refer to health conditions characterised by alterations in thinking, mood or behaviour associated with distress and/or impaired functioning. Mental illness is a leading cause of morbidity worldwide and in the UK. In the UK, it constitutes just under a quarter (22.8%) of the total burden of disability whereas worldwide it accounts for four of the ten leading causes of disability [28, 29]. By 2020, it is projected that mental and neurological disorders will account for 15% of the total disability-adjusted life years lost due to all diseases and injuries. The WHO estimates that a quarter of all people suffer from mental and behavioural disorders at some time during their lives, with a prevalence of about 10% among the adult population at any time [30]. Among adults in Great Britain, these figures are around 1 in 4 and 1 in 6, respectively, with 15% reporting symptoms suggestive of neurotic disorders such as anxiety and depression of which 7.5% were at a level that warranted treatment; the prevalence of psychotic disorders was about 0.5% [28]. There do not appear to be differences in those conditions diagnosed most often (depression, anxiety and substance misuse) in primary care in developed and developing countries [30].

Risk factors

Risk factors for mental disorders are shown in Table 13.6. Age is an important determinant of mental disorders and the prevalence of some mental disorders (for example, depression) rises with age, with a high prevalence among the elderly. Most studies report no difference in overall prevalence of mild to moderate mental disorder by gender. This is also true for severe mental disorders, except depression, which has a higher prevalence among women, and substance misuse, which has a higher prevalence among men [31]. The gender difference in some mental disorders could also be due to a higher exposure to domestic and sexual violence among women. The lifetime prevalence of domestic violence ranges from 16 to 50%. It is estimated that 20% of women suffer rape or attempted rape in their lifetime [30]. Research suggests the existence of a genetic predisposition to mental disorders such as schizophrenia, depression and dementia [30]. Common mental disorders are twice as high among the lowest socio-economic categories as compared to the highest category. This is true for both developing and developed countries. Among prisoners in England, about 90% are estimated to have a diagnosable mental health problem and/or a substance misuse problem [28]. Disorders such as schizophrenia are reported to be higher among British-born ethnic-minority populations. Explanatory factors suggested include increased vulnerability due to social isolation and fewer social networks, and that people from these communities may be more likely to be singled out. Mental and behavioural disorders such as schizophrenia, depression and suicide show an association with life events (job insecurity, bereavement, relationship breakdown, change of residence, business failure, etc.) particularly if they occur in quick succession. War, civil strife and natural disasters affect several million people worldwide and have a huge effect on the mental health of the people affected. Common mental health disorders reported include mental distress, post-traumatic stress disorder, depression and anxiety [30].

Prevention

According to the WHO [30], in countries with sufficient resources, actions required to prevent mental illness include the following: raising public awareness, provision of effective drug therapy and psychosocial interventions, development of good mental health information systems and initiation/extension of research on service delivery and prevention of mental disorders.

Health promotion in the prevention of mental illness is essentially concerned with making changes that will promote people's mental well-being. It covers a variety of strategies, which can be delivered at three levels: individual, community and national. Promotion of interventions that increase coping and life skills work at an individual level. For example, supporting new parents and relationship education helps improve maternal and child mental health [30]. Workplace initiatives, for example raising awareness of mental health issues among employees, can provide opportunities for those suffering from mental health problems to seek help [32, 33]. Increasing social inclusion and cohesion, developing support networks and promoting mental health in workplaces and neighbourhoods are examples of measures that can be undertaken to promote mental health at the community level. Workplace initiatives could include flexible working arrangements, career progression opportunities, increasing employers' awareness of mental health issues, creating a balance between job demands and occupational skills, stress audits, social-skills training, provision of counselling services and early rehabilitation strategies. As unemployment is a significant issue, mental health-promotion strategies could seek to improve employment opportunities, through programmes to create jobs or the provision of vocational training. Reducing barriers to mental health through national policies to reduce discrimination, promote access to employment, and support for vulnerable citizens, are examples of action that can be taken at a national level.

The National Service Framework for mental health [34] sought to improve the quality of adult mental health services through mental health promotion, improved access to mental health services in primary care, effective care for people with severe mental illness, and better support for carers of people with mental illness in England. The initial focus was on improving specialist care, and provision of intensive support for people with the most complex needs with focus then extending to the mental health needs of the whole community. More recently, a new mental health strategy for England has been published with the objective of mainstreaming mental health and establishing parity between services for people with physical and mental health problems [29]. For this to be effective, emphasis on multi-agency working (health and social care; the voluntary and private sectors; housing, employment and training; and the community) is essential – not only to tackle mental illness but also to promote mental well-being and independence.

Implications for policy

In many parts of the world, mental health and mental illness have a low priority as compared to physical health, with only a minority receiving any treatment. Among adults living in Great Britain, around 23% of the population reported receiving some treatment for a mental health problem [28]. However, women were more likely to have received treatment or used services as compared to men (29% versus 17%). The onset and recovery of common mental disorders were associated with unemployment, financial problems and difficulties with activities of daily living. There is a disproportionate relationship between the burden of mental illness and spending on mental health. According to the WHO, although mental and behavioural disorders constitute 12% of the global burden of disease, the mental health budgets of many countries is less than 1% of their total expenditures [30].

Health promotion

It is recognised that primary prevention of conditions important for adult health is a key component of any strategy to tackle these issues. Chapter 8 considers health improvement as a key public health tool and some of the themes of that chapter are illustrated here. There are several approaches to adult health promotion. *Vertical* programmes which tackle a single health condition have already been illustrated. Alternatively, it is possible to address many conditions at once in a particular *setting* (such as workplaces) or to modify an 'up-stream' *determinant* such as housing conditions. One detailed example is given here – healthy workplaces.

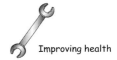
Improving health

Health-promotion settings case-study – healthy workplaces

Initiatives focusing on the workplace can also address the physical and mental health of a large proportion of the adult population and the benefits of a healthy workplace include increased productivity, reduced sickness-absenteeism, and a decrease in injuries and accidents, with a positive impact on staff morale and retention [35].

> **Box 13.1 Sickness-absence in the UK [32]**
> - Sickness costs the economy over £100 billion per year.
> - 150 million days are taken annually in sickness absence.
> - 7% of the population claim incapacity benefit and 25% of the working-age population are not in work.
> - Mental health conditions are an important cause of absence.

There is a fundamental link between health and socio-economic indicators such as job status and income.

In the UK, Dame Carol Black reviewed the health of the working-age population including sickness absence (Box 13.1) [32]. This was followed by a Government policy response the aim of which is as follows:

'We want to create a society where the positive links between work and health are recognised by all, where everyone aspires to a healthy and fulfilling working life, and where health conditions and disabilities are not a bar to enjoying the benefits of work.'

Elements of health promotion that are relevant to this setting are:
- *Normalising wellness not sickness*, for example the creating of fit notes to replace sick notes, and education of general practitioners.
- *Supporting employers to focus on healthy workplaces.* Evaluation studies show that the initial costs of the intervention are outweighed by the gains arising from reduced absenteeism (lost productivity while sick) and presenteeism (lost productivity while at work).
- *Creation of a safe and healthy workplace* through increased awareness of employer responsibilities, carrying out risk assessments, and provision of occupational health services for employees.
- *Good recruitment and retention policies* including options such as flexible working arrangements and policies for managing sickness absence and supporting managed early return to work after absence.
- *Promotion of mental well-being and reduction of stress* through identification of problem areas and taking action to address these, e.g. stress audits, improved recognition of risk factors and raising awareness of mental health issues among employees.
- *Prevention and management of musculo-skeletal disorders* through risk assessment, provision of training, good reporting systems, early identification and follow-up of symptoms.
- *Smoke-free policies* in the workplace to prevent exposure to tobacco smoke and referral to smoking cessation services for those who need it.

- *Prevention and management of substance misuse including alcohol* through the development of policies for the organisation and increasing employee awareness of issues involved.
- *Encouraging physical activity and healthy eating* by increasing awareness, encouraging cycling and walking to work, providing vending machines with healthy options, etc.

Conclusion

This chapter has outlined some diseases and conditions which are public health problems among adults aged 15 to 64 years. Chapter 2 described the epidemiologic transition which explains that as populations change their demographic, economic and social structures they shift towards an age structure with increasing proportions of adults and older people. The conditions outlined in this chapter are of particular relevance in more-developed countries, which are further along this transition process but will become increasing significant worldwide.

Chapter 14 continues this theme and looks in more detail at the public health issues relevant to ageing populations.

REFERENCES

1. Department of Economic and Social Affairs, United Nations, World population prospects: The 2010 revision, United Nations, 2011.
2. Office for National Statistics, *Population Trends* **nr 142**, Winter 2010.
3. World Health Organization, *Global Status Report on Non-communicable Diseases 2010*, Geneva, World Health Organization, 2011.
4. Office for National Statistics, Mortality Statistics: Deaths registered in 2009. Review of the National Statistician on deaths in England and Wales, 2009, Series DR, 2010.
5. World Health Organization, *Cancer* Fact Sheet No. 297, Geneva, World Health Organisation, 2011.
6. Cancer Research UK, Cancer in the UK: April 2011. See: http://info.cancerresearchuk.org/cancerstats.
7. Advisory Committee on breast cancer screening, Screening for breast cancer in England: past and future, NHSBSP Publication No. 61, Sheffield, NHS Cancer Screening Programmes, 2006.
8. National Statistics, Cervical screening programme, England 2004–05 Statistical Bulletin 2005/09/HSCIC, NHS Health and Social Care Information Centre, Health Services Community Statistics, 2005.
9. NHS bowel cancer screening programme, Guidance for Public Health and Commissioners, BCSP Publication no. 3, 2008. See: http://www.cancerscreening.nhs.uk/bowel/about-bowel-cancer-screening.html.
10. Department of Health, The NHS cancer reform strategy, London, Department of Health, 2007.

11. British Heart Foundation Statistics Datbase, Coronary heart disease statistics 2010 edition, Oxford, British Heart Foundation, 2010. See www.heartstats.org.

12. The Health and Social Care Information Centre, Health Survey for England 2006: cardiovascular disease and risk factors in adults, Leeds, Joint Health Surveys Unit, 2007.

13. Office for National Statistics, General Lifestyle Survey 2008, London, Office for National Statistics, 2009.

14. The NHS Atlas of Variation in Healthcare, 2010. See http://www.rightcare.nhs.uk/atlas/qipp_nhsAtlas-LOW_261110c.pdf.

15. R. Doll, R. Peto, J. Borcham and I. Sutherland, Mortality in relation to smoking: 50 years' observation on male British doctors. *British Medical Journal* **328**, 2004, 1519–27.

16. Department of Health, Nutritional aspects of cardiovascular disease, Report of the Cardiovascular Review Group of the Committee on Medical Aspects of Food and Nutrition Policy, London, HMSO, 1994.

17. Chief Medical Officer, At least five a week: evidence on the impact of physical activity and its relationship to health, London, Department of Health, 2004.

18. BMA and NHS Employers, Quality and Outcomes Framework guidance for GMS contract 2011/12, April 2011.

19. Department of Health, The coronary heart disease National Service Framework report: Building on excellence, maintaining progress, London, Department of Health, 2008.

20. Diabetes in the UK 2010, London, Diabetes UK, March 2010.

21. Department of Health, Six years on, delivering the Diabetes National Service Framework, London, Department of Health, 2010.

22. The Health and Social Care Information Centre, Health Survey for England 2009: health and lifestyles. Leeds, Joint Health Surveys Unit, 2010.

23. K. Swanton and M. Frost, Lightening the Load: Tackling Overweight and Obesity, London, Faculty of Public Health and National Heart Forum, 2006.

24. Department of Health, Care pathway for the management of overweight and obesity, London, Department of Health, 2006.

25. NICE, Obesity: the prevention, identification, assessment and management of overweight and obesity in adults and children. Clinical guideline 43, London, National Institute for Health and Clinical Excellence, 2006.

26. Department of Health, The Public Health Responsibility Deal, London, Department of Health, 2011.

27. Department of Health, Healthy Lives Healthy People: Our Strategy for Public Health in England (White Paper), London, HM Government, 2010.

28. S. McManus, H. Meltzer, T. Brugha *et al.*, Adult Psychiatric Morbidity in England, 2007: Results of a household survey, Leeds, Joint Health Surveys Unit, 2009.

29. Department of Health, No health without mental health. A cross-government mental health outcomes strategy for people of all ages, London, Department of Health, 2011.

30. The World Health Report 2001: Mental health: new understanding, new hope, Geneva, World Health Organization, 2002.

31. M. Knapp, D. McDaid and M. Parsonage, Mental health promotion and mental illness prevention: The economic case, London, Department of Health, 2011.

32. Dame Carol Black's Review of the health of Britain's working age population: Working for a healthier tomorrow, London, TSO, 2008.

33. Improving health and work: changing lives. The Government's Response to Dame Carol Black's Review of the health of Britain's working-age population, November, 2008.

34. Department of Health National Service Framework for mental health, London, Department of Health, 1999.

35. Faculty of Public Health and Faculty of Occupational Medicine, Creating a healthy workplace, London, 2006.

Public health and ageing

Lincoln Sargeant and Carol Brayne

Key points

- The population of older people has been increasing in number and as a proportion of populations worldwide.
- The prevalence of physical and cognitive frailty increases with age and as a result older people develop disabilities that prevent them from living independently as they age.
- Primary, secondary and tertiary prevention strategies can be effective for specific conditions that are common among older people.
- Where the scope for prevention is limited, as for example in dementia, provision needs to be made to provide support through health and social care.
- Informal carers, who are often relatives, provide the majority of social care for older people with more formal arrangements possibly becoming necessary as disability levels or health status deteriorate.
- Policy responses to ageing populations need to promote independent living, financial and physical security, as well as health- and social-care provision, in order to encourage older people to be active participants in society.

Introduction

At the start of the twentieth century a child born in the United Kingdom could expect to live for less than 50 years. In the UK, life expectancy at birth was 77.7 years for males and 81.9 years for females in 2009. This substantial change, typical of other developed countries, could well be seen as proof of the triumph of public health (broadly defined); but the success has also brought challenges.

In this chapter we will examine the factors that lead to ageing populations and explore the health, social and economic consequences of the change in the population

Essential Public Health, Second Edition, ed. Stephen Gillam, Jan Yates and Padmanabhan Badrinath.
Published by Cambridge University Press. © Cambridge University Press 2012.

structure. We will then outline the preventive strategies that can lead to healthy ageing and the public health actions that could help to manage the challenges posed by the relative and absolute increase in the numbers of older people.

The demography of old age

'Old age' is often defined as beginning at age 65 years but there is no biological rationale for this cut-off. It may be possible to define old age in terms of economic activity. In the UK, 65 years has been the age of retirement for men since 1908 but before then it was 70 years. Between 1950 and 1995 the average age of retirement in men had fallen in developed countries but in the last decade there has been a small increase. In all Western countries, there is pressure to increase, if not abolish, retirement ages and to increase the age at which state pensions are awarded. In many emerging economies, populations carry on working into old age as provision for older people is minimal or non-existent. Nevertheless, old age is often categorised as shown in Box 14.1.

The proportion of the population living into old age has been increasing worldwide. There are several factors that contribute to the changing structure in populations. Falling fertility rates and increased infant survival since the late nineteenth and early twentieth century have contributed to a larger proportion of the population surviving to middle age. The population structure resembles a pyramid in a young population but becomes more cylindrical as the population ages. See Chapter 2 for more information on population pyramids.

 Demography

Adult survival has also increased since the mid-twentieth century following improvements in the prevention and treatment of major premature causes of death such as heart disease. More people survive to age 65. Improved life expectancy has also occurred in the older age groups. It is estimated that more than 70 per cent of the rise in the maximum age at death in Sweden, which rose from about 101 years during the 1860s to about 108 years during the 1990s, was attributable to reductions in death rates above age 70 [1]. Together these trends have led to relative and absolute increases in the population at older ages, most marked in the oldest old.

Another phenomenon occurring in the mid-twentieth century indicates that further marked increases in the older population can be expected in developed countries in the next few decades. A rapid increase in fertility rates beginning with the end of the

---

Box 14.1 Old-age categories

Young old – 65 to 74 years
Middle old – 75 to 84 years
Oldest old – 85 years and over

Second World War lasting into the 1960s gave rise to the 'baby boom' generation. This generation is now middle aged to young old and will further exaggerate the ageing population profile in those developed countries, bringing with it changing expectations of health- and social-care provision.

The economic activity of the working population supports children and economically inactive adults such as retired older people. Dependency ratios are used to summarise the balance of economically active to inactive members of a society. The total dependency ratio is the ratio of children and people aged 65 and over to economically active adults. One constituent of this, the old-age dependency ratio, averaged 24% for European countries in 2009 and is projected to be over 47% in 2050. All regions of the world are projected to double or treble the old-age dependency ratio by 2050 but this is offset by falls in the proportion of children in less-developed countries. A high dependency ratio has the potential to limit the available funds for pensions and health-care of the elderly, and can have a profound impact on societies, especially those in developing countries where the rate of ageing has been faster than in the West.

However, the experience of old age varies greatly. People over 65 years can and do continue to contribute economically and are not necessarily dependent on the 'working-age population'. Pension and retirement ages are changing in many societies (where they exist). Many older individuals support economically active younger family members through child care and provide social care as unpaid carers for frail or disabled family members. Furthermore, the financial crash of the late 2000s has meant that in some cases older people have been expected to support adult children through the economic downturn. The challenge for public health is to understand the relation between ageing and health, including the wider effects on health, in order to prevent the disability and subsequent dependency that is often associated with growing old.

Ageing and health

Health status
Epidemiology

Ageing is related to ill health in one of three main ways:

- Some conditions are associated with ageing in that they can be expected to occur with all individuals as they age. High-frequency hearing, for example, declines predictably with age.
- Ill health can occur in the elderly because resilience decreases with age. Hence a fall in an elderly person is more likely to lead to fractures because of bone loss than in a young person.
- Some diseases are very closely associated with ageing such as Alzheimer's disease.
  Influences over the life course can also affect health in old age. Events during foetal life affect the risk of conditions such as diabetes and heart disease later in life but there is evidence that these influences can be modified or interrupted by adopting healthy lifestyle choices at any stage.

Box 14.2 Three dimensions of disability

In 1980, the World Health Organization published the International Classification of Impairments, Disabilities and Handicaps, which provides a conceptual framework for disability that is described in three dimensions – impairment, disability and handicap:

- **Impairment**. In the context of health experience an impairment is any loss or abnormality of psychological, physiological or anatomical structure or function.
- **Disability**. In the context of health experience a disability is any restriction or lack (resulting from an impairment) of ability to perform an activity in the manner or within the range considered normal for a human being.
- **Handicap**. In the context of health experience a handicap is a disadvantage for a given individual, resulting from an impairment or a disability, that limits or prevents the fulfilment of a role that is normal (depending on age, sex, and social and cultural factors) for that individual.

Cognitive and physical frailty increase with age and so does the number of chronic conditions that affect an individual. Together, these factors increase the likelihood of disability in the elderly patient (see Box 14.2). The prevalence of disability in the elderly increases steeply with age. This means that increasing proportions of people, as they age, need more support to perform activities of daily living such as bathing and dressing (Box 14.3). Figure 14.1 shows the prevalence by age of disability (difficulty with one or more activities of daily living) from the English Longitudinal Study of Ageing [2].

The strong association of ill health and disability with age has led to concerns that as the population ages so will the burden of ill health. It should be noted, however, that the burden and costs of ill health are concentrated at the end of life, irrespective of the age of death.

There are limited data on the overall effect of a longer life span on time spent in ill health. The worst-case scenario (see Figure 14.2) is that with increased life expectancy a greater proportion of time is spent in ill health. The Office of National Statistics estimates that, for the period 2006–2008, healthy-life expectancy at age 65 for UK men was 58.2% of overall life expectancy at that age. For women, the proportion was 56% [3].

Strategies for healthy ageing have aimed at keeping people in good health as long as possible. Since the 1990s, the World Health Organization has adopted the term 'active ageing' to signal that the ageing process can be so. Active ageing is defined as 'the process of optimizing opportunities for health, participation and security in order to enhance quality of life as people age.' This clearly includes broader themes than just health.

Box 14.3 Activities and instrumental activities of daily living

Activities of daily living
- Dressing, including putting on shoes and socks
- Walking across a room
- Bathing or showering
- Eating, such as cutting up food
- Getting in or out of bed
- Using the toilet, including getting up or down

Instrumental activities of daily living
- Using a map to figure out how to get around in a strange place
- Preparing a hot meal
- Shopping for groceries
- Making telephone calls
- Taking medications
- Doing work around the house or garden
- Managing money such as paying bills and keeping track of expenses

Figure 14.1   Prevalence of difficulty with one or more activities of daily living, in the English Longitudinal Study of Ageing, by age.

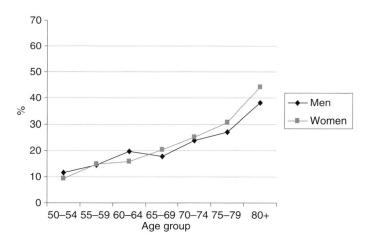

A key factor for promoting active ageing relates to the role of the social and neighbourhood environment. Both individual and neighbourhood deprivation are associated with poor health but the associations are not straightforward and specific mechanisms are not understood. A systematic review found that neighbourhood socio-economic composition was the strongest and most consistent predictor of a variety of health outcomes and that the positive association between physical

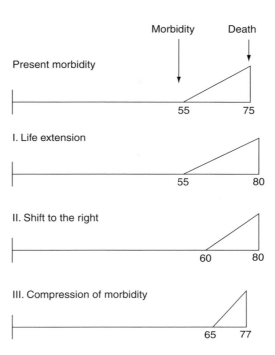

Figure 14.2   Scenarios for healthy-life expectancy.

environment, perceived or objective, and physical-activity behaviour was fairly consistent [4].

Prevention

Promoting active ageing has many facets but any public health approach to active ageing needs to consider the major preventable health threats in old age. The major chronic conditions are listed in Box 14.4.

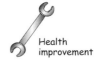

Health improvement

Primary prevention

Prevention of chronic disease starts with promotion of healthy lifestyles in earlier life but is also beneficial in old age. Studies in the United States have identified modifiable predictors for five-year mortality risk in older people living in the community [5,6]. Physical inactivity, a history of smoking, low body mass index and high blood pressure were among the modifiable factors identified to increase risk of death. Promoting physical activity in older people is an effective primary prevention strategy for conditions such as heart disease and diabetes, and may also be for dementia. Other

Box 14.4 Health conditions affecting the elderly

- Cardiovascular disease (such as coronary heart disease)
- Hypertension
- Stroke
- Diabetes
- Cancer
- Chronic obstructive pulmonary disease (COPD)
- Musculo-skeletal conditions (such as arthritis and osteoporosis)
- Mental health conditions (mostly dementia and depression)
- Blindness and visual impairment

Note: The causes of disability in older age are similar for men and women although women are more likely to report musculo-skeletal problems

   Source: the World Health Organization.

primary prevention strategies such as blood-pressure control are also highly effective in the elderly in preventing heart disease and stroke.

   Malnutrition in the elderly is also a concern. The causes in this age group are complex but poor nutrition may be a symptom of social isolation, functional disability and poverty. Vitamin D is important for bone health but may have other beneficial effects. Ensuring adequate nutrition, social engagement and intellectual stimulation are important primary prevention measures in older people.

   Primary prevention is also relevant for acute illnesses in the elderly. During the winter months the number of deaths among older people reaches higher levels than observed in the summer months. This excess winter mortality is mainly due to acute respiratory illnesses, of which influenza is the most important. Primary prevention of excess winter mortality among the elderly is achieved through vaccination against influenza.

Secondary prevention

Screening

For other conditions, the opportunity for primary prevention in old age may be limited. In this context, secondary prevention may be appropriate where the condition can be detected and treated at an early stage. Screening is a public health measure where a suitable test is used to detect a disease before it causes symptoms or signs. The disease is then treated with the expectation of prolonging life expectancy. For example, colorectal cancers develop slowly and prevention in older people often depends on early diagnosis through screening. There is limited evidence for primary prevention of breast cancer, and screening by mammography is the most effective method for reducing breast-cancer mortality in older women (see Chapter 9).

Tertiary prevention

Where primary or secondary prevention are not possible the aim is to reduce the complications of disease. Many chronic illnesses have their onset in middle age but have their greatest impact in old age. Ameliorating or preventing complications of these illnesses as well as rehabilitation are the mainstay of prevention for many older people. Appropriate management of diabetes, for example, aims to reduce disability that can result from lower-limb amputations and blindness.

As mentioned above, disability from physical and cognitive impairment limit the potential of older people to enjoy optimal health. The older population is susceptible to injury from falls and this is a major cause of disability and mortality in those aged over 75 years. Falls-prevention strategies make use of rehabilitation to reduce the disability that can occur with fractures that result from falls in this age group. Dementia, the leading cause of cognitive impairment in the older population, is also a key threat to active ageing. Falls prevention and the management of dementia are examined in greater detail to highlight the different approaches that are necessary to deal with two of the major causes of frailty in the elderly.

Prevention example 1. Falls

The challenges of prevention in the elderly can be illustrated by falls prevention. Falls are common in the older population, estimated to occur in about 30% of the over-65 population. Although less than one fall in ten results in a fracture, a fifth of fall incidents require medical attention.

A Cochrane review [7] has reported that exercise interventions reduced both the rate of falls and the risk of falling. Assessment and multifactorial intervention reduced the rate of falls but not the risk of falling. Overall, home-safety interventions did not reduce falls, but were effective in people with severe visual impairment, and in others at higher risk of falling. An anti-slip shoe device reduced the rate of falls in icy conditions. Gradual withdrawal of psychotropic medication reduced the rate of falls, but not the risk of falling. A prescribing modification programme for primary care physicians significantly reduced the risk of falling. Pacemakers reduced the rate of falls in people with carotid sinus hypersensitivity. First eye cataract surgery reduced the rate of falls. There is some evidence that falls-prevention strategies can be cost saving [8].

Evidence based practice

Health economics

After a hip fracture, many older people are not able to return to independent living, with about 20% requiring nursing-home care. Mortality is high, with estimates of up to 40% within the first year after the fracture. Tertiary prevention seeks to reduce this heavy burden and several approaches to rehabilitation have been investigated. A Cochrane review [8] found that while there was a tendency to a better overall result in patients receiving multidisciplinary in-patient rehabilitation, these results were not statistically significant. The current evidence suggests that multifactorial evaluation and treatment may not be more cost-effective than usual care in older people at risk for falling [8].

Prevention example 2. Dementia

Dementia is another common underlying condition in the elderly and for which there is limited evidence for prevention. In the oldest old the neuropathology is usually Alzheimer's disease and vascular lesions. On the basis of observational studies and short-term trials it is possible that addressing vascular risk factors, for example, by treating high blood pressure, increasing physical activity and memory training may offer benefit in preventing Alzheimer's disease, mixed forms as well as vascular dementia.

There is an on-going debate about the role of secondary prevention in dementia. Population screening is not currently indicated. Mild cognitive impairment (MCI) refers to a subtle impairment in memory, which is not quantified in any standard way but can be detected using cognitive tests that indicate higher risk of future dementia if identified in clinic settings. There is no consensus on which tests should be used and what standardised criteria to use to define the condition. Although some people with MCI progress to dementia and have pathological evidence of Alzheimer's disease at post mortem, studies have shown that up to 40% revert to normal over 2 to 3 years. Furthermore, similar pathological changes may be present in people who showed no signs of dementia during life. Mild cognitive impairment may be valuable in settings where the positive predictive value of cognitive tests is high (see Chapter 9).

Cholinesterase inhibitors show promise in people with mild to moderate Alzheimer's disease but long-term clinical benefit is unproven [9]. It is not clear whether active case finding alters the life course of demented individuals. Cognitive rehabilitation involves recovery of deficits through restoration and compensation through guided therapy to learn (or relearn) ways to cope with cognitive impairment. There is some evidence for non-pharmacological therapies to improve cognition but there is a paucity of high-quality studies on cognitive rehabilitation [10].

With increasing age, the burden of chronic conditions and physical and mental frailty increase and the scope for prevention declines. The oldest old typically need more and more support, initially in their own homes but eventually a substantial proportion require institutional support. This varies between countries and is influenced by policies for social-care provision and the cultural context.

Health and social care

The increasing prevalence of cognitive and physical frailty with age means that older people are more likely than younger age groups to use health- and social-care services. According to the 2002 English Longitudinal Study of Ageing (ELSA), the need for help because of limitations in activities of daily living or mobility increased with age with 42% of those 80 years and over having difficulty with one or more activities of daily living [2]. This pattern of limitation has been found in subsequent waves of ELSA. Assistance with activities of daily living included help with dressing, bathing or showering, eating, getting in or out of bed, preparing a hot meal, shopping for groceries or taking medication. In the Medical Research Council Cognitive Function and Ageing Study [11], the prevalence of severe cognitive impairment rose from 1% in men and 0.9% in women aged 65–69 years, to 18.4% and 40.5%, respectively, in those aged over 90 years.

The support needed can be provided formally by health and social services, voluntary organisations and community projects, or informally by spouses, extended family, neighbours and friends. In the 2002 ELSA, family members accounted for most of the help provided to people aged 60 and over, with spouses or partners most likely to provide help to those aged 60 to 74. For those aged 75 and over, caring was mostly provided by the younger generations such as children, children-in-law or grandchildren. In addition to family, privately paid employees, social- or health-service workers and friends or neighbours provided some help.

The burden of providing care for older people is considerable. The 2001 census in the UK reported 5.7 million unpaid carers, half of whom were caring for someone over 75 years old. Ninety per cent of carers were caring for relatives. A quarter of carers were caring 20 or more hours per week. In addition to the time required to care for an elderly relative there are health consequences for the carer. Carers were more likely than the general population to report health problems and 39% reported that their physical or mental health was affected by caring.

Despite the input of unpaid carers there is a substantial economic cost to supporting older people in their homes as they become increasingly frail. In 2004–5, older people (those aged 65 and over) accounted for 56% of spending by local authorities in England on personal social services, which include home help and home care. This was the single largest portion [12].

The rate of institutionalisation increases from 20% in the first year after diagnosis of dementia to 50% after 5 years [13]. A systematic review of predictors of institutionalisation in people aged 65 years and over found that, among community dwellers, the highest rate of institutionalisation was 17% over 6 years. Predictors with strong evidence were increased age, low self-rated health status, functional and cognitive impairment, dementia, prior nursing-home placement and a high number of prescriptions [14].

A major concern for older people, their families and for governments is the cost of funding care and support in old age. Older people risk spending the majority of their income and assets, including their homes, to pay for social support and residential care. In several countries there is active debate about the most sustainable models for funding long-term social care. Funding for social care through taxation or social insurance schemes is established in some European countries while in others individuals and their families are expected to bear the brunt of the cost for social support and care.

Decision making

End-of-life care

The majority of deaths in most developed countries occur in old age. It is important to recognise and deliver high-quality care to older people with terminal conditions in a way that relieves suffering and maintains the autonomy and dignity of the individual and their families. Cancer, heart failure and dementia are among the most common conditions requiring palliative care among older people.

Most people in the European region die in hospital rather than at home. However, there are variations with age. In the UK, the hospital as place of death is highest among the middle old while among the oldest old it is the care home [15]. There is evidence of lack of access to specialist palliative care for older people in many countries. In the UK, 80% of specialist palliative services beds were provided by voluntary agencies in 2008 [15]. The location of such services is often determined by historical factors rather than by needs assessment. Studies from Australia, the USA and the UK suggest that people with terminal conditions other than cancer are less likely to be admitted to hospices where specialist palliative services are offered. This diverts the provision of specialist care towards younger cancer patients. Heart failure, despite having a 5-year prognosis that is comparable to or worse than several cancers, is more likely to be overlooked as a reason for specialist palliative care.

More on this topic can be found on the internet companion.

Policy responses

The WHO identifies several challenges posed by ageing populations. In developing countries, there is a double burden of disease, where diseases associated with old age are emerging alongside traditional health problems of infectious diseases and malnutrition. The second challenge relates to the increasing prevalence of disability associated with old age and this in turn puts additional pressure on health-care systems to provide adequate care. Women typically outlive their spouses and this places them at great risk, especially where social-support systems are not well developed.

The other challenges arise because of the economic and social sequelae of old age and the associated dependency. The WHO highlights the need for new paradigms that view older people as 'active participants in an age-integrated society and as active contributors as well as beneficiaries of development' [16]. The policy framework for active ageing therefore rests on three pillars: participation, health and security.

In addition to prevention and provision of adequate health- and social-care support, including the needs and training of carers, the WHO advocates steps to increase participation of older people in the wider society. This can be achieved through emphasis on lifelong learning and on opportunities for economic and social participation through formal or informal work and voluntary activities. Security issues are also highlighted to defend the rights of the elderly and to protect against elder abuse. These concerns may become particularly pressing at the end of life if the older person's autonomy is not respected in decisions about their health and financial affairs. In order for older people to age actively, broader issues of housing, transport and income support must also be considered.

Social expectations and attitudes are changing with respect to old age, particularly as the 'baby boom' generation ages. In addition to quality of care, considerations of quality of life have also been prominent. Technologies such as the Internet have increased access to health information and enabled the older population to make more informed choices about their health. An important choice in this population concerns the timing and circumstances of their death. Intergenerational attitudes, financial concerns, the ability and willingness of future societies to provide care and support for its frail, older populations and attention to challenging debates such as assisted death and euthanasia are some of the key challenges for policy makers.

There is the need to provide the appropriate evidence base to underpin policy. This is particularly challenging in the case of older people. The presence of co-morbidity often means that older people are excluded from clinical trials of interventions that could prevent ill health in this population. The Medical Research Council Cognitive Function and Ageing Study (MRC CFAS) found that individuals who refused participation in the follow-up phase were more likely to have poor cognitive ability and had less years of full-time education compared with those followed up [17]. This suggests that long-term studies of ageing and health may under-represent the disadvantaged and disabled.

Epidemiology

Conclusion

Longevity is a reasonable goal for public health but brings about a new set of challenges. Health in old age, as at any age, is not 'merely the absence of disease'. However, age is strongly associated with disease and disability. The role of prevention may be progressively limited at increasing ages and this means that public health must seek to support and care where prevention is not possible. However, policies need to balance investment on immediate care and support against investment on developing and implementing strategies for primary, secondary and tertiary prevention.

The phenomenon of ageing also illustrates the wider determinants of health that must be addressed if older people are to remain active and independent participants in their communities. This demands flexibility in approaching the definition and expectations of 'old age'.

REFERENCES

1. J. R. Wilmoth, L. J. Deegan, H. Lundstrom and S. Horiuchi, Increase of maximum lifespan in Sweden, 1861–1999. *Science* **289**, 2000, 2366–8.

2. M. Marmot, J. Banks, R. Blundell, C. Lessof and J. Nazroo (eds.), *Health, Wealth and Lifestyles of the Older Population in England: The 2002 English Longitudinal Study of Ageing*, London, Institute of Fiscal Studies, 2002.

3. Office of National Statistics, 2010. See: www.statistics.gov.uk.

4. I. H. Yen, Y. L. Michael and L. Perdue, Neighborhood environment in studies of health of older adults: A systematic review. *American Journal of Preventive Medicine* **37**, 2009, 455–63.

5. L. P. Fried, R. A. Kronmal, A. B. Newman *et al.*, Risk factors for 5-year mortality in older adults: the Cardiovascular Health Study. *Journal of the American Medical Association* **279**, 1998, 585–92.

6. M. A. Schonberg, R. B. Davis, E. P. McCarthy and E. R. Marcantonio, Index to predict 5-year mortality of community-dwelling adults aged 65 and older using data from the National Health Interview Survey. *Journal of General Internal Medicine* **24**, 2009, 1115–22.

7. L D. Gillespie, M. C. Robertson, W. J. Gillespie *et al.*, Interventions for preventing falls in older people living in the community. *Cochrane Database of Systematic Reviews* **2**, 2009, CD007146.

8. H. H. Handoll, I. D. Cameron, J. C. Mak and T. P. Finnegan, Multidisciplinary rehabilitation for older patients with hip fractures. *Cochrane Database of Systematic Reviews* **4**, 2009, CD007125.

9. J. Birks, Cholinesterase inhibitors for Alzheimer's disease. *Cochrane Database of Systematic Reviews* **1**, 2006, CD005593.

10. J. Olazarán, B. Reisberg, L. Clare *et al.*, Nonpharmacological therapies in Alzheimer's disease: A systematic review of efficacy. *Dementia and Geriatric Cognitive Disorders* **30**, 2010, 161–78.

11. C. Brayne, F. E. Matthews, M. A. McGee and C. Jagger, Health and ill-health in the older population in England and Wales. The Medical Research Council Cognitive Function and Ageing Study (MRC CFAS). *Age and Ageing* **30**, 2001, 53–62.

12. The Health and Social Care Information Center, Personal Social Services expenditure and unit costs: England 2009–2010. *Social Care Statistics Bulletin: 2011/01/ HSCIC*.

13. M. Luppa, T. Luck, E. Brähler, H. H. König and S. G. Riedel-Heller, Prediction of institutionalisation in dementia. A systematic review. *Dementia and Geriatric Cognitive Disorders* **26**, 2008, 65–78.

14. M. Luppa, T. Luck, S. Weyerer, *et al.*, Prediction of institutionalisation in the elderly. A systematic review. *Age and Ageing* **39**, 2010, 31–8.

15. Department of Health, End of Life Care Strategy, London, Department of Health, 2008.

16. World Health Organization, Active ageing: a policy framework. WHO/NMH/NPH/02.8, World Health Organization, 2002.

17. F. E. Matthews, M. Chatfield, C. Freeman, et al., Attrition and bias in the MRC cognitive function and ageing study: an epidemiological investigation. *BioMed Central Public Health* **4**, 2004, 12.

Health inequalities and public health practice

Chrissie Pickin and Jennie Popay

Key points

- Health and well-being shows a strong and consistent social gradient.
- Socio-economic inequalities in health are widespread in all countries.
- They are caused by the unequal distribution of the social determinants of health such as power, income, goods and services and the impact this has on conditions of daily life.
- At the individual level, the social determinants of health differentially affect people's abilities, or what Armartya Sen has called 'capabilities', to lead a flourishing life.
- They affect individuals across their life course with prenatal and early-life influences having a sustained impact on people's health experience later in life.
- Tackling health inequalities requires action at multiple levels involving many agencies with government playing a pivotal role.
- Resisting the tendency for policy to focus predominantly on individual behaviour change – what has been called lifestyle drift – is important.
- Successfully tackling health inequalities challenges public health practice and calls for a new approach to governance, partnership, leadership and accountability

What are health inequalities?

That my health is better or worse than yours does not necessarily indicate the presence of health inequalities. According to the Global Commission on the Social Determinants of Health, which reported to the World Health Organization in 2008, the term 'health inequality' refers to differences between groups or

Essential Public Health, Second Edition, ed. Stephen Gillam, Jan Yates and Padmanabhan Badrinath. Published by Cambridge University Press. © Cambridge University Press 2012.

Health status

populations defined socially, economically, demographically or geographically' that are 'unfair and avoidable or remedial' rather than to any innate differences between these groups [1]. Statistics used to quantify health inequalities are discussed in Chapter 4 (and see the Internet Companion).

The most commonly discussed dimension of health inequalities and the one focused on here is that between groups living in different socio-economic circumstances. But inequalities may also be observed geographically and between the sexes. In developed countries, men tend to die younger than women although this has been reducing recently, in part due to better treatment of heart disease. However, worldwide, women tend to experience more ill health throughout their lives. The causes of these inequalities are complex but include genetic, social and cultural factors as well as discrimination. There are also health inequalities between different ethnic groups. Work has emphasised the importance of culture in explaining these differences underplaying the importance of discrimination and socio-economic influences [2,3]. There are also differences in health between age groups. However, we would expect the health of 20 year olds to be better on average than 80 year olds, so these are not avoidable health inequalities and comparisons between groups should adjust for age.

Why are health inequalities important for public health practice?

There are consistent and typically large inequalities in health between socio-economic groups in all societies. Despite sustained improvements in life expectancy and average population health, these inequalities have been widening over the last few decades in many countries [4–7]. (See Figures 15.1 to 15.4 for evidence of income inequality and consequent inequalities in life expectancy and mortality in European countries.)

Research has shown that health inequalities show a *gradient* across societies, not a bimodal distribution. Wherever we are in the social hierarchy, apart from the top and bottom, our health will be better than those below and worse than those above us. This means that inequalities in health affect all of the population, not just the poor.

The burden of health inequalities is significant. A review of the evidence published in 2010 [8] suggests that between 1.3 and 2.5 million years of life are lost each year in England as a result of health inequalities in addition to the burden of chronic illness and disability. Tackling health inequalities also contributes to wider societal benefits – including economic growth through increased labour supply and productivity. There are also important synergies between tackling health inequalities and promoting sustainable development (see Chapter 18).

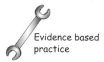

Evidence based practice

Males

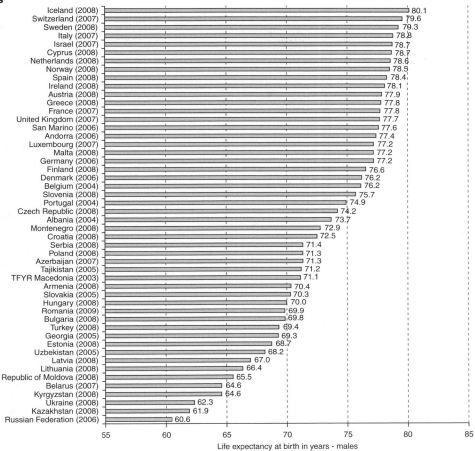

Life expectancy at birth in years - males

Figure 15.1   Life expectancy at birth by sex for countries in the WHO European Region, 2008 or latest available earlier year. Source: the WHO Regional Office for Europe, European Social Determinant and Health Divide Review (interim report), Copenhagen, WHO, 2010.

What causes health inequalities?

According to the Global Commission, the social determinants of health consist of structural factors including social policies, economic arrangements and political systems, and the conditions of daily life these generate. Health inequalities are therefore socially determined: the result of the unequal distribution of power, income, goods, and services, which in turn produce inequalities in people's 'access to healthcare, schools, and education, their conditions of work and leisure, their homes, communities, towns, or cities' [1].

At the individual level, the social determinants of health differentially affect our ability, or what Armartya Sen has called 'capabilities' [9], to lead a flourishing life. The balance between the accumulation and depletion of these capabilities over the

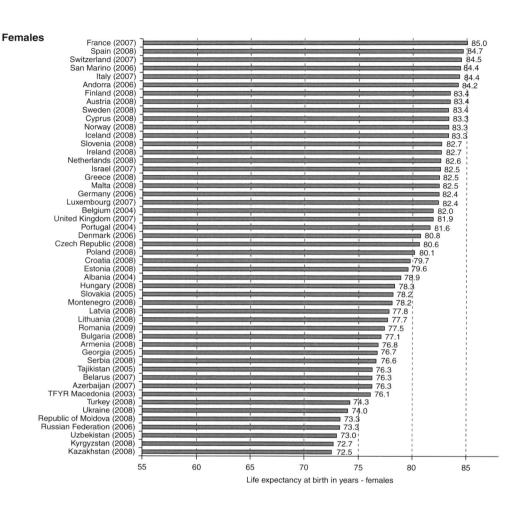

Females

Figure 15.1   (cont.)

individual's life course depends on the inter-relationships between material circumstance, psycho-social conditions and access to essential services.

The impact of material circumstances

Adequate income is required for good health, influencing housing, diet, access to leisure, etc. [1,10]. It is widely accepted that in wealthier countries poverty should be defined in relative terms – you are poor if you cannot afford the standard of living generally accepted as adequate in the society in which you live. There are various ways of measuring poverty but even in a high-income country like England more than 16% of dependent children were living in a household defined as deprived in 2008 [11]. Unemployment is a cause of low income and the risk of unemployment is higher in

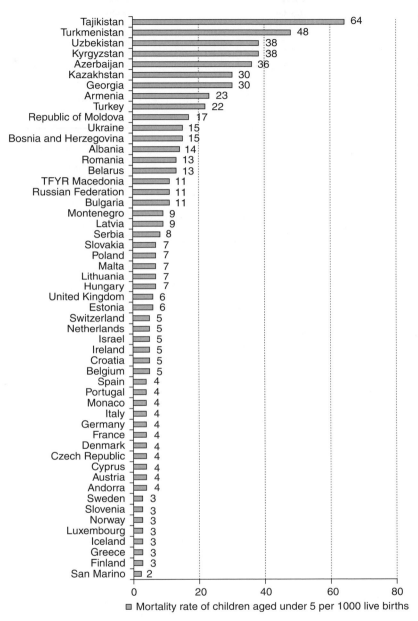

Figure 15.2 Mortality among children younger than 5 years old per 1000 live births for countries in the WHO European Region, 2008. Source as for Figure 15.1.

lower socio-economic groups [12]; however, many employed people also have low incomes. And although having paid employment reduces the risk of poverty it has been estimated that, in 2007, 8% of the employed population in the EU fell into the category of the 'working poor': having an income below 60% of the national average

Figure 15.3   Premature mortality: standard mortality ratios of those aged under 65 years per 100,000 population for regions within EU countries, 2006 or latest available earlier year. Source: I2SARE project: health inequalities indicators in the regions of Europe.

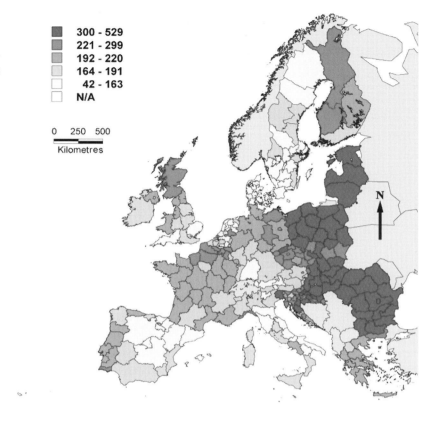

300 - 529
221 - 299
192 - 220
164 - 191
 42 - 163
N/A

0   250   500
Kilometres

[12, 13]. Many aspects of people's material living conditions directly contribute to health. In England, in 2008, a third of all homes were assessed as not decent in the annual government survey of housing standards and more than half of these were assessed as having potentially serious hazards [14].

Social-status differentials and psycho-social conditions

Research has confirmed the protective effect on health of social resources – social support, strong social networks and cohesion, living in a community in which relationships between residents and public agencies are positive (i.e. high 'social capital' [15, 16]. However, research suggests that levels of social cohesion and social capital are lower in societies with more marked income and social-status differentials [17]. At the individual level, people in lower positions in the social hierarchy experience more adverse and unpredictable events and have less control over them as well as more stress during pregnancy and early life [18, 19]. Research suggests that living in a state of sustained tension/stress, particularly in early life, can directly damage health through high levels of circulating stress hormones [20–22]. Similarly, the unequal

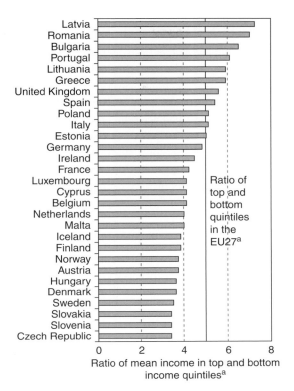

Figure 15.4   EU income distribution indicator: ratio of mean income per person in the top-income quintile to that in the bottom quintile in the EU countries, Iceland and Norway, 2008. Source as for Figure 15.1.

distribution of poor working conditions including exposure to physical hazards makes a significant contribution to health inequalities in adult life. There are also sharp inequalities in the psychosocial conditions of employment – job security, the balance between the demands of a job and control over these and between the efforts and rewards of paid work [23].

Lifestyle and behaviours

The health damage caused by sustained exposure to poor physical conditions and stressful circumstances is also mediated through behaviours such as smoking, diet, alcohol use, physical activity and drug taking. There are systematic differences in these behaviours across the social spectrum which research has shown are shaped by the material and psycho-social contexts in which people live. These behaviours are there-fore 'downstream' risk factors: strategies that help people cope with inadequate access to the social determinants of good health. Their contribution to health inequalities is also relatively modest: sometimes out of proportion to the public health effort directed at changing them (see Chapter 8). The Whitehall studies (see Box 15.1) suggest that lifestyle differences account for only 30% of the health differences between social groups

Epidemiology

Box 15.1 The Whitehall studies

The Whitehall studies (also discussed in Chapter 3) have been very influential in developing our understanding of the social gradient in health and the determinants of socio-economic health inequalities. The first study, which began in 1976, focused on the health experience of 18,000 male British civil servants. The men were classified according to their employment grade – at the lowest end porters and messengers up to the most senior civil servants – the permanent secretaries. The second study (Whitehall II) started in 1985 and included women. Follow-up studies have continued for over 20 years and a large number of papers and reports have been produced [24].

[24]. In addition, Blaxter has shown that unhealthy behaviours do not reinforce the health-damaging effects of social and economic disadvantage to the same extent that healthy behaviour increases the health effects of social advantage [25].

Access to services

Lastly, the ability to access services can impact either positively or negatively on health inequalities. A range of essential services – especially parenting and early-years support, education, housing, social protection, health and social care – help us to develop the capabilities needed to achieve a flourishing healthy life.

Policy approaches to tackling health inequalities

Over the last decade many governments have developed public health policies that aim to tackle health inequalities [26–29]. Three different approaches have been identified [30]. The first focuses narrowly on improving the health of the worst-off in society: health inequalities may stay the same or increase depending on what happens to the health of the rest of the population. The second approach aims to reduce health inequalities by narrowing the health gap between the poorest and the 'average' for the population – 'raising the health of the poorest, fastest'. As Graham has identified [31] both these approaches cast health inequalities as a condition to which only those in disadvantaged circumstances are exposed. The third approach focuses on reducing the social gradient in health across a society.

Whitehead and Popay [32] compared policies aimed at addressing health inequalities in England and Norway. They argue that the English policy, launched in 1998, is a gap approach emphasizing individual lifestyles more than the conditions structuring individual choices. Policy impacts were reduced because programmes were wound down early or key elements of them diluted. This undermined attempts to empower disadvantaged communities [33, 34]. The English attempts to reduce health inequalities were also undermined by global economic forces, which led to a growth in poor working conditions [35] and eroded support for universal welfare systems. In contrast, Norway's policy, published in 2007, takes an explicit social-gradient approach combining universal policies with selective measures to help the most disadvantaged and focusing both upstream on income redistribution and downstream on behaviours. Importantly, Norway's oil revenue has also protected it from the worst effects of the global financial crisis.

The goal of public health policy and practice in aiming to reduce health inequalities

We have already noted the tendency for lifestyle drift in policy and practice aimed at reducing health inequalities: moving from a recognition of the need for action on the wider social determinants of health but, in the course of implementation, drifting downstream to largely focus on individual behaviour [36]. This tendency can be avoided by focusing instead on action aimed at releasing and developing capabilities [37]. Sen [9, 38] has defined capability as the actual or potential freedom an individual has to achieve the level of functioning that they value; but capabilities can also be collective, operating within groups, communities and even nations. From this perspective, key characteristics of public health action to tackle health inequalities would be:

- focusing efforts on releasing and further developing individual and/or collective capabilities to lead flourishing and healthy lives;
- identifying and removing barriers to the release and further development of individual and collective capabilities at the level of individuals, households, communities, society or globally;
- allowing individuals, groups and communities to make choices based on their own concepts of what is of value;
- supporting and enabling inclusive decision making at an individual, community and societal level through participation in and delegation of decision making in social and political life.

The importance of a life-course approach

Policy and practice to address health inequalities must also be informed by a life-course perspective. Disadvantage starts before birth and accumulates throughout life. The effects of material circumstances, early-years experiences, working conditions, adult social position, access to services and the physical environment create a 'probabilistic cascade' of differential exposures and risks over the life course [39]. Understanding that 'history is what you live' [40] is crucial to developing policy and practice that intervenes at the right times and is cognizant of the legacy of these cumulative social processes.

A life-course approach highlights the importance of investment in early-years development, with support here paying dividends well into the future (see Chapter 12). Prenatal and early-life influences cast a long shadow over people's health experience [41]. Low birth weight is a predictor of illness in middle and old age [42] and having poor growth in the first year increases the risk of high blood pressure, heart disease, stroke and diabetes in later life [43]. The Marmot Review of health inequalities policy [8] in the UK called for a 'second revolution in the early years' (page 22) to increase overall spending in this area. However, according to proponents of a life-course perspective, if the accumulation of risks and impacts is to be prevented, action to reduce health inequalities should include interventions at all critical points: prenatally, early years, transition from primary to secondary school, entry into employment, becoming parents and retirement.

Effective action – characteristics and responsibility

Action on the social determinants of health must move beyond the health sector to involve the whole of government, civil society and local communities, non-government organisations, business and global agencies (see Figure 15.5). But the Ministry of Health is critical to change – through championing a social determinants of health approach, demonstrating effective practice and supporting other ministries to create policies that promote health equity (a health-in-all policies approach).

A new approach is needed – one that understands complexity. As Hunter and colleagues argue, health inequalities are 'difficult to define with precision, are interdependent and multi causal, may give rise to solutions which themselves have unforeseen or unintended consequences, are not stable, rarely sit within the boundaries or responsibility of a single organisation and involve changing behaviour – not just of the recipients of support but also of those dispensing it' [44]. Understanding this complexity is vital in ensuring that a sustained, multi-sectoral, systems approach is taken (see Figure 15.6). This is challenging in a political environment that often seeks quick wins and simplistic approaches.

The importance of government action

Government policies have a major impact on the extent and nature of health inequalities. Tackling the social gradient requires universal, high-quality welfare services that promote sustainable, social cohesion by limiting income inequality and differentials in social status. Narrowing income inequalities through taxation, welfare benefits, parental leave and pension entitlements, and the setting of decent wages is likely over time to impact significantly on health inequalities. Recent research has identified that both the nature and generosity of welfare benefits have direct health impacts [45].

A typology of policies and actions to address health inequalities

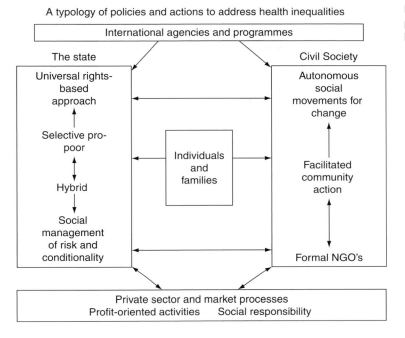

Figure 15.5   A typology of policies and actions to address health inequalities.

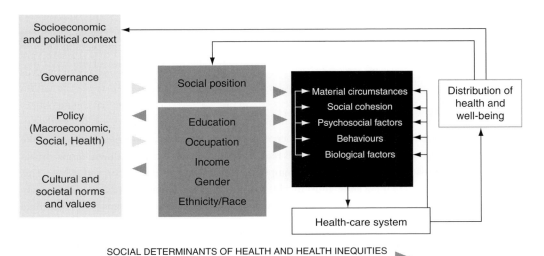

SOCIAL DETERMINANTS OF HEALTH AND HEALTH INEQUITIES

Figure 15.6   Commission on Social Determinants of Health, conceptual framework. Source: the WHO, 2008 [1].

Other legislation with potential to reduce health inequalities includes laws that improve the quality of work and the environment, e.g. the European Working Time Directive; standards for urban planning and housing, particularly social housing; and anti-discrimination laws.

Local governments also have a major role to play in promoting a healthy living environment. Here, action would include ensuring safe play areas and traffic-calming measures in residential areas; well-designed, affordable housing; built environments that reduce the fear of crime and encourage leisure, walking and cycling; and the provision of efficient and affordable public transport and leisure opportunities.

Sustainable economic development is also important if health inequalities are to be reduced: reducing unemployment and job insecurity and ensuring access to high-quality skills training. Governments can also encourage local employers to provide high-quality jobs with appropriate job control, management practices and balance between effort and reward.

A key role of governments is also to ensure universal access to effective and affordable essential services such as family support services (e.g. Sure Start in the UK), child care, pre-school education, schools, facilities for life-long learning, preventative, screening and primary care services, community-based mental health, hospital services and a range of high-quality and affordable services to promote the independence of older people.

But the Marmot review of policies [8] aimed at reducing health inequalities in the UK also highlighted the importance of *proportionate universalism*: combining universal provision with target action to reach those with greatest need. Focusing policies or services solely on disadvantaged groups will not reduce the social gradient but failure to focus action on reducing barriers and releasing the capabilities of the most disadvantaged won't either.

Why working differently is necessary

If public health policy and practice is to create a sustained approach to removing the root causes of inequalities it will require a move away from top-down, target-driven approaches to approaches that emphasise local ownership and 'co-production'. This 'coalition of the willing' must involve the public, practitioners and policy makers working together to identify and implement workable solutions to problems [44]. Traditional needs-based approaches to policy and practice too often present a negative, one-sided view of individuals or communities compromising, rather than contributing to, the release or development of capabilities. In contrast, a capability- or assets-based approach to policy and practice moves away from this 'deficit' mindset to focus instead on enhancing 'the ability of individuals, groups, communities, populations, social systems and/or institutions to maintain and sustain health and well being and to help to reduce health inequalities' [46]. A new style of public health leadership and governance is also required: able and willing to work with complexity and uncertainty, to

 Leadership

Box 15.2 Lessons learned from the Salford Social Action Research Project

Public health work with disadvantaged communities should:

- Focus on identifying existing and potential capabilities in a community rather than simply needs and deficits.
- Move away from the idea that we need to build capability to the idea that we need to identify and release capability within the community. This focuses attention onto the resourcefulness of communities and the barriers to those resources being utilised effectively, including the barriers imposed by traditional public health practice.
- Develop more equal and reciprocal relationships between community members and service providers and local government, e.g. co-mentoring schemes, local exchange trading schemes (LETS), employing community members in various roles including social-action coordinators and researchers.
- Shift from working with individuals and groups to supporting collective community action to identify and address their 'burning issues' themselves.
- Challenge assumptions on all sides through dialogue and enquiry. This means spending time to get to know each other's worlds.
- Move away from offering training to developing shared learning opportunities.
- Recognise that the organisational development to help public agencies and other bodies to change their mindsets and ways of working is as important as community development.

The authors acknowledge the Salford SARP steering group in the development of this learning; in particular Gerry Stone, Anne-Marie Pickup, Emma Rowbottom, Owen Gilliker, Kelly McElroy, Diane Plamping, Julian Pratt, Steve Cropper, Alan Higgins, Steve Young and Diana Martin.

build confidence and trust, to develop and use collective intelligence and multidirectional knowledge transfer, to be accountable for progress to multiple stakeholders, to take risks and innovate and to advocate for equity and social justice.

The Social Action Research Project (SARP) funded by the Health Development Agency (replaced by the Centre for Public Health Excellence in the National Institute for Health and Clinical Effectiveness) aimed to explore the implications of research on the relationship between social capital and health for initiatives aimed at improving the health of disadvantaged communities. In Salford, we found that this meant involving citizens in developing policies that affect them and in designing and delivering the services they use. Doing this in ways that improved the social status of individuals and perceptions of that community by outsiders, required a change of mindset from both community members and public service organisations (see Box 15.2).

Conclusion

So, what are the implications for public health practice? Tackling health inequalities is a challenge as it extends our traditional areas of knowledge, skills and practice. It requires widening our knowledge base beyond demography and epidemiology to encompass the social sciences so that we understand the social constructs within which people's lives and capabilities are shaped. It requires that we extend our actions beyond targeted lifestyle interventions to actions that truly alter the distribution of social determinants. We need to develop effective partnerships that influence the actions of governments, business and the planners and funders of essential services. We need to assess the needs of our communities but in doing so we must focus and report on assets and capabilities and not just deficits. In our health-promotion work we must be sure we understand the lived experience of our communities, that we challenge our assumptions and prejudices and that we always promote reciprocity in our dealings with people.

And crucially, we must understand that the most important thing we can do is to identify and remove the structural, economic and social barriers that prevent people living a healthy and flourishing life.

REFERENCES

1. Commission on Social Determinants of Health – final report. Closing the gap in a generation: Health equity through action on the social determinants of health, Geneva, World Health Organization, 2008.
2. J. Y. Nazroo, Genetic, cultural or socioeconomic vulnerability? Explaining ethnic inequalities in health. *Sociology of Health and Illness* **20**, 1998, 714–34.
3. C. Pickin, S. Karlsen, C. McLean and G. Randhawa, INpho 2: Ethnicity and health inequalities, Cambridge, Eastern Region Public Health Observatory.
4. D. Acheson, *Independent Inquiry into Inequalities in Health Report*, London, The Stationary Office, 1998.
5. NHC (National Health Committee), The social, cultural and economic determinants of health in New Zealand: Action to improve health, Wellington, New Zealand: National Advisory Committee on Health and Disability, 1998.
6. M. Whitehead, P. Townsend and N. Davidson, *Inequalities in Health: the Black Report/the Health Divide*, London, Penguin, 1992.
7. J. P. Mackenbach, Health inequalities: Europe in profile, An independent, expert report commissioned under the auspices of the UK Presidency of the European Union, London, Department of Health, 2006.
8. M. Marmot (Chair), Fair Society, Healthy Lives, Strategic review of health inequalities in England post 2010, London, Local Government Improvement and Development, 2010.
9. A. Sen, *Inequality Re-examined*, Cambridge, MA, Harvard University Press, 1992.
10. R. Wilkinson, K. Pickett, *The Spirit Level: Why More Equal Societies Almost Always Do Better*, London, Allen Lane, 2009.
11. J. Bradshaw, Child Poverty and Health, Background Paper, Marmot Review of Social Determinants of Health in the EURO region, 2011.
12. A. Bethune, Unemployment and mortality. In F. Drever and M. Whitehead M (eds.), *Health Inequalities: Decennial Supplement*, London, The Stationary Office, ONS series DS no. 15, pp. 156–67.

13. Working Poor In Europe, Dublin, European Foundation for the Improvement of Living and Working Conditions, 2010.

14. English Housing Survey: Headline Report, 2010, London, Department of Communities and Local Government, UK.

15. C. Campbell, R. Wood and M. Kelly, *Social Capital and Health*, Oxford, Blackwell, 1999.

16. L. F. Berkman and T. Glass, Social integration, social networks, social support and health. In L. F. Berkman and I. Kawachi (eds.), *Social Epidemiology*, Oxford, Oxford University Press, 2000.

17. I. Kawachi, B. P. Kennedy, K. Lochner and D. Prothrow-Smith, Social capital, income inequality and mortality. *American Journal of Public Health* **87**, 1997, 1491–8.

18. M. Marmot, *Status Syndrome*, London, Bloomsbury Publishing, 2004.

19. R. G. Wilkinson, *The Impact of Inequality: How to Make Sick Societies Healthier*, New York, The New Press, 2005.

20. M. Kristenson, Z. Orth-Gomer, B. Kucinskiene *et al.*, Attenuated cortisol response to a standardised stress test in Lithuania versus Swedish men: the LiVicordia Study. *International Journal of Behavioural Medicine* **591**, 1998, 17–30.

21. E. J. Brunner, M. G. Marmot, K. Nanchahal *et al.*, Social inequality in coronary risk: Central obesity and the metabolic syndrome. Evidence from the Whitehall II study. *Diabetologia* **40**, 1997, 1341–9.

22. D. I. W. Phillips and D. J. P. Barker, Association between low birth weight and high resting pulse in adult life: Is the sympathetic nervous system involved in programming the insulin resistance syndrome? *Diabetic Medicine* **14**, 1997, 673–7.

23. H. Kuper, M. Marmot and H. Hemingway, Psychosocial factors in the aetiology and prognosis of coronary disease. A systematic review. *Seminars in Vascular Medicine* **2**(3), 2002, 267–314.

24. M. G. Marmot and M. J. Shipley, Do socioeconomic differences in mortality persist after retirement? 25 year follow-up of civil servants from the first Whitehall study. *British Medical Journal* **313**, 1996, 1177–80.

25. M. Blaxter, *Health and Lifestyles*, London, Routledge, 1990.

26. Department of Health, Tackling health inequalities: A programme of action, London, Department of Health, 2003.

27. National Strategy to Reduce Social Inequalities in Health, Report No. 20, Oslo, Norwegian Ministry of Health and Care Services, 2007.

28. Minister of Health, *The New Zealand Health Strategy*, Wellington, Ministry of Health, 2000.

29. Government of Denmark, Healthy throughout life: the targets and strategies for public health policy of the Government of Denmark, 2002–2010, Copenhagen, Government of Denmark, 2002.

30. H. Graham and M. P. Kelly, Health inequalities: concepts, frameworks and policy, Briefing paper, NHS Health Development Agency, 2004.

31. H. Graham, Health inequalities, social determinants and public health policy. *Policy and Politics* **37** (4), 2009, 463–79.

32. M. Whitehead and J. Popay, Swimming upstream? Taking action on the social determinants of health inequalities. *Social Science and Medicine* **71**, 2010, 1234–6, doi:10.1016/j.socscimed.2010.07.004.

33. J. Popay, Community engagement for health improvement: questions of definition, outcomes and evaluation. In A. Morgan, R. Barker, M. Davies and E. Ziglio (eds.), *Health Assets in a Global Context: Theory, Methods, Action*, New York, NY, Springer, 2010, pp. 183–197.

34. J. Popay, P. Attree, D. Hornby *et al.*, Community engagement to address the wider social determinants of health: A review of evidence on impact, experience & process. London, National Institute for Health & Clinical Excellence, 2007. Available from: http://www.nice.org.uk/guidance/index.jsp?action=folder&o=34709.

35. S. Poval, M. Whitehead, R. Gosling and B. Barr, *Focusing the Equity Lens: Arguments and Actions on Health Inequalities*, Liverpool, WHO Collaborating Centre, 2008.

36. J. Popay, M. Whitehead and D. Hunter, Injustice is killing people on a large scale but what is to be done about it? *Journal of Public Health* **32**(2), 2010, 148–49.

37. A. P. Ruger, *Health and Social Justice*, Oxford, Oxford University Press, 2010.

38. A. Sen, *Development as Freedom*, New York, NY, Knopf, 1999.

39. M. Bartley, D. Blane and G. Davey-Smith (eds.), *Sociology of Health Inequalities*, Oxford, Blackwell, 1998.

40. G. Williams, History is what you live: understanding health inequalities in Wales. In P. Michael and C. Webster (eds.), *Health and Society in Twentieth-Century Wales*, Cardiff, University of Wales Press, 2006.

41. D. J. P. Barker, *Mothers, Babies and Health in Later Life*, Edinburgh, Churchill Livingston.

42. D. I. W. Phillips, B. R. Walker, D. E. H. Reynolds *et al.*, Low birth weight predicts elevated plasma cortisol concentrations in adults from 3 populations. *Hypertension* **35** (6), 2000, 1301–6.

43. R. Gitau, A. Cameron, N. M. Fisk and V. Glover, Foetal exposure to maternal cortisol. *Lancet* **352**, 1998, 707–8.

44. D. J. Hunter, J. Popay, C. Tannahill, M. Whitehead and T. Elson, Learning lessons from the past: shaping a different future. Cross-cutting sub group report, Marmot Review Working Committee 3, November, 2009.

45. O. Lundberg, M. A. Yngwe, M. K. Stjarne *et al.*, The role of welfare state principles and generosity in social policy programmes for public health: an international comparative study. *The Lancet* **372**, 2008, 1633–40.

46. A. Morgan, M. Davies and Z. Zigli, *Health Assets in a Global Context. Theory, Methods, Action*, New York, NY, Springer, 2010.

16

Health policy

Richard Lewis and Stephen Gillam

Key points

- Rational models of planning and policy making underplay the contingent, ad hoc nature of these processes in practice.
- Policy making is a political process and only ever partially evidence-based.
- Understanding how policy is made can help you influence its development and implementation locally.
- Governments give policy on health services greater precedence over policy on public health although the latter has greater potential to improve population health.

Introduction

An understanding of how policy is made is an important means by which medical and public health practitioners can comprehend the services within which they work – and perhaps change them. The policy process is the means by which particular policies emerge and are pursued by governments and government agencies. There are many competing explanations of the policy process [1]. However, a simple and useful way of understanding how policy is made is as the consequence of the inter-relation of 'actors' (those people or organisations that populate the process), the wider context, the process by which policy is made and the content of the policy itself (i.e. what it is designed to achieve) [2] (Figure 16.1).

Can you think of any unexpected consequences of recent governments' health policies?

What do we mean by policy?

A common-sense approach would equate public policy with the formal decisions or explicit proposals of governments or public agencies. In practice, the process of policy

Essential Public Health, Second Edition, ed. Stephen Gillam, Jan Yates and Padmanabhan Badrinath.
Published by Cambridge University Press. © Cambridge University Press 2012.

Figure 16.1 Walt–Gilson model for policy analysis.

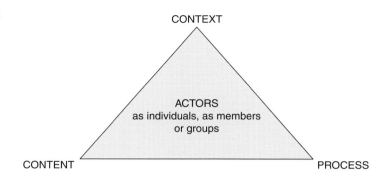

making is subtler and more complex. Policy may emerge from a series of apparently unrelated decisions and governments or public agencies do not control the outcomes of intended policies with any great certainty. In fact, government policy may be as much about what they choose not to do as about what they choose to do [3].

Early theories of the policy process as a system were dominated by two opposing schools of thought – the 'rationalists' and the 'incrementalists'. 'Rational' models of the policy process describe it in terms of a series of linked, but distinct phases and types of activity that together produce 'a policy'. Such an approach is based on the application of a logical and apparently sequential set of functions and technical skills to ensure that an appropriate response is generated to a 'policy problem'. For example, Walt describes four key stages: problem identification and issue recognition; policy formulation; policy implementation; and policy evaluation [2].

This 'rational' approach to the policy process has attractions, not least as it identifies different types of activities that may be involved. However, it has been criticised also for implying that the process is a well-ordered translation of objectives into action. Moreover, critics such as Lindblom opposed the very notion that values and objectives (i.e. the policy 'ends') can be identified separately to any consideration of the policy 'means' [4]. In actual decision making, he suggested, policy makers did not, nor should, set prior aims but should seek only to move from the status quo by small steps and by reaching agreement among competing interest groups – human beings, he felt, simply do not possess the ability to process all necessary information to make 'rational' decisions.

The context for policy making

Policies exist in a 'context' – an environment within which any policy is located, reflecting both constraints and opportunities. Leichter identified four distinct sets of contextual factors that would impact on national health policy [5]:

- situational factors (transient conditions such as war that allow governments to introduce policies otherwise considered out of bounds);

- structural factors (relatively unchanging elements in society such as the political regime);
- cultural factors (reflecting the values within society);
- environmental factors (those that impinge on states from their contact with other countries).

At a more practical level, context will include factors such as the formal and informal relationships between health-care organisations and local interest groups, the wider economy and the local population's health status.

One important contextual factor of particular interest to students of health policy is that of 'professionalism'. As we have seen in Chapter 1, professionals wield power by virtue of their specialist knowledge, ability to control the supply of their membership and to regulate their own affairs. As a result, professionals enjoy high degrees of autonomy and discretion.

Alford's classic study of the New York health system identified key interests within the policy process [6]. 'Professional monopolisers' (the medical profession) were the dominant power, challenged only by 'corporate rationalisers' (managerial interests) who sought to exert control over the medical professionals. The interests of community groups and patients exercised little power within the health-care system and were described by Alford as 'repressed'. Importantly, Alford suggested that professional power allowed the medical interest group to control the ideological and cultural environment that supported their dominant position.

The position of the medical profession within the British policy process has been described as a 'state-licensed elite' [7]. The predominance of medical interests since the formation of the NHS has been held to represent a form of 'ideological corporatism', where governments and the profession share a similar world view [8]. However, a number of conflicts emerged between government and the medical profession. For example, the introduction of market-based reforms to the NHS since the 1980s has been a source of on-going dispute between government and the British Medical Association right up to the present day. Successive governments have also changed the contractual terms which bound both independently contracted and employed professionals to the NHS. The fact that many of these reforms were pursued in the teeth of opposition from professional interests suggests that the prevailing corporatist accommodation between government and professions is weaker now than it once was [9].

Implementation as part of the policy process

In the rational models of the policy process described above, implementation features as a distinct phase that occurs once the formal 'policy' has been created. Implementation is seen as simply a 'technical' or 'managerial' process unconnected to the more vital issue of policy content.

This 'top-down' conceptualisation of the policy process (where managers faithfully execute policy coming down from a political policy-making cadre) has been challenged by a welter of empirical studies. These studies suggest that policy implementation is fundamentally intertwined with policy making. In this view, policy is made 'bottom-up' by those responsible for implementation.

The bottom-up approach is based on two propositions: that the selection of policy solutions may occur during implementation (i.e. policies may not always be clearly defined prior to their operationalisation); and that the behaviour of implementers may mediate the policy content or its outcome. For example, Lipsky, in another classic study, identified a key role for 'street-level bureaucrats' who were able to alter policy outcomes through the way in which they chose to respond to pressures from above [10]. An examination of Dutch policy on heart transplants showed that national policy was deliberately subverted by health-service providers [11].

Health-care institutions therefore may pursue their own organisational strategies and policy-making agenda and are unlikely to see themselves as passive implementers of government policy. Indeed, NHS organisations have their own collective interest group (the NHS Confederation) that actively promotes policy and seeks to influence government opinion. All this means that ministers' ability to achieve change on the ground is rather more constrained than they might wish.

Finally, doctors influence policy both collectively – via their trade union, the British Medical Association – and individually. Think of the recent contribution of Lord Ara Darzi, a surgeon at St Mary's Hospital [12] or Professor Steve Field (chair of the Coalition government's Future Forum – a group established to propose amendments to the much-contested Health and Social Care Bill in 2011). Politicians are all too aware of the power of a profession that makes contact with six million people a week!

Recent English health policy

This section considers briefly some of the main features of health policy in England since the election of the Labour government in 1997. Note that in the post-devolution-era England, Wales and Scotland have adopted very different health policies. However, the substance of all major policy documents and white papers in recent decades can be summarised in terms of a few central themes (Table 16.1).

The Labour government's reforms comprised three overlapping strategies [13]. The first dimension of reform was to improve the provision of care through increased investment in service provision (in the shape of more health professionals, equipment and buildings). As a consequence, health spending has risen from around 7% of gross domestic product (GDP) in 2000 to reach about 10% by 2010, a proportion approaching that of the European average.

The second dimension of reform involved setting national standards and targets and creating a regulatory infrastructure to monitor these standards (such as the

Table 16.1 Common policy concerns

Cost containment and efficiency
Improving access
Variations in quality of care
Increasing user involvement and choice
Information management and technology
Equity
Workforce development

quality regulator now known as the Care Quality Commission). The third dimension of reform involved the development of the commissioning function in local health agencies, giving patients rights to choose their provider and introducing a diverse market of providers supported by new financial incentives.

Markets – the drive for efficiency and cost containment

Perhaps the most contentious policy stream has been the use of market incentives as a means to improve quality and efficiency. This policy began for the NHS in 1990 with the reforms of the Thatcher government. While the Labour Party came to power in 1997 advocating an end to competitive markets and private-sector involvement in clinical services, it soon changed direction and instead introduced a set of initiatives designed to increase competition between health-care providers in the English NHS (devolved government within the UK meant that a divergence in health policy emerged across the four countries).

The main features of this market-based system included:

- new financial incentives (fees for each treatment given) designed to promote competition between providers;
- rights for patients to choose their providers;
- diversification of supply in hospital and primary care to include the independent sector;
- greater autonomy of NHS providers through the replacement of central account-ability of NHS hospitals to the Department of Health with accountability of 'foundation trusts' to local people and to an independent regulator.

So what can explain this apparent volte face? The move towards markets was inspired by a number of concerns [14]. Firstly, the substantial investment in NHS services since 2000 had seen productivity fall, at least as measured by the NHS 'efficiency index' (put simply, rises in clinical activity had not matched the rises in funding). There emerged an increasing concern that an abundance of funds had led to inefficient practices and only modest gains for patients. However, there was also a parallel concern that the public-monopoly nature of the NHS had also led to a lack of responsiveness to the needs of individual patients. Without challenge, and the potential for patients to 'exit' the system, providers might lack motivation to listen to their customers. The 'patient-choice' policy, championed by Tony Blair and underpinned by new financial incentives designed to reward hospitals that attract more patients and punish those that lose custom, was intended to improve responsiveness to the needs of patients.

Labour's broad policy objectives have been maintained by the Coalition government on coming to power in 2010. Indeed, the Coalition's first NHS White Paper on the NHS signalled a further shift towards the marketisation of the NHS. This included plans to liberalise health-care markets so that all 'qualified providers' could ply their trade, supplying more information for consumers to help exercise extended rights to choose their provider, and a new economic regulator with a duty to promote competition [15].

However, the furore that resulted from these proposals – from sections of the public, trades unions (including the BMA) and, importantly, Liberal Democrat Coalition partners – demonstrated clearly that the introduction of market principles to the NHS remains a deeply controversial issue. Some more radical elements of the initial policy were removed or watered down and, at the time of writing, are still being considered by Parliament.

Proponents of health-care competition point to emerging economic evidence suggesting that greater competition may enhance quality [16] and claims that policies of competition and patient choice may be responsible for superior health-system performance in England compared to the other home nations [17]. However, other commentators have also pointed to the risk that competition between providers may impede the delivery of integrated care to patients [18]. The policy conundrum remains of how to harness the positive aspects of competition while promoting 'joined-up' care [19].

Coalition policy and the changing structure of the NHS

The NHS in England has undergone numerous structural reorganisations in the last two decades as successive governments have wrestled with the question as to what organisational form is most conducive to the policy outcomes they seek.

A particularly important issue has been that of the right balance between top-down control by central government, control by arm's-length independent regulators and bottom-up autonomy of local health-care organisations. The accountability of Parliament for such a large publicly funded service has, in practice, limited the ability of governments to 'let go'. However, the scope for central government to dominate the NHS has diminished over time.

The creation of foundation trusts in the last decade has increased the autonomy of providers from central control (such trusts are accountable to an independent regulator, to local commissioners and to locally appointed and elected governors). The Coalition government has signalled, like its predecessors, that all public health-care providers are expected to achieve foundation-trust status by 2014 unless there are compelling local reasons otherwise. New, independent organisational forms have also crept into the provider marketplace, including social enterprises and not-for-profit organisations, which combine the principles of the NHS with an ability to act in a commercial environment.

The reduction of central control over providers has to date been counterbalanced by strong central control over commissioners. However, the Coalition government plans to reduce the degree of political control over the commissioning of health services. This is taking two forms. First, at national level, the Secretary of State and Department of Health is passing direct control of commissioning to an arm's-length National Commissioning Board. Politicians set the objectives of this board but, in theory at least, are not responsible for day-to-day control.

The second form of decentralisation is transferring commissioning powers from primary care trusts to new organisations run by local clinicians (Clinical Commissioning Groups). The government has stressed that it wishes these groups to be more autonomous than their predecessors as long as they can demonstrate commissioning competence (see Introduction to Part 1).

The last decade has also seen a rise in the number and significance of arm's-length bodies and regulators. Three bodies are particularly significant. The Care Quality Commission (CQC) has been given statutory responsibility to license health- and social-care providers on grounds of quality (i.e. give them permission to trade). In addition, the CQC has powers to monitor on-going quality and intervene where quality problems are detected. The National Institute of Health and Clinical Excellence (known as NICE) is responsible for advising government and the NHS on which health-care interventions are cost-effective and on models of best clinical practice. A new regulatory body, Monitor, is responsible for authorising new foundation trusts and for monitoring compliance with the terms of authorisation, intervening if required where there is the risk of non-compliance. Under Coalition plans, the role of Monitor will expand to become that of an economic regulator for health and social care, ensuring that appropriate levels of competition exist to promote efficient and high-quality care.

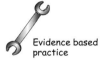

Evidence based practice

Better health as well as better health services?
Public health policy developments

The public health system has been through many changes over recent years, but is a critical part of improving health in communities. Evidence suggests that health services contribute only a third of the improvements we could make in life expectancy while changing lifestyles and addressing determinants of health inequalities (such as education, employment and housing) contribute the remainder [20].

Table 16.2 Government priorities for public health

Priorities for action in choosing health – making healthy choices easier
- Reducing the numbers of people who smoke
- Reducing obesity and improving diet and nutrition
- Increasing exercise
- Encouraging and supporting sensible drinking
- Improving sexual health
- Improving mental health

While much of the public's attention has been drawn towards the debate over how best to improve health services, the Labour government of 1997 to 2010 also developed a substantial public health agenda (Table 16.2). The financial as well as health benefits of securing a healthier population were described by Sir Derek Wanless [21]. In his projection of health expenditure, Wanless calculated that health-care for a population that was not involved in promoting its own health would be significantly more expensive than one that was 'fully engaged'. The government can claim some success: targets for reduced deaths from cancer and heart disease look set to be met. Yet when looked at more critically, many of the achievements are simply in line with longer-term trends in disease prevention and survival.

A further area of commitment is to reduce inequalities in health between the richest and poorest populations. Policies addressing the social determinants of health require working across many sectors (health, education, criminal justice, local government, transport, etc.) and more effective inter-departmental working. This requires what is often referred to as a 'whole systems approach' (although it is not always clear what this means in practice.) Commonly understood characteristics of whole systems working include:
- that services are responsible to the needs of individual patients/clients;
- that all stakeholders accept their inter-dependency;
- that partnerships are advanced by sharing a vision of the service priorities;
- that users of the system do not experience unnecessary gaps or duplication.

The Coalition government from 2010 re-stated a commitment to reduce inequalities, and has made implementation of the Marmot Review (commissioned by the previous Labour administration – see Chapter 15) a part of its public health policy [22]. The Marmot Review 'Fair Society, Healthy Lives' adopted its life-course framework for tackling the wider social determinants of health [23]. Key policy priorities are shown in Table 16.3 demonstrating this life-course approach alongside a settings-based approach to policy implementation (for example, action in schools and workplaces).

The Coalition White Paper ('Healthy Lives, Healthy People') also adopted the Nuffield Council of Bioethics ladder of intervention (see Figure 16.2) to establish a framework for future public health policy development [24].

Table 16.3 Fair Society, Healthy Lives policy objectives

Give every child the best start in life

Enable all children, young people and adults to maximise their capabilities and have control over their lives

Create fair employment and good work for all

Ensure a healthy standard of living for all

Create and develop healthy and sustainable places and communities

Strengthen the role and impact of ill health prevention

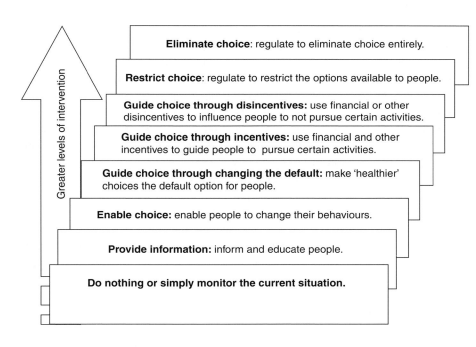

Figure 16.2   Nuffield Council on Bioethics ladder of possible Government action on public health.

The Coalition aims to reduce inequalities, improve health, build self-esteem and resilience from infancy with stronger support in the early years, and intervene at the lowest level of the ladder that is effective, and the key to delivering this is intended to be a new, 'localised' public health system.

Public health has three core elements, improving health (using evidence-based interventions in communities to improve the wider determinants of health), health protection (protecting communities from infectious disease and environmental hazards) and acting to improve health (and other) services, for example by advising commissioners on local health needs and effective interventions.

Currently, health protection is the responsibility of the Health Protection Agency, which supports local NHS organisations, Directors of Public Health (DsPH) and local

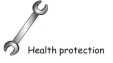
Health improvement

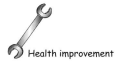
Health protection

government. Health improvement and health service public health are delivered locally through DsPH in PCTs, supported by national programmes such as that on tobacco control. The Coalition government is moving the local DPH role wholly into local government, to act as the 'fount of all wisdom' on the health of the local community. They are supposed to influence NHS and social-care services, children's services, environment, education, economy and health through new health and well-being boards.

This places the strategic leaders for addressing health inequalities, within the local authorities from whence they originally evolved. The first Medical Officers of Health began discharging their responsibilities from municipalities in the middle of the nineteenth century. They are once more closer to those responsible for upstream influences on health, e.g. housing, transport, leisure and the environment.

They will be supported by Public Health England, a dedicated, new service set up as an executive agency of the Department of Health to set public health policy, establish health-improvement commissioning priorities and strengthen emergency preparedness and health protection. Public Health England will take on the functions of the Health Protection Agency, some functions of the Food Standards Agency, and the National Treatment Agency for substance misuse, and will run national programmes for health improvement, develop evidence, support DsPH in their local authority roles, and provide public health support for the new NHS commissioning board.

The centralisation of expertise should allow for more coordinated action on truly national issues, as well as for less duplication of effort. Such proximity to government brings challenges. Restrictions on tobacco display and plain cigarette packs are mentioned, for example, but it takes considerable strength to articulate the case for such measures in the face of fierce political lobbying from industries with vast resources at their disposal.

Conclusion

The NHS in England underwent significant change under the Labour government. It showed a clear preference for market incentives over central planning but these policy solutions have had little impact to date on the familiar problems that they were designed to address: rising demand and indifferent productivity. On the left of the political spectrum, commentators hold this up as evidence that 'markets don't work' [25]; those to the right claim that this illustrates the need to strengthen market mechanisms and the role of private providers.

The incoming Coalition government has pledged another major overhaul of the NHS designed to improve performance and, in part, to remove 'unnecessary' interference by government. It remains to be seen how these new organisations will change relations between politicians and civil servants at the centre and health-service staff at a local level.

REFERENCES

1. P. A Sabatier (ed.), *Theories of the Policy Process*, Cambridge, MA, Westview Press, 2007.
2. G. Walt, *Health Policy: An Introduction to Process and Power*, London, Zed Books, 1994.
3. T. Dye, *Top Down Policymaking*, London, Chatham House Publishers.
4. C. E. Lindblom, The science of muddling through, *Public Administration Review* **19**, 1959, 79–88.
5. H. M. Leichter, *A Comparative Approach to Policy Analysis: Health Care Policy in Four Nations*, Cambridge, Cambridge University Press, 1979.
6. R. R. Alford, *Health Care Politics*, Chicago, IL, University of Chicago Press, 1975.
7. S. Harrison, D. J. Hunter and C. Pollitt, *The Dynamics of British Health Policy*, London, Unwin, 1990.
8. P. Dunleavy, Professions and policy change: notes towards a model of ideological corporatism. *Public Administration Bulletin* **36**, 1981, 3–16.
9. R. Klein, *The New Politics of the NHS*, 3rd edn., London, Longman, 1995.
10. M. Lipsky, Towards a theory of street-level bureaucracy. In W. D. Hawley, M. Lipsky, S. B. Greenberg *et al.* (eds.), *Theoretical Perspectives on Urban Politics*, Englewood Cliffs, NJ, Prentice-Hall, 1976, pp. 196–213.
11. A. De Roo and H. Maarse, Understanding the central–local relationship in health care; a new approach. *International Journal of Health Planning and Management* **5**, 1990, 15–25.
12. A. Darzi, Quality and the NHS next stage review. *Lancet* **371**, 2008, 1563–4.
13. S. Stevens, Reform strategies for the English NHS. *Health Affairs* **23**(3), 2004, 37–44.
14. R. Lewis and J. Dixon, *NHS Market Futures – Exploring the Impact of Health Service Market Reforms*, London, King's Fund, 2005.
15. Department of Health, Equity and excellence; liberating the NHS (White Paper), The Department of Health, 2010.
16. R. Lewis and R. Thorlby, Liberalising the health care market: The new government's ambition for the National Health Service. *International Journal of Health Services* **41**(3), 2011, 565–74.
17. S. Connolly, N. Mays and G. Bevan, *Funding and Performance of Healthcare Systems in the Four Countries of the UK Before and After Devolution*, London, Nuffield Trust, 2010.
18. N. Curry and C. Ham, *Clinical and Service Integration – the Route to Improved Outcomes*, London, KF Publishing, 2010.
19. R. Lewis, R. Rosen, N. Goodwin and J. Dixon, *Where Next for Integrated Care Organisations in the English NHS*, London, Nuffield Trust, 2010.
20. J. Bunker, The role of medical care in contributing to health improvement within society. *International Journal of Epidemiology* **30**, 2001, 1260–3.
21. D. Wanless, Securing our future health: Taking a long-term view, Final report, London, HM Treasury, 2002.
22. Department of Health, Healthy Lives, Healthy People: Our Strategy for Public Health in England (White Paper), London, HM Government, 2010.
23. M. Marmot, Strategic Review of Health Inequalities in England Post-2010 (The Marmot Review), London, University College, 2010. See: http://www.ucl.ac.uk/gheg/marmotreview.
24. Nuffield Council on Bioethics, Public health: ethical issues, London, 2007. See: www.nuffieldbioethics.org/sites/default/files/Public%20health%20-%20ethical%20issues.pdf.
25. A. Pollock, *NHS plc: The Privatisation of Our Health Care*, London, Verso, 2004.

17

International development and public health

Jenny Amery

Key points

- Almost all preventable deaths of children, and of women in pregnancy and child-birth, occur in poor countries. Poor people carry the greatest burden from communicable diseases, and non-communicable diseases are increasing in poor countries.
- Reducing income poverty, through economic development, debt relief and fairer trade, will improve health status, but faster progress will be made by increasing access to health services including affordable medicines.
- Around half of all poor people live in countries where the state institutions are weak or ineffective, including during and after armed conflicts. International agencies have a particular responsibility to address the health needs of such populations.
- Different models of financing and organising health services are appropriate for different contexts. Robust, effective heath systems accessible to and used by poor people are key. There is no one 'right' model.
- The impact of health systems in poor countries must be strengthened by: protecting poor people from large out-of-pocket expenditure on health; improving equity of access to health services; ensuring sustainable health-care worker capacity.
- Better data systems are needed to monitor the impact of health policies and to measure health-service quality.
- There has been a proliferation of agencies and initiatives working to address global health needs since the 1990s. Greater co-ordination is urgently needed to increase the impact of the many agencies and initiatives which aim to improve global health.
- More research is needed in prevention and management of diseases of poverty, including chronic conditions, and ways of reaching the poorest people with proven cost-effective life-saving interventions.

Essential Public Health, Second Edition, ed. Stephen Gillam, Jan Yates and Padmanabhan Badrinath.
Published by Cambridge University Press. © Cambridge University Press 2012.

Introduction

This chapter extends the consideration of the changing global burden of diseases begun in Chapter 2 and discusses what is required to mount an effective response to the public health challenges, particularly in poor countries. It considers the role of international development assistance and the responsibilities of the international community in improving the health of poor people.

The links between poverty and health

Poor health results from poverty: hunger, limited or no access to clean water, sanitation, housing, health and education services; in turn it contributes to poverty and impedes economic growth [1]. A person who is repeatedly ill cannot earn a decent living or contribute to the workforce. Unmet need for modern family-planning methods results in early and repeated pregnancies, closely spaced births, increased risks of illness and death to child and mother. Undernourished and frequently sick children do not learn well at school and often drop out early. When a family member falls sick, poor house-holds may have to make huge payments for health-care, sell their livestock, land or other assets, become indebted to money lenders or enter bonded labour agreements, which may keep the family in poverty. Poverty and ill health cause misery and loss of hope.

There are wide differences between health outcome for the richest and poorest within countries. For example, Figure 17.1 shows inequalities in the under-5 mortality rate in Nigeria in 2008. The large gap between the lowest and highest wealth quintiles has reduced from 178 in 2003 to 132 deaths per 1000 live births in 2008. The gap is widest for mother's education.

The global burden of disease

There have been rapid falls in mortality and overall improvements in health globally in the last half century, but many poor countries have not shared in these benefits, and have fallen behind high-income countries. The number of people living on the equivalent of less than 1.25 US dollars per day fell from 1.8 billion in 1990 to 1.4 billion in 2005. By 2015, the number is projected to be just over 900 million, mostly in south Asia, India and Africa [2] (see Table 17.1). The economic and financial crisis of 2008 slowed economic growth and has serious costs for poverty reduction and human development. Multidimensional poverty measures provide more detailed analysis of trends in multiple aspects of poverty [3].

Poverty and ill health are closely linked. The premature deaths and preventable ill health of millions of poor people present a major contemporary challenge. Poor

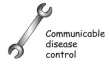

Communicable
disease
control

Table 17.1 Percentage of the population and population numbers (millions) by region living on less than US$ 1.25 per day. 1990, 2005 and projections to 2015 and 2020

Region	1990	2005	2015	2020	1990	2005	2015	2020
	Percentage of the population living on less than $US 1.25 a day				Number of people living on less than $US 1.25 a day (millions)			
East Asia and Pacific	54.7	16.8	5.9	4.0	873	317	120	83
China	60.2	15.9	5.1	4.0	683	208	70	56
Europe and central Asia	2.0	3.7	1.7	1.2	9	16	7	5
Latin America and the Caribbean	11.3	8.2	5.0	4.3	50	45	30	27
Middle East and North Africa	4.3	3.6	1.8	1.5	10	11	6	6
South Asia	51.7	40.3	22.8	19.4	579	595	388	352
India	51.3	41.6	23.6	20.3	435	456	295	268
Sub-Saharan Africa	57.6	50.9	38.0	32.8	296	387	366	352
Total	41.7	25.2	15.0	12.8	1817	1371	918	826

Source: World Bank global monitory report 2010.

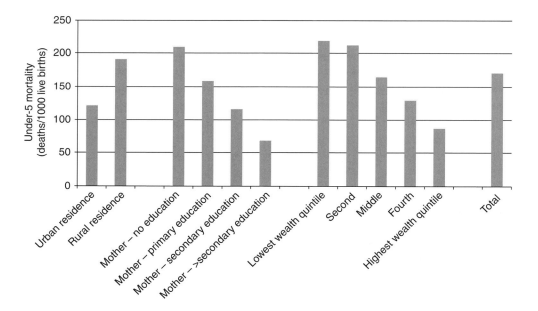

Figure 17.1   Nigeria under-5 mortality rates by socio-economic characteristics. Source: Macro International, 2008 Nigeria Demographic and Health Survey (DHS) report.

people carry the greatest burden from communicable diseases, particularly in Africa where these conditions present acute control challenges and account for over 60% of disease burden, compared to about 30% in the low-income countries of south Asia. Acquired immune deficiency syndrome (AIDS), tuberculosis (TB) and malaria are the three biggest killers, but the so-called neglected tropical diseases such as lymphatic

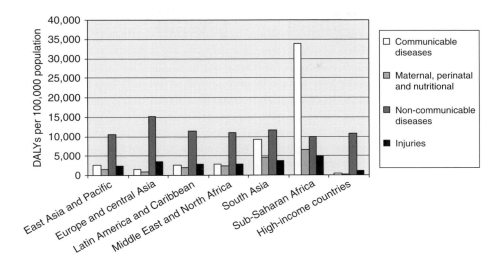

filariasis, onchocerciasis, guinea worm, leprosy and trachoma contribute very significantly to the total burden of disease of poor people in Africa (see Figure 17.2).

Other factors contributing to the changing pattern of disease include international migration, rapid rural-to-urban migration in most poor countries and changing family structures; also, climate change and emerging microbe and vector resistance to drugs and insecticides. New diseases such as severe acute respiratory syndrome (SARS) may emerge, and there is the on-going risk of pandemic human influenza.

Population growth is a major issue, particularly in the face of climate-change impacts and resource scarcity. Total global population exceeds 7 billion. Growth is fastest in some of the poorest countries, for example Nigeria is projected to rise from a total population of 158 million in 2010 to 729 million in 2100, Malawi from 14.9 to 129 million, Tanzania from 44.8 to 316 million, Zambia from 13.1 to 140 million, Somalia from 9 to 73 million [4].

The disability-adjusted life year (DALY) is a measure of the burden of ill health that takes into account both reduced life expectancy and quality of life. It is widely used internationally despite limitations. Values vary widely according to discount rates and weighting of different age groups used. Relatively poor data are available for some countries and conditions, but no better alternative measure has yet been agreed.

Figure 17.2   Burden of disease in DALYs per 100,000 population due to four broad disease categories by region. Source: WHO Global Burden of Disease data for 2002.

Demography

Key health issues and effective interventions

Preventable illness and deaths amongst children

Despite population growth, the number of deaths in children under 5 worldwide declined from 12.4 million in 1990 to 8.1 million in 2009 – a fall in the mortality rate from 89 to 60 per 1000 live births. Ninety per cent of the deaths occurred in only 42 countries. In these countries, serious illnesses commonly occur sequentially or concurrently before death. For example, measles is often complicated by pneumonia or diarrhoea [5]. Underweight and micronutrient deficiencies decrease host defences, and malnutrition is estimated to contribute to over 35% of avoidable childhood deaths [6]. One hundred and ninety-five million children under 5 are chronically undernourished (stunted) from the combined effects of dietary insufficiency, including micronutrient deficiency, and related infections, and this will limit their cognitive as well as physical development if not addressed in the first 2 to 3 years of life. The extent and impact of undernutrition remains a silent emergency, which often only becomes visible when exacerbated by acute famine [6]. Seventy-three per cent of all child deaths in sub-Saharan Africa and 76 per cent in south Asia are from acute respiratory infections, diarrhoeal diseases, perinatal conditions, measles, and – in Africa – malaria (see Chapter 12). The interventions to prevent these deaths are well researched and, with improved coverage, could save many lives (see Table 17.2). Providing sustained access to these interventions by the poorest people remains a major challenge.

Maternal health

Ninety-nine per cent of deaths in pregnancy and childbirth occur in poor countries, and over two thirds in 13 countries: India, Nigeria, Pakistan, Democratic Republic of Congo (DRC), Ethiopia, Tanzania, Afghanistan, Bangladesh, Angola, China, Kenya, Indonesia and Uganda (see Table 17.3).

Overall, the lifetime risk of maternal death for a woman in high-income countries is 1 in 3900. In middle-income countries it is 1 in 190, and in low-income countries 1 in 39. This is the largest disparity in health outcome between the richest and poorest countries. Almost all of these deaths could be prevented if known, cost-effective interventions were available to all women.

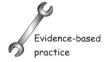

Evidence-based practice

Maternal and child health are linked, but there are fundamental differences in effective approaches to addressing them. While evidence-based, successful approaches to child health deliver services as close to the community as possible [7], the reduction of maternal mortality requires access to hospital-based interventions to deal with life-threatening complications, which mostly develop around the time of delivery. Good maternal health requires functioning health services at community, clinic and hospital levels, and effective referral systems, and is therefore considered an important marker of a functioning health system [8]. The reduction of neonatal deaths is closely linked to maternal health [9].

Reproductive health

Concern at the rapid population growth in the second half of the twentieth century often resulted in population policies focusing on controlling demographic growth, at the expense of the needs and rights of individuals. At the landmark International Conference on Population and Development held in Cairo in 1994, more than 170

Table 17.2 Under-5 deaths that could be prevented in the 42 countries with 90% of worldwide child deaths in 2000 through achievement of universal coverage with individual interventions

	Estimated under-5 deaths prevented	
Preventive interventions	Number of deaths ($\times 10^3$)	Proportion of all deaths
Breast-feeding	1301	13%
Insecticide-treated materials	691	7%
Complementary feeding	587	6%
Zinc	459 (351)	5% (4%)
Clean delivery	411	4%
Hib (*Haemophilus influenzae* type b) vaccine	403	4%
Water, sanitation, hygiene	326	3%
Antenatal steroids	264	3%
Newborn temperature management	227 (0)	2% (0%)
Vitamin A	225 (176)	2% (2%)
Tetanus toxoid	161	2%
Nevirapine and replacement feeding (HIV prevention)	150	2%
Antibiotics for premature rupture of membranes	133 (0)	1% (0%)
Measles vaccine	103	1%
Antimalarial intermittent preventive treatment in pregnancy	22	<1%
Treatment interventions		
Oral rehydration therapy	1477	15%
Antibiotics for sepsis	583	6%
Antibiotics for pneumonia	577	6%
Antimalarials	467	5%
Zinc	394	4%
Newborn resuscitation	359 (0)	4% (0%)
Antibiotics for dysentery	310	3%
Vitamin A	8	<1%

*Numbers represent effect if evidence of both levels 1 (sufficient) and 2 (limited) is included; value in brackets shows effect if only level 1 evidence is accepted. Interventions for which only one value is cited are all classified as level 1.

Source: G. Jones, R. W. Steketee, R. E. Black *et al.* How many child deaths can we prevent this year? *Lancet*, **362**, 2003, 65–71. Reproduced by permission of Elsevier Science.

countries agreed that reproductive health services should be available without coercion to all those who need them, and the conference set out a clear action plan. It defined comprehensive reproductive health-care as:

- voluntary contraceptive and family planning services;
- antenatal care, safe abortion, delivery, post-partum and post-abortion services (or safe motherhood services);
- services for the prevention, detection and treatment of sexually transmitted infections, including HIV.

Table 17.3 Estimates of maternal mortality ratio (MMR: deaths per 100,000 live births), number of maternal deaths and lifetime risk by World Bank regions and income groups, 2008

Region or income group	Estimated MMR	Lower estimate	Upper estimate	No maternal deaths	Lifetime risk of maternal death; 1 in:
Low income	580	420	830	162,000	39
Middle income	200	150	290	195,000	190
Regions with low and middle incomes:					
East Asia and Pacific	89	62	130	26,000	580
Europe and central Asia	32	27	39	1900	1800
Latin America and the Caribbean	86	72	110	200	480
Middle East and North Africa	88	62	130	6700	380
South Asia	290	190	430	109,000	110
Sub-Saharan Africa	650	470	920	203,000	31
High Income	15	14	17	1900	3900
WORLD	260	300	270	358,000	140

Income groups based on 2009 gross national income per capita estimates: low income, US$ 995 or less; middle income, US$ 996–3945; high income, US$ 12,196 or more.

MMR and lifetime risk rounded according to the following scheme: <100, no rounding; 100–999, rounded to nearest 10; and >1000, rounded to nearest 100. The numbers of maternal deaths have been rounded as follows: <1000, rounded to nearest 10; 1000–9999, rounded to nearest 100; and >10,000 rounded to nearest 1000.

Source: Trends in Maternal Mortality 1990–2008. Estimates developed by WHO, UNICEF, UNFPA, World Bank.

It was recognised that many of the issues which impact on reproductive health, including women's empowerment, literacy, poverty and lack of access to health services, could not be resolved quickly, and would require new policies and, in some cases, new legislation. There has been considerable progress in many countries, but about one third of pregnancies worldwide each year, about 80 million, are unwanted or unplanned. Globally, 215 million women who want to delay or avoid pregnancy are not using an effective method of family planning [10]. There are ongoing concerns about how to ensure the future supply of contraceptive methods to those who need them.

Communicable diseases

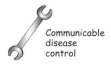
Communicable disease control

Communicable diseases remain a major cause of ill health and death in poor countries, despite advances in vaccine development, diagnosis and available treatment. Most of this disease burden is from malaria, HIV, TB, diarrhoeal and respiratory diseases, and the so-called neglected tropical diseases including leishmaniasis, trypanosomiasis, Chagas disease, lymphatic filariasis, onchocerciasis (river blindness), schistosomiasis, dracunculiasis, soil-transmitted helminth infections, leprosy and tra-choma (which causes 6 million people to go blind each year). Globally, in 2009 there were nearly 1.7 million deaths from TB, close to 1 million from malaria (mostly children in Africa) together with a huge morbidity, and 1.8 million deaths from AIDS, most in Africa. Table 17.4 summarises health-care interventions that address the 'big three'.

HIV and AIDS

Human immunodeficiency virus was first reported in the early 1980s, and has become the first pandemic since that of influenza in 1918. It has stabilised and the number of new infections has been declining since the late 1990s, and there are fewer deaths due to the scale-up of antiretroviral therapy. An estimated 2.6 million people worldwide became newly infected in 2009, nearly one fifth fewer than the peak of 3.1 million in 1999. Sub-Saharan Africa has 10% of the world's population and more than 60% of all those living with HIV. Women are disproportionately affected, especially in sub-Saharan Africa where three women are affected for every two men. People infected with HIV are particularly susceptible to TB and co-infection is very common. Africa remains the global epicentre and even though new infections are decreasing, the lag time between infection and death means the burden of disease will remain high for years to come [11].

In Asia, the epidemics are driven by unsafe sexual practices, particularly commer-cial sex, male-to-male sex and injecting-drug use. Rates of HIV infection continue to rise in Eastern Europe and central Asia, with Ukraine and the Russian Federation most affected.

In high-prevalence countries, AIDS continues to have a huge impact on population structure, family and social life, and economic growth. In many countries, stigma and discrimination prevent people from coming forward for testing or treatment. In parts of Africa, AIDS is reversing improvements in health indicators and average life expectancy.

Non-communicable diseases

Figure 17.2 also shows the burden from non-communicable diseases, which is projected to rise over the next 10 years, and is increasingly affecting poor people in poor countries. Projections to the year 2030 suggest that ischaemic heart disease, stroke, smoking-related cancers, respiratory problems and road traffic accidents will cause proportionately more deaths, although AIDS will remain a significant cause globally [12]. Robust public health measures in sectors other than health are required to address the key risk factors of nutrition, smoking, unsafe sex and the growing epidemic of injury and death from road traffic accidents [13–16]. Fourteen per cent of the disease burden globally is due to mental health disorders, mostly chronically disabling depression and other common disorders, alcohol and sub-stance disorders, and psychoses, and these increase the risk of physical illness. Many

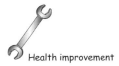
Health improvement

Table 17.4 Summary of effective health-care interventions for reducing illness and death from HIV and AIDS, TB and malaria

Goal	Preventive intervention	Treatment
Prevent and reduce burden of HIV and AIDS	Safe sex including use of male (and female) condoms; injecting drug users have clean needles and oral substitution therapy; safe, screened blood supplies; antiretroviral drugs to prevent mother-to-child transmission; male circumcision.	Prompt treatment of opportunistic infections including TB; cotrimoxazole prophylaxis; highly active antiretroviral therapy; palliative care and support.
Prevent and reduce burden of TB	Directly observed treatment of infectious cases to reduce transmission and emergence of drug-resistant strains; testing of people with AIDS for early diagnosis of TB; preventive isoniazid therapy; BCG (Bacille Calmette Guérin) to reduce childhood TB.	Directly observed treatment to cure symptomatic cases; second-line therapies for multiple drug-resistant cases.
Prevent and reduce burden from malaria	Use of insecticide-treated bed-nets; in epidemic-prone areas indoor residual spraying and intermittent presumptive treatment of pregnant women; prompt identification of drug-resistant strains.	Rapid diagnosis and treatment of cases with locally effective medicines, depending on drug resistance. Increasing use of Artemisin combination treatments (ACTs), and effective parenteral drugs for severe malaria.

low-income countries lack policy or legislation for mental health, have very few trained mental health workers, little or no funding, and any available care is institutionally based. Sufferers are highly stigmatised. Scaling up access to an evidence-based package of interventions for core mental health problems would cost $US 2 per person in low-income countries. There is growing evidence that many interventions can be delivered effectively in decentralised settings by people who are not mental health professionals [17].

Access to medicines

Even when health services reach them, medicines are often not affordable for poor people, who frequently have to pay out-of-pocket for them. Barriers to accessing effective medicines in poor countries include: high prices; insufficient overall financing of health services and poor priority setting with too little money to fund supplies of essential drugs; inappropriate drug selection, weak procurement and distribution systems; and poor-quality or fake medicines. The WHO estimates that 15% of the world's population consumes 91% of the global production of pharmaceuticals, by value [18]. Some pharmaceutical companies are working in private–public partnerships to bring key medicines to poor people, for example the ivermectin donation programme as part of the initiative to eradicate onchocerciasis in Africa [19].

The World Trade Organization agreement on trade-related aspects of intellectual property rights (TRIPS) gives countries the right, under the Doha TRIPS and public health decision of 2003, to protect public health, for example by importing copies of patented medicines, if their own pharmaceutical industry has insufficient capacity to produce them. International trade policy is important to increase poor people's access to medicines [20].

There are a number of public–private product-development partnerships to develop medicines for diseases disproportionately affecting poor people. Advance market commitments (AMCs) for vaccines aim to create a competitive developing-country market for future vaccines that is sufficiently large and credible to stimulate private investment in research and development and manufacturing capacity, that otherwise would not take place. Advance market commitments are being developed initially for the production of new vaccines for pneumococcal disease [21].

How can improvements in health be delivered?

There is a complex inter-relationship between poverty and health which can be a virtuous cycle with a healthier population contributing to economic growth and prosperity, or a vicious cycle of worsening health, increasing indebtedness from health-care expenditure, marginalisation from the economy and slowing economic growth. Orthodox economic arguments highlight the need for macroeconomic growth to reduce levels of poverty, but not all growth benefits poor people, and there are increasing concerns about 'jobless' growth, with millions of poor people remaining at the margins of society. Debt relief, fairer trade with access to markets for poorer countries and communities are also key, and require action from rich-country governments. More predictable aid would enable poor countries to fund sustainable 5- to 10-year health plans and invest in well-trained workforces. Greater investment in new technologies should yield better diagnostics, medicines and vaccines for communicable and other life-threatening diseases. However, none of these will make a significant difference without quality health services, accessible to poor people, staffed by well-trained, supervised, motivated and adequately rewarded health workers.

The framing of numerical goals and targets focuses attention, but also risks a technocratic, top-down approach to the complex challenges facing different countries, populations and cultures [22].

Global knowledge of effective interventions alone is not sufficient to improve health. Governments have a key role, and where a government is unwilling or too weak to implement change, poverty and ill health prevail. The role of the state is, at minimum: first, to maintain borders, provide peace and security; secondly, to create conditions that provide livelihoods and economic growth; and thirdly, to ensure provision of public goods and services such as health and education (see Box 17.1).

Box 17.1 Good governance

Good governance can be summarised as:

- The capacity of the state to raise revenue, use resources and deliver services
- Responsiveness of public policies and institutions to the needs and rights of citizens
- Accountability including free media access to information, opportunity to change leaders through democratic means

Health-care quality

Much poor performance in terms of health-service delivery is due to weaknesses in institutions, budgeting and public-expenditure management, and the fact that governments are not accountable to their people [23]. The quality of private-health-care providers ranges from excellent to dangerous, and is rarely adequately regulated. Governments should be held to account for maintaining fiscal discipline, ensuring resources are allocated and spent in line with stated priorities and not lost through corruption or mismanagement, and are used to achieve maximum impact on health outcomes. Making information more accessible and promoting transparency in fees, budgets and expenditure enable corruption to be tackled more easily, but there are often strong forces at work to avoid such transparency [24].

Emergency planning

Weak or corrupt states, engulfed in armed conflicts or run by repressive military regimes, will not have institutions capable of delivering health services. In such environments, creative, context-specific responses are needed. Donors may wish to work through UN bodies, non-governmental organisations (NGOs), faith-based organisations, for-profit providers and community-based providers to meet the humanitarian needs of the people, and support the long-term development of government institutions that can eventually take on responsibility for service delivery. Exceptional responses for humanitarian and other disasters such as earthquakes, hurricanes and floods need better coordination, and more should be invested in resilience and risk reduction [25].

Improving health through health-care

Organising and financing health systems

There are many ways to promote and sustain health outside the health sector, including housing, water and sanitation, food, security, education and employment. But timely access to a mix of promotion, prevention, treatment, rehabilitation and care is critical, and this needs a well-functioning health system.

One of the reasons for low health-service coverage and poor health outcomes is low per-capita expenditure on health. The Commission on Macroeconomics and Health calculated that US$ 34 per capita in 2002 prices is needed to provide a basic package of services to address the main causes of ill health and premature death in low-income countries [1]. This would require an additional US$ 40–52 billion by 2015 and would save some 8 million lives each year. Increasing taxes on tobacco and alcohol, a foreign-exchange transaction levy and other schemes have been proposed to increase revenues for health [26].

The method of financing health services will influence whether poor people can access them. Tax-financed universal health-care is the most equitable, but may be subject to high administrative cost, poor governance, and disproportionate use by the articulate and well-off. Social insurance can combine risk-pooling and distribute the financial burden according to ability to pay. Prepayment into a community financing scheme tailored to local needs, to pool risk, has to date delivered only limited coverage. Voluntary private insurance benefits those able to pay and will often exclude people with chronic conditions. Out-of-pocket payments at the time of illness is the most regressive form of financing, yet in many low-income countries it is the source of well over half of all financing for health-care. User charges levied by public and private providers of health-care have had mixed impact, but almost universally result in deterring access by poor people or impoverishing those on or near the poverty line [27][28].

Some countries are attaining measurably better levels of service coverage with lower levels of expenditure. Low-income countries, where significant improvements have taken place in the health of the population without high or rapidly rising incomes, include Bangladesh, Costa Rica, Cuba, Sri Lanka and Kerala State in India. Effective policies, well implemented, can greatly improve the health of poor people. The HIV epidemic, and the emergence of new diseases such as SARS, have highlighted the crucial role of governments in strengthening and maintaining core public health functions [29] (see Box 17.2).

Box 17.2 Core public health functions

Core public health functions include:
- Collection and dissemination of evidence for public health policies
- Public health regulation and enforcement
- Pharmaceutical policy regulation and enforcement
- Epidemiological and, where appropriate, behavioural surveillance for risk factors of disease
- Prevention and control of disease
- Health promotion
- Intersectoral action for improving health
- Monitoring and evaluation of public health policy
- Development of human resources and capacity for public health

Box 17.3 Critical issues in financing and organising of health services

- Bringing health-care benefits to those who are currently not accessing services of acceptable quality, including access to essential medicines
- Protecting people from unexpected large financial expenditures (risk protection)
- Creating incentives for appropriate, cost-effective, high-quality health-care
- Strengthening core public health functions
- Regulating and assuring the quality of service providers

To maximise their benefit, health resources must be re-allocated towards more cost-effective services, poorer geographical regions within countries, and services that are used by poor people. The allocation and distribution of resources is an intensely political process, affected by power struggles between competing stakeholders (e.g. different parts of government, external agencies). The ability of the state to set priorities and negotiate the allocation of resources in a way which increases equity and meets the needs of stakeholders is a measure of the state's legitimacy and its commitment to procedural justice [8] (see Box 17.3.)

People-centred or disease-specific services – or both?

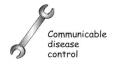

Communicable disease control

Disease- or issue-specific vertical approaches tend to be top-down and controlled by experts. The eradication of smallpox was a success, but efforts to eradicate malaria since the 1960s have failed, and total eradication of malaria is not feasible with current tools. Current examples of vertical programmes include those addressing polio eradication, AIDS and some childhood immunization.

The Alma-Ata Declaration of 1978 [30] rejected such vertical approaches and called on governments to tackle common underlying causes of ill health, with the building of sustainable health-care systems, locally based and locally controlled. Emphasis was given to people's participation in health. There is renewed emphasis on the need for strong primary health-care services, close to the people they serve, and responsive to their needs [31].

Vertical programmes can raise the profile of and funding for specific diseases, and increase access to commodities such as insecticide-treated bed-nets for malaria, and affordable, quality medicines. They can often deliver short-term results against specific targets. But they can weaken the impact of other services, by distorting country priorities, diverting scarce trained staff [32]. Looking ahead, a different focus on delivery systems for chronic conditions as well as acute episodes is needed in low-resource settings [33].

In 2010, there were well over 70 global health partnerships and initiatives addressing disease or other specific health needs, many with private–public financing. This is in addition to the European Commission, World Bank, Regional Development Banks,

WHO and UN technical agencies, private entities such as the Bill and Melinda Gates Foundation, and many bilateral donors (see the Internet Companion). There are concerns that this 'international health architecture' may be undermining poor countries' own capacity to deliver essential health services. International efforts must be better channelled, in line with emerging evidence on the effectiveness of international aid [34]. China, India and other emerging donors in health are increasingly influential in low-income countries' health services.

What else hinders access to health-care?

Other factors prevent poor people from using health services. Complex social, cultural and political factors make it difficult to break the intergenerational poverty, which affects hundreds of millions of people.

Social exclusion

Social exclusion is a process causing systematic disadvantage on the basis of ethnicity, religion, caste, descent, disability, HIV status, i.e. who you are and where you live. Excluded groups and individuals are denied equal rights and opportunities compared with others. Some people may suffer multiple forms of exclusion, for example low-caste women living in isolated rural areas [35].

Gender inequalities

Gender inequalities are a manifestation of one form of exclusion. Sex disparities are higher in south Asia than anywhere else in the world. A girl in India is greater than 40% more likely to die between her first and fifth birthday than is a boy. Child mortality would drop by 20% if girls had the same mortality rate as boys between the ages of 1 month and 5 years. The reasons for this are both environmental and behavioural. Girls are less likely to be brought for timely treatment and have less money spent on them when they are sick than boys [36].

Cost

Cost is a major obstacle. Both formal and informal charges and transport costs will prevent poor people from using services, and may plunge them further into poverty if charges for drugs or treatments require selling assets or borrowing money at inflated rates.

Human resources for health

Adequate numbers of well-trained, motivated health workers are essential for effective service delivery. Many countries face a deep crisis in staffing their health services, resulting from chronic under-investment in staff and health systems. This is exacerbated by outward migration and, especially in southern African countries, by the impact of AIDS on health services and staff. Low-income countries are currently subsidising high-income ones by supplying them with trained staff. From Africa, the net outflow is equivalent to about US$ 500 million a year. Changes to international recruitment practice may help to manage the flow of migrants, but migration is the result of low pay, lack of career prospects and poor working conditions in 'source' countries, as well as the inability of the high-income 'destination' countries to train and meet their own workforce requirements [37].

Measuring progress, increasing success

The millennium development goals (MDGs) and targets collectively address the different dimensions of poverty. They are documented in the Millennium Declaration signed by 189 countries in September 2000, and progress towards them is under regular review. There are 8 goals, 21 targets and 48 indicators. Countries, with the support of international agencies and donors, are intensifying efforts to make faster progress on the MDGs, particularly in Africa and south Asia. The MDG indicators measure average progress for a country, but do not reflect inequalities or widening gaps if poor people are left further behind.

Progress towards the health-related MDGs and respective indicators is being monitored closely, but is limited by incomplete vital registration of births and deaths, and poor-quality data [38].

Key outcomes are listed in Table 17.5.

Table 17.5 The millennium development goals and health-related targets: progress at 2011 in sub-Saharan Africa and south Asia

Goal	Target by 2015	Selected indicators	Progress in sub-Saharan Africa	Progress in south Asia
1. Eradicate extreme poverty and hunger	Reduce extreme poverty by half	Proportion of people living on equivalent of less than US$ 1 per day; % children under 5 underweight	High rates – slow progress	On track
	Reduce hunger by half		High rates – little change	High rates, progress but poorest left behind
2. Achieve universal primary education	Universal primary schooling	Net enrolment in primary education Completion rate at Grade 5	Progress in enrolment but lagging; conflict limits progress	Progress but lagging

Table 17.5

Goal	Target by 2015	Selected indicators	Progress in sub-Saharan Africa	Progress in south Asia
3. Promote gender equality and empower women	Girls equal enrolment in primary, secondary and tertiary education	Ratio of girls to boys in primary, secondary and tertiary education	Progress but lagging especially in secondary education	Progress but lagging
4. Reduce child mortality	Reduce under-5 mortality rate by two thirds	Under-5 mortality rate. Infant mortality rate	Very high rates; progress slower than other regions: especially diarrhoea, malaria and pneumonia	Overall progress but lagging for neonatal deaths
		Percentage of 1 year olds immunised against measles	Improving – poorest children lack access	Progress but lagging
5. Improve maternal health	Reduce maternal mortality ratio by three quarters Achieve universel access to reproductive health	Maternal mortality ratio. Births attended by skilled health worker	Very high; progress since 2000; high unmet need for family planning	Progress from high rates
6. Combat HIV/AIDS, malaria and other diseases	Halt and reverse spread of HIV and AIDS	HIV prevalence amongst 15–24-year-old pregnant women (generalised epidemics)	New infections falling; number of people living with HIV rising	Infections increasing in some vulnerable groups
	Halt and reverse spread of malaria Halt and reverse spread of TB	Prevalence and death rates associated with malaria	High; some remarkable reductions	Moderate; threat of emerging drug resistance
		Prevalence and death rates associated with TB	High; rates rising	High; deaths declining
7. Ensure environmental sustainability	Halve the proportion without access to safe drinking water		Some progress but lagging	On track
	Halve the proportion without access to sanitation		Low access – small increase	Progress but lagging
8. A global partnership for development	Multiple targets on aid, trade and debt, includes access to essential drugs			

There is an urgent need for better data systems to guide result-based performance monitoring, better disaggregation to allow analysis of equity and distributional issues, and improved capture of health-service quality measures. Governments and international organisations do not always use the same data sources or definitions. The demand for high-quality data has grown in response to the need to monitor progress against the MDGs, to monitor and evaluate health-system interventions, to show that increased funding is having the desired impact and delivering value-for-money, and to hold governments and international donors to account for the money spent on health. Priorities include accurate reporting on mortality, morbidity, health status, service coverage and risk-prevalence. For this to happen in a sustainable way, efforts must be made to strengthen poor countries' own capacity to collect and analyse data. Vital registration systems (of births and deaths), household surveys, and analysis at sub-national level wherever feasible, are priorities. The World Health Organization can play a key role in this.

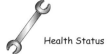

Health Status

Post 2015–priorities for poverty reduction and international health

The MDGs have been successful in encouraging global consensus and challenging rich countries to do more to reduce poverty. They were built on targets set in the 1990s. Criticisms include the lack of synergy between them, the absence of any measure of equity, and the exclusion of many issues (selectivity is also seen as a strength) [39]. Looking ahead, future goals could be set for a vision of development shared by low-income countries as well as the rich ones and the donors, and the actions required by rich as well as poor countries. Issues of public health importance that are likely to feature in the forthcoming agenda include: action on climate change, both adaptation and mitigation; urbanisation; vulnerability to disasters; population growth; emerging resistance to medicines and its global spread; emerging new diseases and efforts to improve disease surveillance and early action; and the rising burden of chronic diseases amongst poor populations as well as the richer ones.

Conclusion

Only 10% of the annual US$ 70 billion spent on global health research targets the diseases responsible for 90% of the world's health problems. Further research is needed into neglected health problems. In addition to increased global investment, new ways of stimulating research into the diseases of poverty and the development of commodities including vaccines, diagnostics and medicines are required. Research is urgently needed on the best way of delivering health interventions, and more rigorous impact evaluations of new approaches to better understand what works and why.

REFERENCES

1. J. Sachs (chairman), Macroeconomics and health: investing in health for economic development. Report of the Commission on Macroeconomics and Health, Geneva, World Health Organization, 2001.
2. Global Monitoring Report, World Bank, 2010.
3. S. Alkire and M. Santos, Acute Multidimensional Poverty: a new index for developing countries, OPHI Working Paper 38, July 2010.
4. United Nations Population Division, World Population Prospects 2010 Revision, United Nations, 2010.
5. R. E. Black, S. S. Morris and J. Bryce, Where and why are 10 million children dying every year? *Lancet* **361**, 2003, 2226–34.
6. R. E. Black, L. H. Allen, Z. A. Bhutta *et al.*, Maternal and child undernutrition: global and regional exposures and health consequences. *Lancet* **371**, 2008, 243–60.
7. J. Bryce, S. el Arifen, G. Pariyo *et al.*, Reducing child mortality: can public health deliver? *Lancet* **362**, 2003, 159–64.
8. United Nations Millennium Project Task Force on Child Health and Maternal Health, *Who's Got the Power? Transforming Health Systems for Women and Children*, London, Earthscan, 2005.
9. J. Lawn, S. Cousens and J. Zupan, for the Lancet Neonatal Survival Steering Team, Why are 4 million newborn babies dying each year? *Lancet* **364**, 2004, 399–401.
10. S. Singh, J. E. Darroch, L. S. Ashford and M. Vlassoff, Adding it up: the costs and benefits of investing in family planning and maternal and newborn health. Guttmacher Institute and UNFPA, 2009.
11. Report of the Global AIDS Epidemic, Geneva, Joint United Nations Programme on HIV/AIDS (UNAIDS), 2010.
12. C. D. Mathers and D. Loncar, Updated projections of global mortality and burden of disease, 2002–2030: data sources, methods and results, Geneva, World Health Organization, 2005.
13. Disease Control Priorities Project, *The Global Burden of Disease and Risk Factors*, Washington, DC, World Bank, 2006.
14. Institute for Health Metrics and Evaluation, Global Burden of Disease Study. See: http://globalburden.org/design.html.
15. R. Beaglehole, R. Banita, R. Horton *et al.*, Priority actions for the non-communicable disease crisis. *Lancet* **337**, 2011, 1438–47.
16. S. Ameratunga, M. Hijar and R. Norton, Road traffic injuries: confronting disparities to address a global health priority. *Lancet* **367**, 2006, 1533–40.
17. J. Eaton, L. McCay, et al. Scale up of services for mental health in low-income and middle-income countries. *Lancet* **378**, 2011, 1592–603.
18. World Health Organization, *World Health Report: Shaping the Future*, Geneva, WHO, 2003.
19. D. Molyneux, P. Hotez and A. Fenwick, Rapid-impact interventions; how a policy of integrated control for Africa's neglected tropical diseases could benefit the poor. *PLoS Medicine* **2**(11), 2005, 1064–70.
20. J. C. Kohler and G. Baghdadi-Sabeti G. The world medicine situation 2011: Good governance for the pharmaceutical sector, Geneva, World Health Organization, 2011.

21. Bill and Melinda Gates Foundation, Advanced market commitments: saving lives with affordable vaccines. See http://www.gatesfoundation.org/vaccines/Pages/advanced-market-commitments-vaccines.aspx.

22. L. Freedman, Achieving the millennium development goals: health systems as core social institutions. *Development* **48** (1), 2005, 19–24.

23. M. Grindle, Good enough governance: poverty reduction and reform in developing countries, Cambridge, MA, Kennedy School of Government, Harvard University, 2002.

24. Commission for Africa, Our Common Interest. Report of the Commission for Africa 2005. See: www.commissionforafrica.org.

25. Department for International Development, Humanitarian Emergency Response Review UK, London, March 2011.

26. Taskforce on innovative financing for health systems, More money for health, and more health for the money, March, 2009.

27. N. Palmer, D. Mueller, L. Gilson *et al.*, Health financing to promote access in low income settings – how much do we know? *Lancet* **364**, 2004, 1365–70.

28. World Health Organization. *World Health Report: Health Systems Financing: The Path to Universal Coverage*, Geneva, WHO, 2010.

29. A. Wagstaff and M. Claeson, *The Millennium Development Goals for Health, Rising to the Challenges*, Washington, DC, World Bank, 2004.

30. World Health Organization, Primary Health Care. Report of the International Conference on Primary Health Care, Alma-Ata, USSR, 6–12 September 1978, Geneva, WHO, 1978.

31. The World Health Organization, Global Health Report 2008.

32. WHO Maximising positive synergies collaborative group, An assessment of interactions between global health initiatives and country health systems. *Lancet* **373**, 2009, 2137–69.

33. P. Allotey, D. Reidpath, S. Yasin *et al.*, Rethinking health-care systems: a focus on chronicity. *Lancet* **377**, 2011, 450–1.

34. R. Manning, *Organisation for Economic Cooperation and Development (OECD) Development Co-operation Report 2005*, Paris, OECD, 2005.

35. N. Kabeer, Poverty, social exclusion and the MDGs: the challenge of "durable inequalities" in the Asian context. *IDS Bulletin* **37** (3), 2006, 64–78.

36. C. Victora, A. Wagstaff, J. A. Schellerberg *et al.*, Applying an equity lens to child health and mortality: more of the same is not enough. *Lancet* **362**, 2003, 233–41.

37. World Health Organization, *World Health Report: Working Together for Health*, Geneva, WHO, 2006.

38. United Nations, The Millenium Development Goals Report 2011, New York, NY, United Nations, 2011.

39. J. Waage, R. Banerji, O. Campbell *et al.* for the Lancet and London International Development Centre Commission. The Millenium Development Goals: a cross-sectoral analysis and principles for goal setting after 2015. *Lancet* **376**, 2010, 991–1023.

Jenny Amery works for the UK Department for International Development (DFID). The views expressed are not necessarily those of DFID.

18

Sustainable development – the opportunities and the challenges for the public's health

David Pencheon

Key points

- Sustainable development can be defined as development that meets the needs of the present without compromising the ability of future generations or people elsewhere to meet their own needs.
- Encouraging sustainability in general and tackling climate change specifically brings significant benefits for health in both the short and longer term.
- The National Health Service in England has developed an approach to sustainable development which can be used as an example of how policy and practice can be shaped within the health sector.
- Creating a sustainable future requires public health professionals to use their skills and the application of public health knowledge in a rapidly changing world.

The only thing we can be certain about the future is that our predictions will be wrong. It is easy to predict the future; it is just difficult to get it right. This last chapter is therefore not a 'crystal-ball' exercise into trying to guess exactly what the future holds. Instead, it aims to describe some of the most important transitions, challenges and opportunities that are already with us, and how we should be trying to shape them, for the benefit of all. Public health skills, knowledge and attitudes are essential elements of helping to shape a sustainable health system as part of a sustainable world. This public health approach has a crucial part to play in shaping a future-proof system, in the same way as other global challenges have been addressed: from cholera to tobacco to AIDS. Such challenges make public health frustrating, fascinating, challenging and rewarding.

Essential Public Health, Second Edition, ed. Stephen Gillam, Jan Yates and Padmanabhan Badrinath.
Published by Cambridge University Press. © Cambridge University Press 2012.

Sustainable development – our greatest challenge – and our greatest opportunity

If another (more) intelligent life form were to circulate our planet and could see what we are doing, they might be struck by two strange things. First, despite being a global village, there are extraordinarily high variations in opportunity, empowerment, and health around the world: differences that harm us all [1]. Secondly, we are consuming resources with a dangerous and selfish lack of consideration for the consequences. The consumption per person and the growing population make the present way of life on Earth completely unsustainable. Climate change, as the most dangerous and obvious manifestation of an unsustainable way of life, is the largest strategic public health threat we face [2]. All material resources on this planet are limited – and yet growing aspirations, globalisation, and a mass addiction to carbon-based energy and lifestyles mean we feel ourselves locked into the current paradigm. If you think heroin is addictive, consider carbon. We have yet to adopt a global policy of living as if tomorrow matters. Inherited economic systems do not help, despite highly credible alternatives [3].

Sustainable development is exactly that: a complete way of thinking and acting that improves the lives and welfare of people and populations today but which avoids prejudicing the lives and welfare of future generations; a whole-system approach to prosperity and equity without unsustainable material growth [3]. This is the essence of Gro Harem Brundtland's definition [4]:

development that meets the needs of the present ...
    ... without compromising the ability of future generations to meet their own needs.

For public health practitioners, who think in terms of both time and space, the definition can be usefully expanded to:

development that meets the needs of the present ...
    ... without compromising the ability of *others elsewhere and* future generations to meet their own needs.

This second definition highlights the fact that there are populations under even greater risk from adverse life events (drought, war, famine...) today as a result of climate change.

Yet, although there is the temptation to preach doom and gloom, there are some important steps that can be taken to promote the large-scale change that is needed, and much of the evidence of how to do this already exists. It largely comes from transdisciplinary sources that depend on an understanding of how large-scale change actually happens [5–7]. Most positively, and most important to understand for population health, is that most climate-change interventions that improve the long-term health of the world's population improve the health of the population today [8,9]. These co-benefits can be classified under three headings, see Box 18.1.

> **Box 18.1 Health co-benefits of taking action on climate change**
>
> 1. For people
>   More physical activity, better diet, improved mental health, less road trauma,
>   less air pollution, less obesity/heart disease/cancer, more social inclusion.
> 2. For the health-care system
>   More prevention, care closer to home, more empowered/self care,
>   better use of drugs, better use of information technology, better skill mix,
>   better models of care for long-term conditions
> 3. For global fairness/social justice
>   A fairer distribution of the world's resources between communities,
>   now and inter-generationally

Consider three examples:

Moving

Never before have our bodies moved around our world so much without our bodies doing that actual moving. The consequences are that we burn carbon-based fuel and not our own internal fuel. We accelerate climate change and we accelerate our own obesity. Active travel addresses both public health issues, with both immediate and long-term health gains [10].

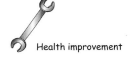
Health improvement

Eating

Too many people can afford to eat too much, and too many people cannot afford to eat enough. Making food consumption globally sustainable would have major co-benefits for many of us who eat too much saturated fat, often from animal sources, and for those where too much land is used inefficiently for meat production. Eating less red processed meat is good for our health today and tomorrow [11].

Redistributing resources

Food (above) is a good example of how we can redistribute resources in the interests of everyone, both now and in the future. Sadly, too many people seem to believe that one person's (*their*) good fortune relies on another's misfortune – often someone far away of whom they know little and care less. The obvious (and growing) interdependence of us all, both with each other and the biosphere that supports us, should make us understand that it is in no-one's interest to have gross disparities in needs and opportunities. Water, the lack of which kills most quickly, is perhaps the resource that is (and will) cause most conflict, as there is no alternative. But oil is the resource where we have the most potential to address our dangerous dependency. Decarbonising the global energy supply means a range of renewable resources. One of these (concentrated solar power from the world's deserts coupled with a global electricity grid) has the potential to move energy from the warmest (and often poorest communities) in the world to the more industrialised countries, and crucially to move resources to pay for it back again, whilst promoting energy security; see, for example, the work of the the Desertec Foundation (www.desertec.org/). This is possibly the only practical strategy that improves health, promotes social justice, and is integrated with workable economic models such as Contraction and Convergence (a proposed global framework for reducing greenhouse gas emissions that combats climate change at the same time as promoting social justice; see www.gci.org.uk/contconv/cc.html).

Within health services globally, health professionals and health systems have huge potential to exploit some of these opportunities for the health of people today and the health of populations in the future (and elsewhere now).

A framework for action

Sustainable development, like many other public health topics, is a very broad area, much more than just dealing with climate change and carbon reduction. Living within our means implies sustainability within all areas of our lives.

The most important areas of knowledge can be subdivided:
- the reasons why humankind is causing climate change and an unsustainable future, and the case for sustainable development being an important solution [12];
- the health effects of climate change on human health, and the public health benefits of taking action [13];
- the importance of developing policies and implementing systems of governance at every level that promote adaptation to (managing the unavoidable) and mitigation (avoiding the unmanageable) of climate change [13];
- the practical steps that can be taken at an
    (i) individual level (as a citizen or health professional [14,15])
    (ii) organisational level (such as a health-care organisation or a whole health system [16–18] (see below)).
    (iii) national/international level (as in international climate-change negotiations) [19].

Case study: an approach to sustainable development by one national health system
a. Measure and develop a strategy which can be monitored and reported on

Since 2008, the National Health Service (NHS) in England has been developing policy, instigating research, and engaging policy makers, clinicians and other staff in how a health service should take seriously its responsibility for high-quality health-care, both now and in the future. A non-mandatory consultation yielded a high-level mandate for this work, which started with a carbon-reduction strategy and the measuring of the carbon footprint of the entire health service with the best available methods and metrics [17].

There are particularly good reasons to engage the health service in making sustainable development a core part of its quality agenda [20].

These reasons include:
- saving money;
- complying with legislation (in the 2008 Climate Change Act and the subsequent Carbon Reduction Commitment [21]);
- improving the resilience of the service (the capacity of a system to absorb [sudden and unpredicted] disturbance and still retain function);
- improving the reputation of the service;
- engaging health professionals and empowering them to be important exemplars to the public;
- direct improvements in health, both immediately and in the future [22].

Like any strategy which can be monitored and reported on, the research needs to be repeated to track progress [18].

b. Develop a clear vision for the future

It is both futile and dangerous to predict the details of what the future holds. However, it is crucial to be able to articulate some of the likely features of a future, both good and bad. Again, with wide engagement, public health professionals can convene relevant groups to ensure there is a broad acceptance for the need for action [23].

Leadership

c. Get agreement for a route map for action

Most public health actions: reducing tobacco consumption, addressing child poverty, mitigating climate change, will need a broad coalition of people and actions. Hence the need for a clear set of actions in multiple areas. This was achieved in the NHS in England in 2010 where a Route Map for Sustainable Health was developed, the result being a set of actions in three main areas: behaviours, governance and technology [24]. A different process may have come up with a different way of grouping the actions needed. What is crucial is that there is some kind of common framework for action whereby both duplication and gaps in action and research are avoided.

A distillation of the route map can be seen in Figure 18.1.

d. Monitor the impact of action

The measuring of our environmental impact should be routine with appropriate levels of discounting to take into account the future. Discounting is an economic concept which quantifies the difference in value between benefits received now or in the future (for example, how much more valuable would we consider a benefit such as £100 received today than we would if we had to wait for 5 years to receive it?). It is a way of putting a value on the future.

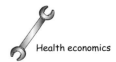
Health economics

This measurement should be done in internationally recognised ways using not just direct (e.g. direct energy usage) but also indirect metrics (e.g. energy usage of procurement practice down the complete supply chain). These data should be analysed in absolute terms, not relative terms. The NHS in England has an annual carbon

Figure 18.1 A framework for sustainable health-care. (see Internet Companion)

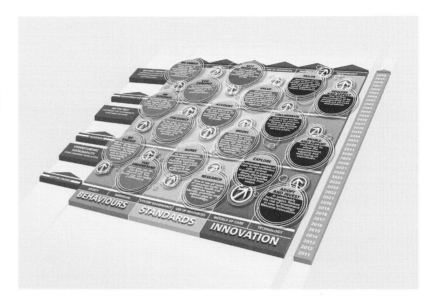

Figure 18.2 The NHS Carbon Footprint (NHS Sustainable Development Unit. Saving Carbon, Improving Health, UPDATE NHS Carbon Reduction Strategy. January 2010).

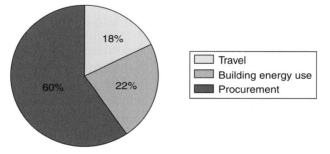

footprint of approximately 21 million tonnes of carbon dioxide [15] which is broken down as shown in Figure 18.2.

Measuring such an impact is necessary as a baseline, but needs to be repeated and compared with the calculated trajectory that shows what the system needs to do to develop sustainably. For the NHS in England [18] some of the necessary levers have been provided by, in this case, the UK's Climate Change Act [21] (see Figure 18.3).

Creating a sustainable future – how does public health fit in?

What causes health today?

It does not take long for any health professional to realise that a huge burden of ill health in any part of the world is best addressed through prevention at a societal level

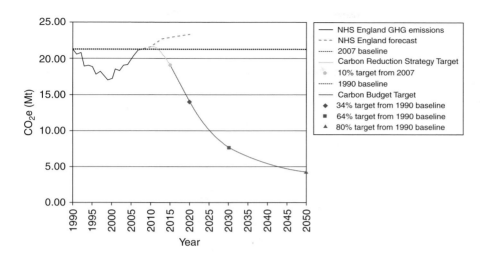

Figure 18.3 Measuring UK environmental impact. NHS England carbon dioxide emissions (CO_2e) footprint 1990–2020 with Climate Change Act targets.

rather than ignoring the causes (or even the 'causes of the causes' [25]) and working only at an individual level. Most action to restore health at a personal level is necessary because we have failed elsewhere to preserve and improve health at a population level. It quickly becomes apparent that most health protection and promotion is not done just through programmes such as screening and immunisation, but also in a more profound way by enabling all of us to take more control over our current and future health. The real causes of health and illness are not just the bacteria which cause infectious diseases, but how one's place in society determines one's life chances, and, crucially, what can be done to help oneself and others through the organised efforts of society.

These wider societal changes include the ageing and expansion of nearly all populations worldwide, the technology that we have (and are likely to develop) in preventing and curing diseases, the changing shape of how communities and countries govern themselves, and the dangerously short-sighted way in which we are using finite resources (and the consequences in terms of climate chaos and social injustice). The expectations of nearly everyone on the planet are increasing, quite out of proportion to either personal need or material availability. These are fuelled by a global information system that shows what might be possible rather than what is currently affordable or ethically acceptable.

Although many illnesses (such as infectious diseases) are preventable and curable, far too many people, especially in economically poorer countries, still die from these preventable diseases. If preventable, why not prevented? In many societies (often the poor in rich countries and the rich in poor countries), there is the additional burden of other causes of illness and death: cancer, heart disease and many other lifestyle-related conditions. Many of us, across the globe, live longer with multiple conditions rather than die younger of one specific cause. Lastly, we live on an increasingly fragile and highly interdependent planet in a highly unsustainable way. Nobody is immune from the global effects of viruses, warfare, migration, economic collapse or human-induced climate chaos.

Despite these profound and global changes, there are at least two eternal truths in the struggle for social justice and public health. The first is that social justice never happens by accident. It requires organised and coordinated analysis and action. It is the result of the relentless struggle of individuals (usually engaging others and working together) to assess and address inequities of health, welfare and opportunity. The natural order is that opportunities and services tend to be more available to those with the least need (the "Inverse Care Law" [26]). The practice of public health is a constant struggle to demonstrate this and to do all that is possible to ensure that the resources and opportunities are directed and available to those with the most need. It used to be said that 'there was enough for everyone's need but not enough for everyone's greed.' Sadly, at the rate we are increasing global consumption, very soon there will be insufficient even for everyone's need [27]. Secondly, it should be understood that, everywhere in the world, the health of individuals and populations is won largely outside the formal health-care system (described by Maslow as a 'hierarchy of needs' in his classic 1943 paper [28] (see Figure 18.4)), especially outside the hospital system. Hospitals are hugely important, and are an essential part of any health system, but they contribute less to population health and fairness per unit investment than most other health-related interventions. Good health depends on absence of war, clean water, sanitation, food, education, jobs, lack of corruption, equitable and sustainable resource use, accountability and good governance – and many of these are ultimately determined by an informed and empowered population.

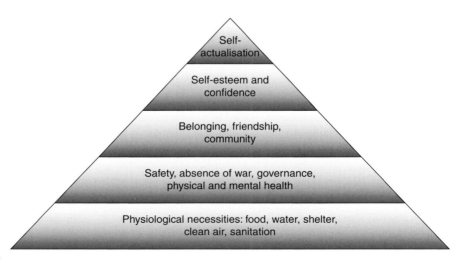

Figure 18.4   Maslow's hierarchy of needs.

There is nothing more empowering in the twenty-first century than high-quality information (for public, patients, policy makers, practitioners and politicians). However, this access to information needs to be coupled with an ability both to 'sort the wheat from the chaff,' and the opportunity to actually use the information appropriately, avoiding vested interests and historical imbalances of power and opportunity.

The right knowledge, accessed and used in the right way by the right people at the right time is a crucial cause of health. Knowledge is the greatest enemy of disease (J. Muir Gray, personal communication, 2009) whether it comes over the radio to women in rural communities, or whether it helps scientists share expertise globally to develop an effective vaccine for malaria.

The world is less easily divided into the more-developed and the less-developed countries of the globe. Industrialised countries face public health challenges that sometimes differ from those of more resource-poor countries. However, many of the public health challenges will either be similar (at least in type if not scale) and need to be addressed with similar approaches. Globalisation itself poses significant challenges as well as opportunities for health (see Chapter 17). Multinational companies wield huge influence and the health of their present customers may not be their biggest concern.

However, the most pressing global public health concerns must be the glaring inequities in health. In 2009, life expectancy was 48 in Chad and 83 in Japan [29]. These disparities are surely unacceptable.

Causes of health: using information, evidence and knowledge – key skills for public health professionals

Just as knowledge is an increasingly important cause of health, so the use of knowledge is a central competence for health professionals, especially public health professions. All effective change is based on having sufficient knowledge and information. Oratory is the other vital tool for change – but oratory without knowledge is merely Leadership

rhetoric. Together, they can, and have, changed the world. The practice of public health depends on individuals, teams, and organisations keeping abreast of the knowledge (e.g. of effective interventions to protect and improve health) and speaking out. There is increasing pressure and need to move away from simplistic approaches towards evidence of effectiveness to a more integrated approach where evidence of multiple types and from multiple sources are assessed and appropriately combined (e.g. evidence of need, evidence of effectiveness, public acceptability, and evidence of cost-effectiveness and cost-benefit (Chapter 5)). Politics of all types will inevitably still play a large part in decision making (Chapter 7). However, without being able to say: "...this is the need, this is the burden, this is how it compares and is changing, and these are the costed and publicly acceptable interventions that are potentially available," your contribution to strategy and tactics will be marginal and marginalised. These sorts of knowledge are vital to governments and organisations if they are to

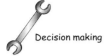

Decision making

justify their decisions, priorities and actions to support an increasingly empowered population. Such decisions will be challenged and will therefore need to be transparent and defensible [9]. The evaluation, availability and affordability of information and communications technology have a significant effect on how professionals can and should work. However, the speed at which the public are being similarly empowered is equally important. The Internet, and particularly social networking, has already made rapid debate, mobilisation and action a part of the mainstream political process. If we, as members of the public, can shop, lobby, and debate 24/7, then we may not find a public health report, which uses 3-year-old data, is jargon-filled and only available in hard copy, either engaging, empowering, or relevant. Public health professionals serve an increasingly diverse and demanding set of people and organisations. As the public are increasingly faced by bewildering choice, these decisions will be influenced by many factors. Within health, we increasingly choose everything from our carers or our food, to whether we spend our income (if we have any) on the pleasures of today (e.g. more food) rather than the security of tomorrow (e.g. more health insurance, or action on climate change). Such decisions are based on many factors. The role of public health professionals is, for instance, to ensure that food choices are not influenced solely by the food industry. Similarly, an empowered and vocal population will look somewhere, anywhere, for credible information on health-care professionals and health-care facilities. Good-hospital guides and good-doctor guides will be increasingly common, and will need to be written in a comprehensive and unbiased way, acknowledging that different people will have different requirements and priorities for themselves and their families.

Developing competencies in the key skills for public health

Public health professionals, as in all areas which are broad and multidisciplinary, need to be jacks of all trades and masters of many. Professionals need breadth and depth, and need to have good insight into exactly what they need for their present and future roles. This is not simply an annual process of ritual bureaucracy, but should be about constant self-reflection and critique of fitness to practice and deliver. If we profess to be competent, we need to demonstrate evolving competence in a changing world. We need to provide an evidence-based assessment of competency to practice: for our profession, for our employer, for our regulator, but most important for the people we purport to serve.

People who are professionally responsible for maintaining and improving public health (and who do not usually have the words in their job title) are well placed to understand and take action on helping to develop a more sustainable world – a world where we do more good than harm, a world where we live within environmental limits, and a world where we are not stealing from each other or from the future. This is a world where we should meet our needs today without jeopardising the needs of others elsewhere in place or in time. Already, we have compelling visions of what a future health system could look like with some scenarios much more attractive than others [23]. The added value of public health professionals is that they are in a potentially powerful position to communicate the health co-benefits and to align policies and practices [30].

Conclusion

Sustainability is one of a series of ever-increasing threats to human welfare – the tobacco or cholera of our time [31]. We have the knowledge and expertise to address it. But do we have the commitment to do this together, now? The challenges and opportunities are happening on our watch and will be our legacy.

REFERENCES

1. R. Wilkinson and K. Pickett, *The Spirit Level: Why More Equal Societies Almost Always Do Better*, London, Penguin, 2010.
2. A. Costello, M. Abbas and A. Allen, Managing the health effects of climate change. *Lancet* **373**, 2009, 1693–733.
3. T. Jackson, *Prosperity without Growth, Economics for a Finite Planet*, London, Earthscan, 2009.
4. G. H. Brundtland, Our Common Future (The Brundtland Report): World Commission on Environment and Development, United Nations, 1987.
5. J. Kotter, *Leading Change*, Boston, MA, Harvard Business School Press, 1996.
6. P. E. Plsek and T. Greenhalgh, The challenge of complexity in health care. *British Medical Journal* **323**, 2001, 625–8.
7. P. E. Plsek and T. Wilson, Complexity, leadership, and management in healthcare organisations. *British Medical Journal* **323**, 2001, 746–9.
8. D. Ganten, A. Haines and R. Souhami, Health co-benefits of policies to tackle climate change. *Lancet* **376**, 2011, 1802–4.
9. A. Haines, A. McMichael, K. Smith *et al.*, Public health benefits of strategies to reduce greenhouse-gas emissions: overview and implications for policy makers. *Lancet* **374**, 2009, 2104–14.
10. I. Roberts and P. Edwards, *The Energy Glut: The Politics of Fatness in an Overheating World*, London, Zen Books, 2010.
11. S. Friel, A. D. Dangour, T. Garnett *et al.*, Public health benefits of strategies to reduce greenhouse-gas emissions: food and agriculture. *Lancet* **374**, 2009, 2016–25.
12. P. Wilkinson, Climate change and health: the case for sustainable development. *Medicine, Conflict and Survival* **24** (Suppl 1), 2008, S26–S35.
13. L. F. Wiley. Mitigation/adaptation and health: health policymaking in the global response to climate change and implications for other upstream determinants. *Journal of Law Medicine and Ethics* **38**, 2010, 629–39.
14. M. Gill and R. Stott, Health professionals must act to tackle climate change. *Lancet* **374**, 2009, 1953–5.

15. A. Coote, How should health professionals take action against climate change? *British Medical Journal* **336**, 2008, 733–4.

16. A. Coote, What health services could do about climate change. *British Medical Journal* **332**, 2006, 1343–4.

17. NHS Sustainable Development Unit, Carbon Reduction Strategy for NHS England, Cambridge, NHS Sustainable Development Unit, 2008.

18. NHS Sustainable Development Unit, Saving Carbon, Improving Health; UPDATE NHS Carbon Reduction Strategy, Cambridge, NHS Sustainable Development Unit, 2010.

19. S. Singh, U. Mushtaq, C. Holm-Hansen *et al.*, The importance of climate change to health, *Lancet* **378**, 2011, 29–30.

20. A. Haines, K. R. Smith, D. Anderson *et al.*, Policies for accelerating access to clean energy, improving health, advancing development, and mitigating climate change. *Lancet* **370**, 2007, 1264–81.

21. Department of Energy and Climate Change, UK Climate Change Act, 2008.

22. A. Coote, *Claiming the Health Dividend, Unlocking the Benefits of NHS Spending.* London, King's Fund, 2002.

23. NHS Sustainable Development Unit, Forum for the Future. Fit for the Future. Scenarios for low-carbon healthcare 2030, Cambridge, NHS Sustainable Development Unit, 2009.

24. NHS Sustainable Development Unit, Route Map for Sustainable Health. Cambridge, NHS Sustainable Development Unit, 2011.

25. M. Marmot, Achieving health equity: from root causes to fair outcomes. *Lancet* **370**, 2007, 1153–63.

26. J. T. Hart, The Inverse Care Law. *Lancet* **297**, 1971, 405–12.

27. J. Guillebaud and P. Hayes, Population growth and climate change. *British Medical Journal* **337**, 2008, 247–8.

28. A. Maslow, A theory of human motivation. *Psychological Review* **50**, 1943, 370–96.

29. World Health Organization, World Health Statistics Report 2011, Geneva, WHO, 2011.

30. A. Haines, P. Wilkinson, C. Tonne and I. Roberts, Aligning climate change and public health policies. *Lancet* **374**, 2009, 2035–8.

31. J. Muir Gray, Climate change is the cholera of our era. *The Times*, **25** May, 2009.

Absolute risk reduction (ARR)   The difference in the absolute risk (rates of adverse events) between study and control populations.

Absolute risk   The observed or calculated probability of an event in the population under study.

Acquired immunity   Resistance acquired by a host to a pathogen as a result of previous exposure from natural infection or immunisation. It is the result of the production of antibodies (immunoglobulins) targeted to specific antigens.

Adjustment   A summarising procedure for a statistical measure in which the effects of differences in composition of the populations being compared have been minimised by statistical methods.

Aetiology   The study of the causes of disease.

Agent (of disease)   A term used to imply the organism that causes a disease.

Antibody   Protein molecule formed in response to a foreign substance (antigen). It has the capacity to bind to the antigen to allow its removal or destruction.

Antigen   A foreign molecule which elicits an antibody response.

Association   Statistical dependence between two or more events, characteristics, or other variables. An association may be fortuitous or may be produced by various other circumstances; the presence of an association does not necessarily imply a causal relationship.

Attributable risk   The proportion of the risk of a disease which can be attributed to a named causal factor.

Audit (clinical)   A planned assessment of a clinical process against predefined standards.

Bias (syn: systematic error)   Deviation of results or inferences from the truth, or processes leading to such deviation. See also selection bias.

Blind(ed) study (syn: masked study)   A study in which observer(s) and/or subjects are kept ignorant of the group to which the subjects are assigned, as in an experimental study, or of the population from which the subjects come, as in a non-experimental or observational study. Where both observer and subjects are kept ignorant, the study is termed a double-blind study. If the statistical analysis is also done in ignorance of the group to which subjects belong, the study is sometimes described as triple blind. The purpose of 'blinding' is to eliminate sources of bias.

Carriage/carrier   When a host is infected but shows no signs of disease it is termed a carrier. It may transmit infection so is a potential source of infection.

Case fatality rate   The proportion of people with a disease who die within a defined period from diagnosis.

Case–control study   Retrospective comparison of exposures of persons with disease (cases) with those of persons without the disease (controls) – see retrospective study.

Case series   Report of a number of cases of disease.

Causality   The relating of causes to the effects they produce. Most of epidemiology concerns causality and several types of causes can be distinguished. It must be emphasised, however, that epidemiological evidence by itself is insufficient to establish causality, although it can provide powerful circumstantial evidence.

Clinical governance   The framework through which NHS organisations and their staff are accountable for the quality of patient care.

Cohort study   Follow-up of exposed and non-exposed defined groups, with a comparison of disease rates during the time covered.

Commensalism   A neutral relationship between host and another organism. Often used to describe the bacteria which live in the human gut harmlessly.

Co-morbidity   Co-existence of a disease or diseases in a study participant in addition to the index condition that is the subject of study.

Comparison group   Any group to which the index group is compared. Usually synonymous with control group.

Confidence interval (CI)   The range of numerical values in which we can be confident (to a computed probability, such as 90 or 95%) that the population value being estimated will be found. Confidence intervals indicate the strength of evidence; where confidence intervals are wide, they indicate less-precise estimates of effect. The larger the trial's sample size, the larger the number of outcome events and the greater becomes the confidence that the true relative risk reduction is close to the value stated. Thus, the confidence interval is narrow and 'precision' is increased. In a 'positive finding' study the lower boundary of the confidence interval, or lower confidence limit, should still remain important or clinically significant if the results are to be accepted. In a 'negative finding' study, the upper boundary of the confidence interval should not be clinically significant if you are to accept this result confidently.

Confounding variable, confounder   A variable that can cause or prevent the outcome of interest, is not an intermediate variable, and is associated with the factor under investigation. A confounding variable may be due to chance or bias. Unless it is possible to adjust for confounding variables, their effects cannot be distinguished from those of factor(s) being studied.

Contamination   The presence of an infectious agent on the body of a host or on inanimate articles. A contaminated host does not always become infected but may be a possible source of infection for others.

Demography   The study of human populations.

Determinant   Any definable factor that effects a change in a health condition or other characteristic.

Disability   In the context of health experience, a disability is any restriction or lack (resulting from an impairment) of ability to perform an activity in the manner or within the range considered normal for a human being.

Disability-adjusted life year (DALY)   A method of calculating the health impact of a disease in terms of the cases of premature death, disability and days of infirmity due to illness from a specific disease or condition.

Dose–response relationship   A relationship in which change in amount, intensity or duration of exposure is associated with a change – either an increase or decrease – in risk of a specified outcome.

Dynamic population   A population in which there is turnover of membership during the study period.

Effectiveness   A measure of the benefit resulting from an intervention for a given health problem under usual conditions of clinical care for a particular group; this form of evaluation considers both the efficacy of an intervention and its acceptance by those to whom it is offered, answering the question, 'Does the practice do more good than harm to people to whom it is offered?' See intention to treat.

Efficacy   A measure of the benefit resulting from an intervention for a given health problem under the ideal conditions of an investigation; it answers the question, 'Does the practice do more good than harm to people who fully comply with the recommendations?'

Endemic   The constant presence of a disease or infectious agent within a given geographic area or population group.

Environmental health   The theory and practice of assessing, correcting, controlling and preventing those factors in the environment that can potentially affect adversely the health of present and future generations.

Epidemic   The occurrence of disease at higher than expected levels. This could be an endemic disease at higher than usual levels or non-endemic disease at any level.

Epidemiology   The study of the distribution and determinants of health-related states or events in specified populations, and the application of this study to control of health problems.

Evaluation   A process that attempts to determine as systematically and objectively as possible the relevance, effectiveness and impact of activities in the light of their objectives.

Evidence-based health-care/medicine/public health   Systematic use of evidence derived from published research and other sources for management and practice.

Exclusion criteria   Conditions which preclude entrance of candidates into an investigation even if they meet the inclusion criteria.

Fertility   The childbearing capability of a woman, couple or population.

Follow-up   Observation over a period of time of an individual, group, or initially defined population whose relevant characteristics have been assessed in order to observe changes in health status or health-related variables.

Gold standard   A method, procedure, or measurement that is widely accepted as being the best available.

Handicap   In the context of health experience, a handicap is a disadvantage for a given individual, resulting from an impairment or a disability, that limits or prevents the fulfilment of a role that is normal (depending on age, sex and social and cultural factors) for that individual.

Health   The extent to which an individual or a group is able to realise aspirations and satisfy needs, and to change or cope with the environment. Health is a resource for everyday life, not the objective of living; it is a positive concept, emphasising social and personal resources as well as physical capabilities. Your health is related to how much you feel your potential to be a meaningful part of the society in which you find yourself is adequately realised.

Health equity audit   A technique to identify how fairly services or other resources are distributed in relation to the health needs of different population groups or geographical areas.

Health improvement   The theory and practice of promoting the health of populations by influencing lifestyle and socio-economic, physical and cultural environment through methods of health promotion, directed towards populations, communities and individuals.

Health inequality   Differences observed between groups due to one group experiencing an advantage over the other group rather than to any innate differences between them.

Health inequity   The presence of unfair and avoidable or remedial differences in health among populations or groups defined socially.

Health promotion   The process of enabling people to exert control over and to improve their health. As well as covering actions aimed at strengthening people's skills and capabilities, it also includes actions directed towards changing social and environmental conditions, to prevent or to improve their impact on individual and public health.

High-risk strategy   This targets preventative interventions at people most at risk of a disease.

Host   A living organism on or in which an infectious agent can subsist.

Impairment   In the context of health experience an impairment is any loss or abnormality of psychological, physiological or anatomical structure or function.

Incidence   The number of new cases of illness commencing, or of persons falling ill, during a specified time period in a given population. See also prevalence.

Incidence rate   The rate at which new cases occur in a population.

Incubation period   The interval from exposure to onset of clinical disease.

Index case   The first case identified in an outbreak.

Infant mortality   The proportion of live births that die up to one year of age.

Infection (colonisation)   This occurs when an organism enters the body and multiplies. It may be termed infection when damage is caused and colonisation when no damage is caused to the host. Acute infection implies a short-lived infection with a short period of infectivity. Chronic infection refers to a persistent condition with on-going replication of the organism. Latent infection refers to a persistent infection with intermittent replication of the organism.

Infectivity   The proportion of exposed, susceptible persons who become infected (for a given number of organisms).

Intention-to-treat analysis   A method for data analysis in a randomised clinical trial in which individual outcomes are analysed according to the group to which they have been randomised, even if they never received the treatment they were assigned. By simulating practical experience it provides a better measure of effectiveness (versus efficacy).

Interviewer bias   Systematic error due to interviewer's subconscious or conscious gathering of selective data.

Koch's (Henle–Koch's) postulates   These postulates should be met before a causal relationship can be inferred between an organism and a disease:
1. The agent must be shown to be present in every case of the disease by isolation in pure culture.
2. The agent must not be found in cases of other disease.
3. Once isolated, the agent must be able to reproduce disease in experimental animals.
4. The agent must be recovered from this experimental disease.

Lead time bias   If prognosis study patients are not all enrolled at similar, well-defined points in the course of their disease, differences in outcome over time may merely reflect differences in duration of illness. Lead time bias occurs when detection by screening seems to increase disease-free survival but this is only because disease has been detected earlier and not because screening is delaying death or disease.

Length time bias   Length time bias occurs if a screening programme is better at picking up milder forms of the disease. This means that people who develop a disease that progresses more quickly or is more likely to be fatal are less likely to be picked up by screening and their outcomes may not be included in evaluations of the programme. Thus the programme looks to be more effective than it is.

Life expectancy   The average number of additional years a person could expect to live if current mortality trends were to continue for the rest of that person's life. Generally given as a life expectancy from birth.

Likelihood ratio   Ratio of the probability that a given diagnostic test result will be expected for a patient with the target disorder rather than for a patient without the disorder.

Maternal mortality ratio   The number of deaths during pregnancy and up to 42 days after delivery, per 1000 live births.

Morbidity   The impact of a disease which is not death. Measures of morbidity include incidence and prevalence rates.

Mortality (rate)   The number of deaths in an area as a proportion of the number of people in that area.

Needs   These may be expressed by action, e.g. visiting a doctor; or felt needs, e.g. what people consider and/or say they need. The need for health-care is often defined as the capacity to benefit from that care.

Negative predictive value (of a diagnostic or screening test)   The proportion of persons testing negative for a disease who, as measured by the gold standard, are identified as non-diseased.

Neonatal mortality   The proportion of live births who die within the first 28 days.

Non-specific immunity   This is the natural barriers a host has to pathogens. It includes mechanical barriers, body secretions, physical removal of organisms, phagocytosis and inflammatory response.

Normal distribution   Many biological variables show a normal distribution of ranges between individuals within a population. A probability density graph of the normal distributions takes the shape of a bell-shaped curve.

Number needed to treat (NNT)   The number of patients who must be exposed to an intervention before the clinical outcome of interest occurred; for example, the number of patients needed to treat to prevent one adverse outcome.

Odds   A proportion in which the numerator contains the number of times an event occurs and the denominator includes the number of times the event does not occur.

Odds Ratio   A measure of the degree of association; for example, the odds of exposure among the cases compared with the odds of exposure among the controls.

Outbreak   A localised epidemic. Health-protection professionals often look for two or more cases linked in time and place.

P value   The probability (ranging from zero to one) that the results observed in a study (or results more extreme) could have occurred by chance.

Pandemic   A global epidemic. This term is sometimes used for a very large-scale epidemic.

Perinatal mortality   The proportion of all births that die before birth or in the first week.

Placebo   A substance that has no therapeutic effect, used as a control in interventional studies.

Policy   An overall statement of the aims of an organisation within a particular context.

Population strategy   Targets preventative interventions at the whole population.

Positive predictive value (of a diagnostic or screening test)   The proportion of persons testing positive for a disease who, as measured by the gold standard, are identified as diseased.

Poverty   Absolute poverty – a family's ability to purchase essential goods (such as housing, heating, food, clothing and transport). Relative poverty – poverty in relation to the average income in a particular population (such as below 50% of the national average).

Precision   The range in which the best estimates of a true value approximate the true value. See confidence interval.

Predictive value   In screening and diagnostic tests, the probability that a person with a positive test is a true positive (i.e. does have the disease) or that a person with a negative test truly does not have the disease. The predictive value of a screening test is determined by the sensitivity and specificity of the test, and by the prevalence of the condition for which the test is used.

Prevalence   The proportion of persons with a particular disease within a given population at a given time. Point prevalence is the prevalence at one single point in time. Period prevalence is the proportion of persons with a particular disease over a specified period of time.

Prevention   Primary prevention – actions designed to prevent the occurrence of the problem, e.g. health education, immunisation.
Secondary prevention – actions designed to detect and treat the occurrence of a problem before symptoms have developed, e.g. screening, early diagnosis.
Tertiary prevention – actions designed to limit disability once a condition is manifest, e.g. limitation of disability, rehabilitation.

Prevention paradox   Preventive measures bringing large benefits to the community offer little to each participating individual.

Primary health-care   First-contact care provided by a range of health-care professionals: general practiioners, nurses, dentists, pharmacists, optometrists, and complementary therapists working in the community.

Prognosis   The possible outcomes of a disease or condition and the likelihood that each one will occur.

Prognostic factor   Demographic, disease-specific, or co-morbid characteristics associated strongly enough with a condition's outcomes to predict accurately the eventual development of those outcomes. Compare with risk factors. Neither prognostic nor risk factors necessarily imply a cause-and-effect relationship.

Prospective study   Study design where one or more groups (cohorts) of individuals, who have not yet had the outcome event in question, are monitored for the number of such events which occur over time.

Public health   The science and art of preventing disease, prolonging life and promoting health through the organised efforts and informed choices of society, organisations, public and private, communities and individuals. Public health practice is the emphasis in this book, while public health may also be considered as a discipline or a social institution.

Public health practitioner   In this book, includes anyone working in the broad field of public health, neither defined by formal qualifications nor restricted to a professional group.

Quality-adjusted life year (QALY)   A health measure which combines the quantity and quality of life. It takes 1 year of perfect-health life expectancy to be worth 1 and regards 1 year of less than perfect life expectancy as less than 1.

Randomised controlled trial   Study design where treatments, interventions or enrolment into different study groups are assigned by random allocation rather than by conscious decisions of clinicians or patients. If the sample size is large enough, this study design avoids problems of bias and confounding variables by assuring that both known and unknown determinants of outcome are evenly distributed between treatment and control groups.

Recall bias   Systematic error due to the differences in accuracy or completeness of recall to memory of past events or experiences.

Relative risk   The ratio of the probability of developing, in a specified period of time, an outcome among those receiving the treatment of interest or exposed to a risk factor, compared with the probability of developing the outcome if the risk factor or intervention is not present.

Reproducibility (repeatability, reliability)   The results of a test or measure are identical or closely similar each time it is conducted.

Retrospective study   Study design in which cases where individuals who had an outcome event in question are collected and analysed after the outcomes have occurred (see also case–control study).

Risk   The number of cases of a disease that occur in a defined period of time as a proportion of the number of people in the population at the beginning of the period.

Risk factor   Patient characteristics or factors associated with an increased probability of developing a condition or disease in the first place. Compare with prognostic factors. Neither risk nor prognostic factors necessarily imply a cause-and-effect relationship.

Screening   A public health service in which members of a defined population, who do not necessarily perceive they are at risk of, or are already affected by, a disease or its complications, are asked a question or offered a test. The aim is to identify those individuals who are more likely to be helped than harmed by further tests or treatment to reduce the risk of a disease or its complications.

Secular trend   A trend over time, also termed temporal trend.

Selection bias   A bias in assignment or a confounding variable that arises from study design rather than by chance. These can occur when the study and control groups are chosen so that they differ from each other by one or more factors that may affect the outcome of the study. In screening, selection bias occurs when the screening programme attracts people who are more or less likely to have the condition being screened for than the general population.

Sensitivity (of a diagnostic or screening test)   The proportion of truly diseased persons, as measured by the gold standard, who are identified as diseased by the test under study.

Social capital   Networks, together with shared norms, values and understandings, which facilitate co-operation within or among groups and which may thereby improve health.

Specificity (of a diagnostic or screening test)   The proportion of truly non-diseased persons, as measured by the gold standard, who are identified as non-diseased by the test under study.

Strategy   A plan of action designed to achieve a series of objectives.

Stratification   Division into groups. Stratification may also refer to a process to control for differences in confounding variables, by making separate estimates for groups of individuals who have the same values for the confounding variable.

Strength of inference   The likelihood that an observed difference between groups within a study represents a real difference rather than mere chance or the influence of confounding factors, based on both P values and confidence intervals. Strength of inference is weakened by various forms of bias and by small sample sizes.

Surveillance   The on-going, systematic collection, collation and analysis of data and the prompt dissemination of the resulting information to those who need to know so that an action can result.

Sustainability   Requires the reconciliation of environmental, social and economic demands. Sustainable development meets the needs of the present without compromising the ability of future generations to meet their own needs.

Survival curve   A graph of the number of events occurring over time or the chance of being free of these events over time. The events must be discrete and the time at which they occur must be precisely known. In most clinical situations, the chance of an outcome changes with time. In most survival curves, the earlier follow-up periods usually include results from more patients than the later periods and are therefore more precise.

Validity   The extent to which a variable or intervention measures what it is supposed to measure or accomplishes what it is supposed to accomplish. The internal validity of a study refers to the integrity of the experimental design. The external validity (generalisability) of a study refers to the appropriateness by which its results can be applied to non-study patients or populations.

Years of life lost (YLL)   Years of potential life relate to the average age at which deaths occur and the expected life span of the population. Therefore, a measure of how many potential years are lost due to early death and provides a measure of the relative importance of conditions in causing mortality.

Index